BREASTFEEDING MADE EASY

About the author

Carlos González, a father of three, studied medicine at the Universidad Autónoma de Barcelona and trained as a paediatrician at the Hospital de Sant Joan de Déu. The founder and president of the Catalan Breastfeeding Association (ACPAM), he currently gives courses on breastfeeding for medical professionals. Since 1996 he has been breastfeeding correspondent for *Ser Padres* (*Being Parents*) magazine.

His books *Kiss Me! How to raise your children with love* and *My Child Won't Eat! How to enjoy mealtimes without worry* are also published by Pinter & Martin.

BREASTFEEDING MADE EASY

A gift for life for you and your baby

Carlos González

translated by Lorenza Garcia

The information in this book is general and should not be taken as specific medical advice for individuals. If you are having problems breastfeeding, or are concerned about your baby, contact your midwife, health visitor or GP, or call the National Breastfeeding Helpline on 0300 100 0212 (UK).

Breastfeeding made easy: a gift for life for you and your baby
First published as *Un regalo para toda la vida* by Ediciones Planeta Madrid, S.A.

This English edition first published by Pinter & Martin Ltd 2014

© Carlos González 2006, 2009, 2014

© Ediciones Planeta, Av. Diagonal 662-664, 08034 Barcelona, Spain

Translated by Lorenza Garcia

Edited by Susan Last

Index Helen Bilton

All rights reserved

ISBN 978-1-78066-020-2

The right of Carlos González to be identified as the author of this work has been asserted by him in accordance with the Copyright, Designs and Patent Act of 1988

British Library Cataloguing-in-Publication Data
A catalogue record for this book is available from the British Library

This book is sold subject to the condition that it shall not, by way of trade and otherwise, be lent, resold, hired out, or otherwise circulated without the publisher's prior consent in any form or binding or cover other than that in which it is published and without a similar condition being imposed on the subsequent purchaser

Printed in Great Britain by TJ International Ltd, Padstow, Cornwall

This book has been printed on paper that is sourced and harvested from sustainable forests and is FSC accredited

Pinter & Martin Ltd
6 Effra Parade
London SW2 1PS

www.pinterandmartin.com

CONTENTS

'Her Highness María Victoria is so good and kind that she seems more like an ordinary woman than a queen. I doff my hat when she goes by, and forgive her for being an Italian. She nurses her children herself, you know. I hear that this summer, whilst strolling in the grounds of the Escorial Palace, she came across an abandoned child clamouring to be fed. She gathered him up, and began to suckle him, not from a bottle, Tito, but from her own breast.'

Benito Pérez Galdós, *Amadeo 1*

INTRODUCTION

My interest in breastfeeding began when I first started studying medicine. I have my professor of practical anatomy to thank for this. His name, if I remember correctly, was Joaquin, and in a faculty containing thousands of students, to whom none of the professors paid much attention, he stood out as someone with a passion for teaching. As soon as he had a few students gathered round him, he would give a rousing lecture, and one of his favourite subjects was breastfeeding.

For many years I regarded breastfeeding from a doctor's point of view, as the best form of nutrition, which protects against a legion of illnesses and saves thousands of lives. I thought that advocating it was in the interests of public health, and that a good mother should make every effort to breastfeed her child, because it is best for him.

Then I had three children of my own, and something changed. I saw my children nursing, being breastfed by their mother, and I had feelings of… pride, admiration, astonishment, fascination, envy? I have read a great deal since then, about how fathers feel in those circumstances, and yet I still find it impossible to describe that feeling. Some things in life are too deep for words.

I understood then that breastfeeding isn't a tool for achieving health, but rather an integral part of health itself. Not a means, but an end. Telling people to 'avoid artificial breastfeeding because it causes diarrhoea' now seems to me as absurd as exhorting them to 'avoid blindness because blind people are more likely to get run over'. Breastfeeding is no more a way of avoiding infection than being able to see is a way of avoiding accidents. They are both normal parts of a healthy life. I know now that breastfeeding is not an effort, much less a sacrifice, that a woman makes for the good of her child, but rather that it is part of her life, of her own sexual and reproductive cycle. It is a right that no one can take away from her.

I am aware that some women don't want to breastfeed. This is fine. A right isn't the same as a duty. Many people don't go on marches or vote in elections, but they still have that right.

I didn't write this book in order to attempt to convince mothers to breastfeed, but rather to help those who want to do so to achieve their aim. I make this very clear in the title, and those who prefer to bottle feed can buy other books.

Some might find it surprising that a man should write about breastfeeding. I won't for a moment try to conceal the fact that I've never breastfed. People who know how to do something do it, people who don't write books.

Chapter 1
HOW THE BREAST WORKS

To the consumer's taste

Fifty years ago, it was a commonly held and mistaken belief that women produced a fixed amount of breastmilk, and that some had a lot while others had a little. Some had a week's worth, others two month's worth, but when it stopped that meant the well had run dry. And of course a mother's milk could also be good or bad. These were things you simply had or didn't have; if you were lucky you had plenty of good-quality milk and could breastfeed, and your child would grow up to be strong and handsome. If you didn't have much milk, or it was watery, then there was nothing you could do. How fortunate that they invented the bottle! Nothing a mother did or didn't do would change the outcome: if you knew a mother who had breastfed for three months (which in those days was an achievement), or for more than six months (which was downright eccentric), it would never have occurred to you to say: 'I wish I could breastfeed my baby, tell me how you do it!' You would simply declare, with a measure of envy: 'You're so lucky to have milk! I wish I'd had enough to breastfeed my baby!' (In fact, to tell the truth, the most frequent remark was: 'I don't know why you put yourself through breastfeeding, I bottle fed mine and he's a picture of health').

And yet, wasn't it a huge coincidence that while European women had almost no milk, African mothers had plenty? Of course, it was a question of race; black women produced more milk, as did gypsies, while white women simply didn't (there were those, of course, who argued that this was because blacks and gypsies were *primitive races*). In that case, how was it that the European mothers' grandmothers, who belonged to the same race, had plenty of milk? Opinion here was divided. Some believed the stresses of modern life had put an end to lactation (I will talk more about this on page 27), others that this was an example of evolution in action: an organ that wasn't used would atrophy and soon little girls would be born without breasts (as if little girls were ever born *with* breasts), like in a cartoon, where animals mutate in five minutes.

However, evolution doesn't work like that; acquired characteristics aren't inherited. This means that even if women stopped breastfeeding for a hundred generations, the hundred and first generation would still have the same genes and the same breasts, and they would still work if the woman knew how to use them. And even if a mutant gene produced one woman who could not secrete milk (something which could, and has happened – see page 156), and she had a daughter or two, and two or three granddaughters, it would take thousands of years for a significant percentage of the population to inherit the mutant gene. But above all, it would require a reproductive advantage: women who secreted no milk would need to give birth to a lot more children, or their children would have to have a higher survival rate. When a mutation has no clear evolutionary advantage, there is no reason for it to flourish, and after thousands of years that woman might have only a handful of descendants. During the last third of the twentieth century, among the middle classes of the industrialised countries, there was no reproductive advantage for a supposed *non-secretion of milk* gene. On the contrary, for millions of years, and still today in most parts of the world, if a mother produces insufficient or poor-quality milk, her children will probably die (unless another woman nurses them). Any possible mutant gene, far from proliferating, would have been eliminated. This is why there are so few women who don't secrete milk.

So we haven't evolved. We have the same genes as our great-great-grandparents. The same genes as the Altamira cave dwellers. And a fixed amount of milk, or an amount that only lasts for a limited time, doesn't fit with the widely observed facts.

Perhaps this mistaken belief came about because we tried comparing humans to cows. Some breeds of cow produce more milk than others; country-dwellers have known this for centuries. Why shouldn't there be a *dairy breed* among women? Because dairy cows aren't like other mammals. They are mutations, carefully selected over thousands of years to produce more milk than they need to feed their young. A female deer that produced as much milk as a dairy cow would be one sick deer.

It is obvious that growing babies consume more and more milk (until they begin on solids, after which the amount stabilises and then begins to reduce). It makes no difference whether they are breastfed or bottle fed, they all need more milk as they grow bigger.

Let us suppose that a newborn needs 500ml of milk, and a four-month-old needs 700ml (these are approximate figures, so don't worry; breastfeeding doesn't require knowing exactly how much milk a baby needs or drinks). If the amount of milk a woman produces were fixed at 500ml a day, when her baby reached a month old he would start to go hungry, and she would need to give him a supplement. 'Exactly!' more than one woman will be thinking, 'That's what happened to a friend of mine. And some women can't produce 500ml, they only manage 300ml, and their babies need a supplement from day one.' Yet we also know of women who breastfeed for several months and their milk never 'dries up'. They even existed when the 'ten minutes every four hours rule' was in full force; nowadays they are growing in number. And we know that in our great-grandparents' time, all babies breastfed for months, or years, as they do today in most parts of the world. So, how do they work, the breasts of those fortunate women, who, in increasing numbers, breastfeed for four months or more without giving their babies supplements? Do they produce 700ml of milk from day one? And in that case, where did the extra 200ml of milk go during the first few months? Did the baby drink it? That is impossible. A baby who only needs 500ml of milk will only drink 500ml. A lot of mothers who bottle feed have tried making their babies take just a little bit more (raise your hand anyone who hasn't). 'Just a little, so she is chubby, and healthy-looking.' But the babies won't take it. If they did, nearly all one-year olds would weigh more than twenty kilos and some more than thirty.

So, the baby only takes 500ml, yet his mother produces 700ml. What happens to the extra 200ml? That 200ml is a whole glassful. Does it leak out of her breast? If so, she would need buckets not breast pads in her bra. Does it remains inside the breast, accumulating? After a week she would have accumulated 1,400ml, and after a month she would have six litres of milk, three in each breast. All mothers would be forced to express and discard 200ml of breastmilk every day, for weeks and weeks, otherwise their breasts would explode.

The amount of milk a mother produces isn't fixed: *her milk production increases as her baby's needs grow*. The same mother who started off producing 500ml will, in time, produce 700ml.

Is this increased production to do with time, then? In other words, are mothers programmed, like washing machines, to produce 500ml in the first month, 700ml after four months, a bit more after six months, and then less and less? Is that why we start babies on solids at six months, because milk production drops off? And, worse still, are some women's programmes set at *whites* while others are set at *delicates*, so that some women produce as much as 800ml of milk for two years while others never go above 600ml, and their milk dries up after three months?

This is impossible. Human beings can't be that badly designed; our bodies don't work that way. If the variations in milk production were pre-programmed, what would happen when a baby died? For thousands of years, and still today in many parts of the world, the death of a baby was commonplace, and an experience that many mothers went through at one time or another. If a baby died during delivery, or at two months old from meningitis, do you suppose the mother went on producing milk for six months, and in lesser amounts for the next two or three years? What an ordeal, what a waste!

And what about wet nurses? For hundreds of years, throughout Europe, the majority of wealthy women didn't breastfeed. Do you suppose wet nurses retired after two years because they stopped producing milk, that their professional careers were shorter than those of a footballer? No. When a wet nurse finished with one child, she would go on to the next, and so on for decades.

And what about changes in supplementary feeding guidelines? At the start of the twentieth century, paediatricians recommended exclusive breastfeeding for the first twelve months; then ten, then eight, then six, then three, then up to a month old… and then suddenly it was three months again, then four, then six. If milk production dropped off after six months, how did our grandparents survive between the ages of six and twelve months? Or does a woman's milk production setting automatically change in accordance with the latest recommendations of the Paediatric Association, the way the clock on your computer adjusts when you connect to the Internet? On the contrary. We don't start feeding babies solids at six months because milk production drops off when they reach that age; milk production begins to drop off at six months because we begin feeding babies solids.

It is a matter of design. We need a system that adapts constantly to the baby's needs, producing more milk when the baby wants more, and less when the baby wants less. A system that goes on producing milk for as long as the baby needs it, and then stops producing it when the baby stops nursing, that produces enough milk for one if there is only one baby, and for three if the the mother has triplets.

The solution is wonderfully simple: the amount of milk a woman produces doesn't depend on her race, or on how much time has elapsed since she gave birth, but rather on how much her baby feeds. If he feeds a lot, then she will secrete a lot of milk; if he stops feeding, the milk will stop. The first mammals developed this mechanism over 200 million years ago; nature tends to hang on to solutions that work well.

We could refine this even further. In nature, if a baby doesn't feed, its mother stops producing breastmilk and that is that. However, many mothers of babies who can't nurse because they are ill or premature, and many working mothers, will express their milk and feed it to their children by other means. What really makes the breast produce milk is not the baby feeding, but milk being taken from the breast either by the baby, or by expressing manually or with a pump.

The breast: how it works and what it is it for

The only thing most TV owners need to know about the working of their set is how to switch it on and off and how to change channels. If we are asked for more information, we have to resort to a generalisation: 'It works on electricity'. In order to be able to watch our TV, we don't need to know all its component parts or what they are for.

Similarly, the only thing we need to know in order to breastfeed is how to place the nipple in the baby's mouth. If we are asked for more information, we can now proudly declare: 'the more milk you take out, the more milk you will produce'; animals don't even know this, and they are rather good at breastfeeding. It is quite another thing knowing about the inside of the breast, how it works, and why it produces more milk when more is taken out. Although it isn't necessary to know these things in order to breastfeed, I will go into a little more detail in the following pages, because it is interesting (to some), and because it gives the book a more lofty tone, and, well, because I have to pad it out with something.

But first of all we must make an important distinction. Your television was designed and manufactured by a handful of people who know exactly what components it contains (the ones they put there!) and what each is for. We can't say the same about the breast, or about any other part of our bodies. Although our knowledge is expanding, nature is still able to surprise us. We only know a fraction of what actually goes on in the breast, and some of what we think we know is probably wrong. What I know about the breast is only a fraction of what a handful of scientists worldwide know. The following explanations are therefore intended as no more than a summary.

The breast from the outside

Generally, women have two breasts. This hasn't always been the case: you only need look at your dog or cat to see that other mammals have several pairs. As a throwback to those distant relatives, some people have more than two breasts. This usually presents itself as a third nipple located somewhere between the armpit and the groin. In some cases, the nipple is so rudimentary that the owner thinks it is a mole or a wart. In others, there is glandular tissue at varying stages of development, which can lead to swelling and leakage when lactation begins. Don't be alarmed by this, it won't last; keep breastfeeding normally, apply cold packs if this helps, and in two or three days the discomfort will pass.

In the centre of the breast is the nipple, a structure that can be either protruding or sunken, and from which milk is secreted. Around the nipple is a coloured area of varying size, known as the *areola*, not to be confused with the *aureola*, which refers to the celestial crown worn by saints and martyrs depicted in sacred art.

The areola contains tiny lumps, known as Montgomery's tubercles, which grow during pregnancy and lactation. Each of them contains a huge sebaceous gland and a tiny mammary gland (the total size is about a millimetre). Our skin is covered in sebaceous glands, which secrete protective substances; the ones in the areola are bigger and so offer more protection. The tiny mammary gland produces milk, of course, which contains antibodies and epidermal growth factor, as well as having numerous anti-inflammatory effects – a veritable balm for the skin.

Beneath the nipple and the areola are a series of involuntary muscle fibres, cleverly interlaced so that when they contract the nipple becomes erect – i.e., the areola contracts, causing the nipple to stick out. Touch, cold or sexual arousal can produce this effect.

The unseen parts

Few things are more boring than a breast seen from the outside. If you have seen one you have seen them all.

Inside, however, there is far greater variety. The breast contains glands, ducts, connective tissue, ligaments, arteries, veins, nerves, lymph nodes and so on.

The glands are made up of various lobules, mixed together with fatty tissue. It is the varying amount of fatty tissue that produces different-sized breasts; the glands are always more or less the same size, and size has nothing to do with the breast's ability to produce milk. Women are unique among mammals for this capacity to accumulate fatty tissue in the breast. If you have ever seen a dog or cat with its young, you will recall that the mother is almost flat-chested.

Curiously enough, the number of lobules in the breast is a matter for debate. Some say there are around twenty, the ducts from which sometimes merge before reaching the nipple; others say there are ten, which branch out as they leave the nipple. It seems to me that in the end they are saying the same thing. In any event, several ducts, known as lactiferous ducts, converge in the nipple, and when the breast is squeezed, the milk is secreted from several holes, as from a watering can.

The part of the lactiferous duct that is close to the nipple has the capacity to dilate and fill with milk, forming lactiferous sinuses. Each breast contains about a dozen of these sinuses. Often, when the baby is feeding, it is possible to feel the lactiferous sinuses filled with milk, a centimetre or two from the nipple, beneath the areola.

The ducts go on branching out exponentially from the nipple, until a microscopic duct reaches a microscopic sac of cells known as the acinus. Each acinus is surrounded by myoepithelial and contractile cells.

A hormone acts on each of these cells. Prolactin causes the secretory cell to produce milk; oxytocin causes the contractile cell to contract and eject the milk.

Lactation hormones

The pituitary gland is situated at the base of the brain. It produces oxytocin and prolactin in response to a neuroendocrine reflex. The most commonly known reflexes, such as the leg lifting when tapped below the knee, are purely neurological: there is a sensory receptor in the rotulian tendon, a nerve that conveys the signal to the spinal cord, a central processor that decides what needs to happen next, and a motor neuron that relays the message to the muscle, commanding it to contract. The nipple and the areola also contain sensory receptors and neurons that convey information to the hypothalamus. Only instead of transmitting messages via a neuron, the central processor sends them via a hormone, which is carried in the bloodstream. This is a *neuroendocrine* reflex.

Prolactin

Prolactin levels are extremely low before pregnancy. They start to increase after the first trimester, but no milk is produced because the progesterone and oestrogen produced by the placenta inhibit the action of prolactin.

After the birth, prolactin levels remain high for several months, but if the mother doesn't breastfeed, they go down again after a couple of weeks. Following the expulsion of the placenta, progesterone and estrogen levels fall spectacularly, allowing the prolactin to do its job. Placental expulsion is what triggers milk production.

So, prolactin levels remain high for several months. But they go up much more, ten or twenty times, each time the baby nurses. These prolactin peaks only occur in response to the breast being stimulated. If the baby nurses a lot, there will be lots of prolactin, and lots of milk. If the baby doesn't nurse much there won't be much milk. If the child stops nursing altogether, milk production will stop.

Some people mistakenly think it is necessary to wait a few hours between feeds to allow the breast to fill up again. This isn't true. The breast doesn't work like a toilet cistern that has to fill up again before it can be flushed. It is more like a tap: when you want more water you open the tap more.

For two or three hours after the baby nurses, prolactin levels slowly go down until they reach a basal level (which, remember, is already high after delivery). Let us imagine a baby who nurses for ten minutes every four hours (ten minutes every four hours? Yes, we are talking about a completely imaginary baby!). Let us suppose that, for whatever reason (perhaps simply because she is growing older) our baby wants more milk. What does she do? Does she nurse for fifteen minutes every four hours? Unlikely. This wouldn't be a very effective method. Nursing for longer would produce more or less the same levels of prolactin, and therefore of milk. If on the other hand she decided to nurse for ten minutes every *two* hours, this would produce more prolactin peaks throughout the day. And, as prolactin levels wouldn't have returned to the basal level, the fresh peak would be even higher (let us say that instead of rising from 50 to 500 it would rise from 100 to 550). More frequent nursing produces spectacular increases in prolactin, and therefore in milk supply.

So, there is no better way of inhibiting lactation than by reducing the number of feeds. Each time we tell a mother to wait for four or three hours, or never to feed her baby before two-thirty, or that he can't possibly be hungry again, or that there is no point in feeding him now because she has no milk, or that his tummy needs a rest, or that she shouldn't nurse him during the night, we are placing major obstacles in the way of breastfeeding.

During the night, both basal levels and prolactin peaks are higher. This means that the baby can take more milk with less effort. This is one reason (among others) why advising mothers not to nurse their baby at night is complete nonsense.

Oxytocin

Oxytocin controls various aspects of a woman's sexual life. It is the hormone that is released during orgasm, during labour, and each time the baby nurses. The main effect of oxytocin is to cause various muscle fibres to contract: those in the womb, in the vagina, those surrounding the breast acini, and those beneath the nipple and the areola. During orgasm the womb and the vagina contract, and the nipples become erect. During labour, a woman's womb and vagina contract, and I imagine her nipples also become erect, although no one usually notices this. When the baby is nursing, the nipple is erect, and there are contractions in the womb and vagina: the famous afterpains.

Afterpains are more or less painful contractions, which occur during the first few days after childbirth whenever the baby nurses. They are a nuisance, but remember they are *good for you*: the contractions help your womb return to its normal size, probably reducing the risk of bleeding or infection. They say afterpains are worse with each new child (just as giving birth is usually easier: you win some and you lose some!).

The body's response to oxytocin may be very similar during sexual activity and childbirth, but the effect it has on women is often very different, because her sensations not only depend on the hormone, but also on her state of mind. The majority of women don't feel sexually aroused while giving birth or breastfeeding, but some do.

Some mothers notice sexual feelings while breastfeeding their baby, and can even reach orgasm. This is quite rare, and I only mention it so that any mothers reading this book who have experienced those feelings will know that there is nothing wrong with them. You aren't sexual perverts, you aren't having 'bad thoughts', it doesn't constitute child abuse, or incestuous behaviour, and there is no reason for you to stop breastfeeding. If you are fortunate enough to find breastfeeding particularly pleasant, enjoy it while it lasts. Why deprive yourself of one of life's few pleasures?

As well as producing muscular contractions, oxytocin affects behaviour. If you place a baby rat in the cage of a virgin female rat she will eat it. But if you first give her an injection of oxytocin, she will try to look after it as if she were its mother and even try to nurse it (although, needless to say, she has no milk).

When lactation begins, most mothers notice the effects of oxytocin: a slight contraction or tingling sensation in the breast, the feeling that their milk is 'coming in', the appearance of drops or even a stream of milk. This is the milk ejection reflex, also referred to as 'the let-down'. I say 'when lactation begins' and 'most mothers', because some mothers never feel their milk coming in. This doesn't mean they have no milk, or that their milk hasn't come in. In fact, after two or three months, most mothers no longer feel the let-down, yet their milk keeps coming without any problem. Don't worry if you don't feel your milk coming in, it doesn't mean it has dried up.

Those of you who do experience the effect of oxytocin will have noticed that the let-down often begins long before your baby begins nursing. It is enough just to think of breastfeeding your baby, hear her cry, or picture her when she isn't there, for your nipples to contract and start to leak milk. How is this reflex possible without a physical stimulus? Because it is what is known as a *conditioned reflex*. Do you remember Pavlov's famous dog, which salivated when a bell rang? Salivation occurs as a result of the stimulus of food entering the mouth. By ringing a bell each time he gave the dog food, Pavlov managed to train the animal to associate the two stimuli, so that hearing the bell was enough to make it salivate. In fact, all dogs have this conditioned reflex: show them a juicy bit of meat and they will start drooling before the food reaches their mouth. The sight or even the thought of delicious food will also make our own mouths water. Pavlov's genius lay in substituting a bit of meat for a bell; if he had told the members of the Moscow Science Academy: 'See how my dog drools when I show him this bit of meat', the learned professors would have replied disdainfully: 'What of it? So does my dog'. But the bell left them all fascinated.

Just as salivation is automatically conditioned in dogs (and in people), so the milk ejection reflex is automatically conditioned in all mothers. The effects of this are still noticeable years after lactation; some mothers feel a tingling in their breasts when they hear a baby cry, or when they see images of starving or destitute children. This has been referred to as *postlactation phantom let-down*, analogous with the phantom limb sensation some people experience after losing an arm or a leg.

It could be that this conditioned reflex exists in order to speed things up: this way, the baby doesn't even need to suck for the milk to come; it is enough for him to latch on and the milk is already there. However, the English physiologist Michael Woolridge believes that the primary usefulness of this conditioning is not to trigger the reflex, but to inhibit it, as a protective mechanism for female mammals. Because it is a conditioned reflex, it no longer depends on the physical stimulation of the baby's mouth on the breast, but on the mother hearing her baby, seeing her baby, thinking about her baby... In brief, it depends on the cerebral cortex. The mother's thoughts can trigger the reflex, and they can also inhibit it. Thence the familiar story: 'She had a shock, and her milk dried up'.

Imagine a doe peacefully feeding her young. Suddenly she smells a wolf. She flees, concealing her fawn, which is unable to run, in the thicket. The fawn gives off no scent (because its mother spends all day licking it clean) and it remains motionless. The doe does give off a scent, and she makes a noise as she flees, so the wolf is more likely to follow her, and not look for her fawn. If the wolf catches the mother, then her hapless offspring will also perish in a matter of hours. But if the mother escapes, she will quickly return to her young and continue nursing it. If the doe's teats were leaking milk, no wolf worth its salt would lose her trail. However, the let-down reflex is conditioned, and the secretion of oxytocin stops when the doe is frightened. Unlike prolactin, which takes several hours to disappear, oxytocin only remains in the blood for a few minutes: when the pituitary gland stops producing it, it is quickly destroyed. This is why, when oxytocin is used to speed up labour, it has to be given through a drip; administering an injection of oxytocin every three hours would be pointless. For extra security, the adrenaline produced by a frightened animal directly inhibits the effects of oxytocin. The same mechanism can probably prevent a mother from giving birth when she is frightened. Hyenas present no threat to a female hippo, rhino or giraffe, but their newborn offspring would be easy meat. The presence of danger can inhibit oxytocin production and delay labour by several hours, until the threat has passed. Perhaps this is why labour can be so difficult in the unfamiliar setting of the hospital, surrounded by strangers. Most women feel better when they are accompanied by their husband or another close relative, while others prefer to give birth at home with the help of a midwife they know well.

But I digress. Let us consider our friend the doe, who is now returning to her fawn: because she is no longer afraid, the adrenaline has left her blood, her conditioned reflexes have been triggered again, her milk has reappeared and her baby fawn has started happily nursing. But if we were talking about a woman, and not a female deer, things might not be so simple. Besides the mother and baby, there is the baby's grandmother in the mix, as well as the husband, the mother-in-law, the friend, the doctor and the nurse, and one, if not all of them, will begin catastrophising: 'You had a shock and your milk dried up? That happened to a cousin of mine, her baby almost died of hunger; her husband had to rush out to an all-night chemist on a Saturday to buy formula.'

It is no longer fear of the wolf, but fear of not having any milk that causes adrenalin levels to go up and oxytocin levels to go down. The baby tries to nurse, but almost no milk comes out; the baby gets frustrated and cries, and the mother-in-law takes the opportunity to score a point: 'You see? Now you're making him nervous. I told you that in your present state you should stop fussing and give him a bottle'. The mother bursts into tears and grows even more alarmed…

One of the best ways to upset lactation is by upsetting the mother, convincing her she won't be able to breastfeed and that breastfeeding is a tricky business. It is a common strategy among producers of artificial baby milk. But this is not what I am arguing. I am not suggesting that anxious or stressed mothers can't breastfeed. Of course they can! Lactation isn't a fragile hothouse bloom, it is one of the body's most solid functions, and one that is vital (not for the mother, but for her baby). Any of our organs can fail (we have to die of something), but for a mother's milk to suddenly dry up is as rare as having a heart attack or suffering kidney failure. Those who talk of the stresses of modern life forget that we in Western civilisations belong to the first generation able to go to sleep at night knowing there will be food on the table the next day. Women have breastfed their babies for thousands of years in far worse situations: when reaching the age of thirty-five was considered 'living to a ripe old age', when droughts meant starvation, when war razed homes, when women worked like slaves, when epidemics decimated whole towns and cities. The effect of stress on lactation is temporary: the milk doesn't come out immediately, and the baby gets frustrated and cries. He keeps nursing because he is hungry, and in the end, despite the mother's stress, the milk begins to flow again. What happens nowadays, which didn't happen before, is that when the baby gets frustrated and cries, the mother gives him a bottle. It is bottle feeding, not stress and anxiety, that causes the mother's milk to dry up.

Feedback Inhibitor of Lactation (FIL)

For a long time it was thought that the way lactation works could be explained, at least superficially, by oxytocin and prolactin. I say superficially because there are other hormones involved which we haven't even mentioned.

When a baby nurses, why does more milk come out? Because suckling stimulates the production of prolactin? Why does milk leak from one nipple when the baby is feeding from the other? Because oxytocin is transported via the bloodstream, arriving at both breasts at the same time. Why did women who tried to follow the ten minutes every four hours rule find that their milk dried up? Because there wasn't much stimulation and therefore not enough prolactin. Why do mothers of twins produce enough milk for two babies, and mothers of triplets enough milk for three babies? Because when there are three times as many babies there is three times as much prolactin.

However, there was a strange phenomenon that couldn't be explained by those two hormones alone. There was a tribe in Hong Kong whose women always fed their babies from the same breast. Their babies always nursed from the right breast, never from the left (and, in fact, there were more cases of cancer in the left breast). But we needn't go as far as Hong Kong to find children who, for one reason or another, stop feeding from one breast. This can be temporary, and after a few days the mother is able to persuade her baby to nurse from both breasts again. But, from time to time, a child will refuse outright and there is nothing the mother can do. I sometimes come across a mother who has been feeding from the same breast for two weeks or two months.

As the oxytocin and prolactin arrive via the bloodstream to both breasts in equal amounts, so both should respond in the same way and produce more or less the same amount of milk. Imagine a breast that produces half a litre or more of milk every day, which the baby refuses to drink. After a day, the pain would already be unbearable; after three days the mother would have to be hospitalised; after two weeks, with an accumulation of seven litres, her breast would literally burst.

And yet this never happens. When a child refuses to feed from one side, that breast swells up and is painful, and sometimes the mother has to express some of her milk to relieve the feeling of fullness, but after a few days the pain goes away, the milk dries up and the breast shrinks and remains empty. The left breast then compensates by producing twice the amount (naturally; if the baby doesn't starve, it is because he is getting as much milk from one breast as other babies get from two), while the right breast remains dry, and this can go on for weeks or months. How can this be explained? There has to be a localised control mechanism that acts on each individual breast.

At first it was thought that this mechanism was purely physical. The breast is overfull and the pressure constricts the blood vessels, stopping the blood supply, and with it the supply of oxytocin, prolactin and nutrients necessary for the gland to continue producing milk. The breast comes to a standstill, like an airport during an air traffic controller's strike.

Undoubtedly the physical mechanism plays a part. However, a few years ago scientists discovered another hormone that acts locally to control milk secretion. This hormone is a peptide (a tiny protein), and is called Feedback Inhibitor of Lactation (FIL). It has been found in the milk of goats, women and other mammals (and, to my knowledge, everywhere it has been looked for).

FIL is a fine example of end-product inhibition. Milk contains a milk production inhibitor. If the baby feeds a lot, the inhibitor is removed from the breast via the milk, and so more milk is produced. But if the baby only feeds a little, the inhibitor stays inside the breast, and milk production slows.

A group of Australian scientists have shown how this works by serial measurements of breast volume. A camera takes photographs of the breast from different angles, and based on this information a computer calculates the breast volume (similar to the ultrasound method used to measure your baby's growth prenatally). The procedure is painless and relatively comfortable, and can be repeated several times an hour if necessary. (The old method consisted of dipping the breast in a tub of water and measuring the displaced water. It was rather uncomfortable and not very accurate). The Australian team were able to observe that breast volume gradually increases between feeds as the milk accumulates. After the baby feeds, there is a sharp decrease in breast volume, and then the cycle starts again. If for any reason the baby takes less milk at one feed, milk production slows down during the following hours. If the baby takes more (because he took less during the previous feed and is now hungry, for example) milk production will speed up. If the baby only feeds from one breast, milk production in that breast will rise sharply, while in the other, which is still full, it will almost come to a halt. Milk production, then, adapts instantly to the baby's needs, from one feed to the next, and separately in each breast. Providing, of course, that the baby is allowed to nurse as much or as little as he wants, when he wants. If one day the baby has to wait for an hour or two because his mother is out, he will simply nurse more when she gets back to compensate, and all will be well. On the other hand, if the baby is systematically denied the breast when he wants it, morning, noon and night, day after day, if his mother has been persuaded by the advice commonly given to mothers, 'to space out his feeds' or to nurse him 'ten minutes every four hours', he won't be able to give the breast instructions, and as a result it won't know how much milk to produce. When the mother waits for hours for her breasts to fill up before nursing her baby ('why feed him now if your breasts are empty?') she will gradually produce less and less milk, because the inhibitory factor will steadily accumulate as the breast fills with milk.

Any doctor or nurse will have observed the effects of FIL hundreds of times, long before it was discovered. How and when does lactation normally end? In Western countries it doesn't usually end when mother or baby choose. In a survey of mothers, the majority said they would have liked to nurse for longer, but unfortunately their milk dried up. How is this possible?

A mother is happily nursing her baby, when suddenly, for

some reason or other, the baby (or someone else) decides that he is still hungry. Perhaps because he can't go for three or four hours without feeding, or because he cries, or wakes up, or chews his fingers, or because he doesn't do a poo, or he nurses a lot, or he doesn't nurse enough. The reason is unimportant. The fact is that the unfortunate day arrives when he receives his first bottle. A lot of babies, especially if they are older than two or three months, won't take it because they aren't hungry. But the younger ones, the poor little things, are sometimes bamboozled. And occasionally the mother will go on insisting, or she will be advised to withhold the breast until the baby is hungry enough to take the bottle.

If the baby takes the bottle, which in fact he didn't need, he will overfeed. He is used to taking 500ml of breastmilk a day, and today he has drunk 50ml or 100ml more. This isn't slightly more than usual, it is 10-20 per cent more. Do you feel like moving around much after eating Xmas lunch? If the baby wasn't sleeping he will now sleep for several hours; if he was crying, he will stop crying; if he was sucking his fingers, he will stop sucking them, and so on. 'You see, the poor little chap was hungry! All he needed was a bottle and now he's fast asleep.' Fast asleep indeed! The poor baby is stuffed!

Christmas in Spain (where I live) is an ordeal for the digestion. We eat at least two big meals one after the other. What do we do the following day? We eat fruit. No one can manage three big meals in a row. Our baby will do the same: if one day he let himself be taken in and was overfed, it won't happen again. The next day he will not feel like over-eating, and he will take less milk. The mother may or may not notice; but, even if he nurses from her breast as often and for the same length of time as before, he will have taken less milk, because he was overfull from the previous day. And so the bottle, which came to the rescue on the first day, by the third day will no longer work; if the baby was crying, he will start crying again; if he was waking up he will wake up again; if he was sucking his fingers, he will suck them again. The mother will think: 'My milk is drying up, I must give him another bottle'; and she is partly right. Her milk is drying up, but what she doesn't realise is that it is drying up because of the bottle. The solution is not to give the baby a second bottle, but to refrain from giving him the first. But she gives him a second bottle, and then a third, and a fourth and so on. I have seen it happen hundreds of times: within a few weeks of starting the baby on the bottle, the breast will stop working. In the words of a famous doctor a hundred years ago: the bottle spells the end for of the breast.

As a result, the baby who was taking 500ml of breastmilk will now take 400ml, 300ml, 200ml… If the mother went on producing 500ml, where would the excess milk go? Within two weeks she would be taken to casualty, her breasts swollen and inflamed from carrying around several excess kilos, cursing her fate: 'I started bottle feeding him a fortnight ago, and look how my breasts have filled up!' But this never happens, quite the opposite: 'I started bottle feeding him, and now he refuses to nurse and my milk has dried up.'

The less a baby breastfeeds, the less milk his mother secretes. FIL is a fail-safe. We never see women with breasts filled to bursting with one, two, three, four litres of excess milk. So FIL is like a lift: it either works or it doesn't work. If it goes up it will also go down. If you reduce the number of bottle feeds you give your baby, he will breastfeed more and more, and you will produce more and more milk. Within a few days you will be able to throw the bottles away.

A few months after childbirth, prolactin levels go down. The basal level falls drastically, and the prolactin peak, which occurs with each feed, also decreases. And yet, milk production continues to increase. We don't know exactly how or why, but it seems that this localised control, or FIL, plays an increasingly important role in regulating lactation.

→ Ing, R., Petrakis, N.L., Ho, J.H. 'Unilateral breastfeeding and breast cancer', *Lancet* 1977 Jul;2:124–7

Control of milk volume

In some respects the way the breast works is comparable to the way the lungs work. Normally, we don't even realise we are breathing: we inhale some air and exhale some air. But not all the air that could go in does go in, and not all the air that could go out goes out. If we take a very deep breath, we can fill our lungs with more air than usual, for example when we go underwater. We can also try to exhale as much air as possible, for example when we blow out the candles on a cake. Likewise, if necessary a breast can produce more milk than usual, and if he is hungry a baby can have a bigger feed than usual.

In healthy people, the amount of air inhaled and exhaled in a normal breathing cycle (the tidal volume), is much lower than the maximum lung capacity. There is always a big reserve that allows us to breathe more deeply and quickly if we are obliged to make an unusual effort. If this reserve diminishes, it means we are ill: we are suffering from respiratory failure. First we get breathless when we run, then when we climb the stairs, and in severe cases when we get up from a chair; this happens when the tidal volume and the full lung capacity are the same.

All our organs and our body systems work on the same principle. Providing a person isn't seriously ill, they have a lot of room for forcing the machine to work harder. If necessary, our hearts can beat faster, our stomachs can digest more food, our kidneys can eliminate more liquid and toxins, and our livers can metabolise more substances. This is how living beings function.

The same is true of the breast. Any woman is able to produce milk for three, or even four or five babies. Besides the residual milk (which it is physically impossible to extract, and which we will call the *anatomical* reserve), there is always a certain amount of milk, which the baby could take if he wanted, but which he almost never does. We will call this the *functional* reserve.

No one has measured the precise volume of these reserves, so for the purposes of illustration I will use an arbitrary figure. Let us imagine that the breast contains 100ml of milk: 10ml of this makes up the anatomical reserve, and 20ml the functional reserve; under normal circumstances, the baby will take 70ml and the breast will produce another 70ml. One day, the baby is hungrier and takes 80ml. Because there is a decrease in FIL, milk is secreted at a faster rate, and the breast produces 90ml for the next feed. If this change is permanent (if from then on the baby decides to take 80ml at each feed) a new balance will be reached: from now on the breast will contain 110ml: 10ml for the anatomical reserve, 20ml for the functional reserve, and 80ml which the baby will take each time he feeds, and which the breast will then continue to produce after each feed. If, on the contrary, the baby taking 80ml is a *one off*, and at the next feed he goes back to taking 70ml, the breast will suddenly have more reserves than usual. The amount of FIL in the breast will be higher, milk production will slow down, and there will be 100ml waiting for the baby at his next feed.

Does this sound complicated? It was only a practical example, in real life things are far more complex. Why? Because no baby takes exactly the same amount of milk at each feed or from each breast. Real life is so complex and unpredictable that it can't be subjected to rules. No book, or doctor, or grandmother, not even the all-seeing eye, can tell you exactly when or for how long to breastfeed your baby. Only your baby knows this.

Control of milk composition

The way in which a baby feeds determines not only the amount of milk produced, but also its composition. The baby controls the breast to obtain the type of milk he needs at any given moment. The fat content in the milk increases during the course of the feed. This increase isn't small, and the concentration of fat in the milk has been shown to be as much as five times higher towards the end of the feed than at the start of the feed. People sometimes talk about *foremilk* and *hindmilk*, but these aren't two different types of milk: there is no moment at which the skimmed milk is finished and the whole milk begins. The amount of fat (and therefore calories) increases gradually, as shown in *Figure 1*.

To start with, the baby takes fewer calories from more milk; at the end, more calories from less milk. You will see that time

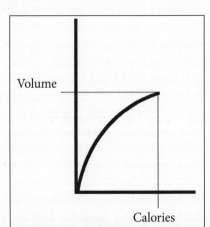

Figure 1: To start with, the baby takes fewer calories from more milk; at the end, more calories from less milk.

doesn't factor in the graph. The time depends on the speed at which the baby feeds; he may take two or three minutes to get as much milk as he needs, or more than twenty minutes.

Accordingly, the more milk the baby takes in one feed, the higher the concentration of fat in the milk (there is, of course, a maximum limit, but this limit is never reached because, as we have already seen, the baby never empties the breast completely). The last drops that leak out when he releases the breast have a very high fat content. When he feeds again a few hours later, the first drops of milk will contain very little fat. During those few hours, the high fat content milk from the end of the last feed will have been diluted into the freshly secreted, more watery milk. It is thought that there is a self-regulating system at work here as well, and that if the baby leaves a lot of fat inside the breast, this inhibits the production of further lipids, so that the next lot of milk will be more watery than usual. It is as if the baby had said: 'I can't finish that macaroni dish, Mum, it's too oily,' and his mother had replied, 'Don't worry, I won't use as much oil next time.'

Let us suppose that the baby feeds, and then releases the breast, but that five minutes later he changes his mind and starts feeding again. Will the milk that comes out contain fewer lipids? Obviously not. Not enough time has passed for the freshly secreted milk to dilute the milk from the end of the last feed. The first milk that comes out will be the *hindmilk* from a few moments before. The amount of lipids in the milk at the beginning of the feed depends on the level that was reached during the previous feed, and the time that has passed between feeds.

I have been talking about 'the breast', as if there were only one, when of course there are two. Taking 100ml of milk from one breast isn't the same as taking 50ml from each breast, which would mean the baby would get a lot less fat and far fewer calories. It isn't the same either to take 70ml and 30ml or 85ml and 15ml...

If this is the case, then when is it best to take the baby off the one breast and put him on the other? I have no idea. We don't know how many lipids a baby needs. You may read a book on nutrition that says: 'Babies of between six and nine months need between x or y mgs/kilo/per day of lipids', but it can't tell you how many lipids eight-month-old Laura Smith will need this afternoon at 4.28pm. We don't know exactly how much fat the milk contained at the beginning of her feed, we can't measure how many millilitres of milk she has actually taken, we have no idea how fast the fat content of the milk has increased during this particular feed, we don't know how high the fat content of the milk is in her mother's other breast, and we don't know how much milk from that breast will fit in Laura's tummy. How is it that people still manage to say things like: 'Give your baby ten minutes on one breast, then take her off and put her on the other'? It beats me. Ignorance sometimes makes for bold assertions.

Every baby, then, uses three control mechanisms for modifying the composition of the milk she takes at any given moment: she can decide how much milk she takes, how long it is before she feeds again, and whether she feeds from one breast or from both. Experiments have shown, by analysing the milk in each case, that these three factors affect the composition of breastmilk. The amount of milk ingested ought to depend on how long the baby feeds, but the relationship is so variable as to be statistically irrelevant (some babies feed quickly, others slowly); we can't say categorically 'If she has fed for five minutes she has taken 80ml, if she has fed for ten minutes she has taken 130ml'. The fat content of the milk doesn't depend on how long the baby feeds, but rather on how much milk she has taken during this time. Obviously if during a particular feed we take a particular baby off the breast sooner, she will have taken less milk. In addition, although it is easy to measure the length of a feed, it is very difficult to know how much milk the baby has taken. For purely didactic purposes, then, we could say that the three control mechanisms a baby uses are: the length of feed, the frequency of feeds, and feeding from one or both breasts. All babies modify these three factors day and night to get the nutrition they need.

If you take your baby off the first breast before she has finished feeding (perhaps because some well-meaning person has said: 'Make sure you let her feed from the second breast before she falls asleep'), she will be taking the first milk from the second breast rather than the last milk from the first breast. As shown in *Figure 2* this means she will need a bigger quantity in order to obtain the same number of calories. If it is a matter of a minute, then a short feed from the second breast will probably suffice. But if she is taken off the first breast much too soon (for example, after ten minutes when she needs fifteen or twenty), the amount she will need from the second breast will be so great that it won't fit into her stomach. Adults use only part of the full capacity of their stomach; drinking a litre of water after a meal wouldn't be much of a problem for us. But a baby's stomach is very small, and has almost no reserve capacity. The baby is forced to release the second breast, because her stomach won't take any more milk, even though she is still hungry. A similar situation occurs when the breastfeeding position is wrong (see page 51).

In 1988, Michael Woolridge and Chloe Fisher published in *The Lancet*, a leading medical journal, five case studies of babies who suffered from incessant crying, colic, diarrhoea and other symptoms. It was enough to instruct the mothers not to take their babies off the first breast, but to wait until they released the breast of their own accord when they had finished feeding, for all the symptoms to disappear. Shortly afterwards, Woolridge and coworkers tried to reproduce the situation experimentally with a group of healthy babies who had no problems with breastfeeding. Half of the mothers were told to take their babies off the first breast after ten minutes, and the other half to wait until the babies released the breast of their own accord. The researchers were expecting the babies from the first group to take too much liquid containing too much lactose and not enough fat, which would produce colic, vomiting and wind. And, indeed, to begin with they did take less fat. But as the day wore on, the babies

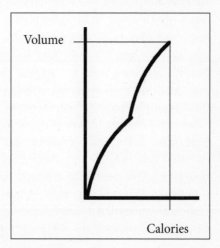

Figure 2: If she is taken off the first breast before she has finished feeding, the milk she takes from both breasts will have a lower fat content, and she will need a much bigger quantity in order to obtain the same amount of calories.

themselves began to modify the two other factors – the length of the feed and whether to feed from one or both breasts – so that in the end they were able to take the same amount of fat as the other group, and didn't suffer any adverse symptoms.

Because the baby has those three ways of controlling the milk's composition (remember: frequency of feeds, length of feeds, one breast or two), even when we have fixed the third arbitrarily they are still able to control the other two. Perhaps the five babies who had problems when their feeding time was curtailed were exceptions. Perhaps they (or their mothers) were less physiologically capable of adaptation: we are all able to walk, but when it comes to running, some people move more slowly and tire more quickly than others.

The capacity of living beings to adapt is sometimes astonishing, but we can't ask for miracles. Throughout the twentieth century, many doctors insisted on controlling all three factors simultaneously: the baby has to feed for precisely ten minutes on each breast every four hours. Precision became almost an obsession: even today some mothers ask whether they should count the time between feeds from the beginning or the end of the feed. A lot of books and a lot of experts provided exact times (eight o'clock, twelve o'clock, four o'clock, eight o'clock, twelve o'clock,) rather than specifying 'every four hours'. Don't nurse him at nine o'clock, one o'clock and five o'clock, whatever you do! Between midnight and eight in the morning there was an eight-hour rest (spending half the night listening to your baby cry without being able to nurse him was called *the nocturnal rest*). The four-hour rule came from the German school. There was also a French school that recommended feeding at three-hourly intervals, with a six-hour pause during the night. We may ask ourselves whether nursing five or seven times a day influenced the national character of those respective countries! Some schools were in favour of giving one or both breasts at each feed (most advocated the latter), so that all in all there were four theories: one breast every three hours, both breasts every three hours, one breast every four hours, both breasts every four hours. But generally speaking, each doctor espoused one theory and vigorously defended it. The result was that babies were completely defenceless: they could no longer choose the frequency and duration of each feed, or how many breasts they nursed from. They could no longer control the amount or the composition of the milk they took, and had to accept whatever they were given. In most cases, the amount was insufficient and the composition was inadequate; the babies cried, protested, were sick and failed to gain weight. A few years ago, it was unusual in Spain to still be breastfeeding a baby of three months, and breastfeeding without the 'help' of a bottle was considered almost heroic.

Of course, there are cases where, by some unbelievable stroke of luck, the baby manages to obtain the necessary amount of milk with the right composition by nursing every four hours. Those rare exceptions only strengthened doctors' faith in keeping to a strict time schedule: 'Breastfeeding on demand is a lot of hot air. I knew a mother who stuck rigidly to the four-hour rule, and it worked perfectly; she breastfed her baby for nine months, the baby slept like an angel and was plump and healthy. The problem is that women nowadays can't be bothered to make the effort, they prefer the ease of the bottle.'

→ Woolridge, M.W., Fisher, C. 'Colic, "overfeeding", and symptoms of lactose malabsorption in the breastfed baby: a possible artifact of feed management?' *Lancet* 1988;2:382-4

→ Woolridge, M.W. 'Baby-controlled breastfeeding: biocultural implications', in Stuart-Macadam, P., Dettwyler, K.A., eds.: *Breastfeeding. Biocultural perspectives*. New York: Aldine de Gruyter, 1995

→ Woolridge, M.W., Ingram, J.C., Baum, J.D. 'Do changes in pattern of breast usage alter the baby's nutrient intake?' *Lancet* 1990;336:395-397

Chapter 2
HOW TO BREASTFEED

My wife used to say to me sometimes: 'I don't know what all the fuss is about breastfeeding. You have a baby, you have a breast, and that's all there is to it.'

And she is right. In the vast majority of cases, in order to be able to breastfeed you only need to know two things: the meaning of breastfeeding on demand, and how to breastfeed in the correct position. And under normal circumstances it wouldn't be necessary to explain either of those things to any mother. It wouldn't be necessary to talk about breastfeeding on demand if certain people hadn't taken it into their heads to recommend strict feeding regimes. And it wouldn't be necessary to teach correct positioning if little girls learned, as they have since time immemorial, from watching other women breastfeed, and if we hadn't interfered in certain processes, which I will discuss further on. Women have been breastfeeding for a million years without the need for courses or books, and this remains true in most parts of the world. Out of the several thousand other species of mammal on the planet, none needs lessons in breastfeeding.

There is one exception: some primates in captivity. For most mammals, suckling and rearing their young is a totally instinctive activity. A gazelle or a lion in captivity is perfectly able to rear its young. But with primates, particularly those most closely related to us, it is a different matter. Females born into captivity (and reared by humans instead of by their mothers in zoos, for example) are incapable of looking after their young. They either ignore them or don't know how to look after them. I remember a photo of a female gorilla, who put her offspring on her head like a hat instead of holding him in her lap. And a female orang-utan, who kissed her young on the lips instead of placing him on her breast; she seemed very surprised when this method didn't work. Often the only solution is to separate the young from their mothers and rear them artificially. There are two possible explanations for this type of behaviour: one is that female primates born in captivity haven't been able to learn from observing their own mothers; the other is that deprived of a normal emotional bond with their mothers, the females are unable to relate properly to their own offspring. Perhaps it is a mixture of both those things. Some zoos have resorted to showing educational videos to pregnant apes, or to recruiting human mothers to breastfeed in front of their cages.

Hygiene

Cleaning your breasts with soap and/or water before or after feeding is unnecessary, unless you happen to have dragged yourself naked across the floor. You will be clean enough from showering in the morning (and you shouldn't rub your nipples too hard with the sponge). An excess of soap can remove substances that naturally protect the nipples, and probably promotes cracks.

Frequency and duration of feeds

No doubt you have heard people talk about breastfeeding on demand. But the idea probably wasn't explained properly.

It is extremely difficult in our society to get rid of the collective obsession with scheduled feeds. It is as though they had *always* existed. Some people, when they hear about breastfeeding on demand, think that it is something invented by hippies, a fad that will breed a generation of wild children. And yet it is exactly the other way round; breastfeeding on demand has *always* existed, and scheduled feeds are a modern invention. It is true that a Roman doctor once mentioned the word schedule, but this was an isolated case, and mothers then didn't ask doctors how to breastfeed. Nearly all doctors prior to the eighteenth century recommended breastfeeding on demand (or they didn't recommend anything, because, as breastfeeding isn't an illness, doctors weren't particularly concerned about it). It was only at the start of the twentieth century that nearly all doctors began recommending scheduled feeds, and even then few mothers followed the rule, because there was no free health service, and poor people never went to the doctor unless they were seriously ill. Only in the middle of the last century, when visits to the doctor became more common, did mothers begin to attempt to feed according to a schedule, without much success.

Let us think for a moment. Up until eighty years ago, only wealthy people owned watches. Up until 200 years ago, not many people had a clock in their house, and they were obliged to tell the time by the chimes of the church bell. Six hundred years ago, clocks were sundials and most people had never seen one, and wouldn't know how to read it. Do you think it is possible to count ten minutes every four hours using a sundial? Roman soldiers, Vikings, and Columbus's sailors were all breastfed on demand; do you imagine they were spoiled or tied to their mothers' apron strings?

A lot of people (mothers, doctors, nurses) read or hear about breastfeeding 'on demand' and think: 'Of course, there's no need to be rigid about the three-hour rule; if your baby starts to cry fifteen minutes before his feed is due, then go ahead and feed him, and if he's asleep, you don't need to wake him right away'. Or alternatively: 'Of course, like I said, breastfeed him on demand: never before two and a half hours or after four hours'. None of the above is 'on demand'; they are simply more flexible schedules, which obviously aren't as bad as strict ones, but still cause problems. On demand means any time, without looking at the clock, and regardless of whether the baby nursed five hours ago or five minutes ago.

But how can he be hungry again after five minutes? Imagine that you are bottle feeding your baby. He usually takes 150ml, and then, one afternoon, he only takes 70ml. If after five minutes he is hungry again, will you give him the remaining 80ml or will you say: 'You can't be hungry, you had a bottle only five minutes ago'? I am certain that every mother would give him the remainder of the bottle without thinking twice about it. And many would spend more than an hour trying to stick the bottle in his mouth every five minutes. So if a baby releases the breast, and then five minutes later he seems hungry again, is it not equally possible that he has only taken half the amount of milk he usually takes? Perhaps he swallowed some air and felt uncomfortable, but now he has burped he can resume feeding. Perhaps he got distracted by a fly, but the fly has gone now and he realises he is still hungry.

Perhaps he made a mistake and thought he'd had enough, but now he has changed his mind. Whatever the case, that baby, at that precise moment in time, is the only one capable of deciding whether or not he needs to feed more. An expert sitting at home and writing a book a year ago or a hundred years ago, or the doctor who saw your baby last Thursday and recommended you stick to a schedule, can't possibly know whether your baby will be hungry today at 2.25pm. In order to know that, they would need to be endowed with supernatural powers. If you know someone able to predict when your baby will be hungry, don't bother asking them such a useless question, ask them for the winning lottery numbers for this Saturday's draw.

'Won't he get a tummy ache if he feeds again so soon?' 'Shouldn't I wait until his stomach is empty, doesn't his digestive system need a rest?' Of course it doesn't.

There has been much discussion about the idea that stomachs need to 'rest'. The way some people talk about it, anyone would think they were in danger of overheating and exploding. What about our hearts? When do our hearts ever rest? Or our lungs or kidneys? There isn't a single organ in our body that needs a rest. On the contrary, it is better for us that they never rest. Our brains don't rest (we dream at night, and in any case the brain carries on controlling the body), neither do our muscles (we twitch when we dream). Why should our stomachs need a rest?

The idea that the stomach should be purged is another absurd myth, which unfortunately is very widespread among doctors. Doctors do their practical training in hospitals, not health centres. They spend four years specialising, but they spend most of their time in hospitals. This means they have come across many babies with meningitis and tuberculosis, but very few with colds, and almost none that are healthy. Their knowledge of infant nutrition is purely theoretical; when a baby is admitted to hospital they only have to note down 'normal age-appropriate diet', and the kitchens will know what food to provide. The only time a doctor is required to oversee a baby's nutrition in person is when he or she is dealing with premature babies. You will understand that feeding a premature baby, especially a severely premature baby (which means a very small baby weighing less than a kilo), is no easy task. You have to work out exactly how many millilitres of milk to give her, and how often, and you mustn't give her a drop too much. The smallest babies are unable to suck, and need a nasogastric tube. And sometimes their digestive tracts haven't even started working yet, because they should still be in their mother's womb, where they don't need to digest anything. To begin with, before you give them milk, you must suck through the tube to make sure there is no milk left in their stomach from the previous feed. Excessive retention is a bad sign, and pumping milk into the stomach when it is not emptying properly can be very dangerous. Unfortunately, some paediatricians forget that this problem is specific to severely premature babies, and they leave hospital with the idea that babies shouldn't feed until their stomachs are empty.

And yet, at best, the baby's stomach is only empty before she begins to nurse. After one minute of feeding, her stomach is no longer empty. When we tuck in to our second course, our stomachs aren't empty. They are full of soup or salad; how can we eat a steak on top of all that? When a baby is nursing on one breast, it burps (or not), and then begins nursing from the other breast, despite having only just finished feeding. If a baby can nurse again after only one minute, why can't she nurse again after five or fifteen minutes, or half an hour or an hour and a half?

'What if she wasn't hungry at all, what if she was crying for some other reason, won't it be bad for her feed again?' Of course not. First of all, a baby will want to nurse for reasons other than hunger. Secondly, if she doesn't want to feed, she won't. The simplest way of finding out whether a baby is hungry or not is to offer her your breast and see what happens.

'Should I wake her up to nurse her?' 'What is the longest time she can go without feeding?' In theory, as long as she likes. There is no need to wake up a healthy baby who is gaining weight normally. She will feed when she is hungry. Her sugar levels won't plummet because she goes a few hours without milk. In fact, thirty-odd years ago babies were *obliged* not to feed for eight hours every night; oddly enough, nowadays some mothers are told that it is *obligatory* to wake them up every four hours.

When a baby is sick or isn't gaining weight normally, this is a different matter. A baby may be so weak she is unable to ask for the breast. In such cases, it is necessary to give her the breast more often. The same can also apply to newborns (see page 86).

When the baby sleeps too much, often there is no need to wake her; just be attentive to any signs that she is hungry. 'On demand' doesn't mean 'nursing her every time she cries'. On the one hand, babies cry for many different reasons; if it is obvious she is crying for some other reason, then there is no need to give her your breast (if in doubt, breastfeed just in case; even when babies are crying out of fear or pain, giving them your breast is often the best way to calm them down). On the other hand, crying is a delayed response to hunger. If an adult went without food for three or four days, he or she would probably also cry from hunger. But we eat long before this happens, don't we? Older babies, when they are hungry, will go several hours before starting to cry. In the case of small babies, depending on their disposition it may take several minutes or more from when they are hungry to when they start to cry. But it is rare for a baby to start crying the moment she feels hungry. She will usually show other signs first: waking up, moving, making mouthing motions and searching movements with her head, gurgling, lifting her hands to her mouth… Give her your breast straight away, don't wait until she starts crying. If a baby who is weak from losing weight is left alone in a room, out of sight of her parents, she will doubtless show all these signs, but no one will notice, and she will fall asleep again from exhaustion. It is best to keep her near you at all times, or better still, to hold her so that you can give her your breast immediately.

A passing comment. When babies want to feed, why do they open their mouths and move their heads from side to side? Is it a gesture, a way of communicating? I don't think so. For millions of years, babies were constantly cradled in their mothers' arms. While in many cultures mothers carry their babies on their backs, until our ancestors learned how to weave fabric or cord, this was impossible. Prior to this, babies were held with one arm, at the front not the back. And the mother wore no clothes, so that asleep or awake, her nipples were always within easy reach of the baby's mouth. When the baby searched for the breast he invariably found it. When babies make these movements, *as if they were searching*, they really are searching.

Breastfeeding on demand doesn't mean that however much or little a baby feeds he is always 'normal'. Blood sugar and blood pressure are also 'on demand', meaning that everyone has the level they have. But not all these levels are normal; high blood pressure is a sign of ill health. A doctor won't say to a patient: 'Why is your blood pressure so high? Didn't I tell you it has to be lower? From now on make sure it doesn't go above 140/90'. It isn't up to the patient; he didn't choose to have high blood pressure. The doctor's job is to recommend the appropriate treatment that will make his blood pressure go down.

There are also normal values for the length and frequency of feeds. In order to know what these are in any given species of mammal, you only have to observe a few females with their young. (Amazing isn't it, the way zoologists and vets allow mothers and babies to do what they want, and then they decide that this is *normal*. It would never occur to them to write in a book: 'Female giraffes must feed their young for twelve minutes every five hours', and then try to persuade mothers giraffes to conform. This only happens in the human species.) Obviously other species don't breastfeed by the clock, but they still have normal values; if we knew that the baby unicorn (an imaginary animal!) nurses three to five times a day, one that nurses six times a day might be a bit 'odd', whereas one that nurses fourteen times a day might be abnormal.

The problem is that we don't know exactly what the normal value for human babies is, because humans no longer live in the wild. We all live in societies, in civilizations that have their own beliefs and norms. Thirty years ago, Spanish women nursed their babies for ten minutes every four hours. They didn't do what they wanted, what was 'normal'; they followed the recommendations given by a doctor or a book. If a tribe from the upper Orinoco nurses for five minutes every hour and a half, are they doing what is natural, or what the tribe's witch doctor recommended? And so, unlike with animals, where humans are concerned it isn't enough to observe in order to establish what the norm is in breastfeeding. We must also apply a criterion of efficiency: if mothers do it *this way* and it works, then we have to acknowledge that although it may not be exactly 'normal', it is at least compatible with our needs.

In the West, babies who breastfeed on demand initially nurse at irregular intervals approximately ten times every twenty-four hours (most nurse between eight and twelve times, some more, some less). The feeds often come in clusters: the baby may nurse two or three times in fairly quick succession then sleep a little longer. Newborns, who still don't know how to breastfeed properly, sometimes nurse for fifteen or twenty minutes, but once they have got the hang of it they nurse a lot faster, and at around three months many babies will only nurse for five or seven minutes, or even as little as two or less. The ten or so feeds a day will continue for the first year, and for part of the second. There comes a time when the child nurses less and less, perhaps once or twice a day; but at around two or three, children often experience a sort of feeding frenzy when they want to nurse all the time, sometimes every fifteen minutes. (This doesn't go on all day long, of course; they might nurse several times in a row then stop for several hours). It is almost as if they are 'play-nursing'. Kindly friends and relatives will usually take the opportunity to undermine your morale by saying things like: 'I tell you, you've spoiled that child, he'll still be nursing when he's walking to the altar'. (One of the reasons for children this age wanting to nurse all the time is the presence of strangers, so relatives and friends have ample opportunities to observe the phenomenon!) There is no need to worry. You have reached the final leg; after a few turbulent weeks (or months) most children will automatically wean themselves, while others may keep up a kind of 'token' nursing (once or twice a day) for a few more years.

In other cultures, babies nurse far more frequently. The world record appears to be held by the !Kung or bush people of the Kalahari, who nurse approximately six times an hour during the day, although each feed only lasts an average of ninety seconds. To give you an idea: a group of anthropologists observed children under two for periods of fifteen minutes to see how they behaved with their mothers. In only 25 per cent of the observations did the children go the entire fifteen minutes without nursing. Children under three always nursed at night. The figures for traditional peoples in Africa, Asia, and Latin America are lower, but on the whole they breastfeed more often than Western mothers.

So we can say that there are two patterns of breastfeeding that work well in human beings: few (meaning ten a day) but relatively long feeds, or frequent but shorter feeds – with all the variations in between. What is not normal, here or in the Kalahari, is for the baby to feed frequently *and* for long periods; for him to be constantly latched on to the breast. When this occurs, it is usually a sign of incorrect positioning, tongue-tie, or both, as we will see later on.

Even within Europe variations exist. Surprisingly, a multi-country study of child growth found that the average number of feeds per day at two months ranged from 5.7 in Rostock through to 8.5 in Porto, 6.5 in Madrid and 7.2 in Barcelona. How is it possible that babies of women from such similar cultures, who are supposedly being breastfed on demand, want to nurse more in some countries than in others?

The answer is simple, but alarming. It turns out that breastfeeding on demand, the idea on which this, and any other contemporary book on the subject, is based, doesn't actually exist. It doesn't exist because babies aren't able to talk.

If babies could talk, an independent observer could confirm: 'this mother is indeed breastfeeding on demand'; or 'this mother isn't breastfeeding on demand, because at 11.23 her little boy said: "Mama, milk", and then again at 11.41, but his mother didn't feed him until he had asked a third time at 11.57'. Since babies can't talk, it is up to the mother to decide when her baby is asking to be fed and when not. Two babies are crying: one mother immediately nurses hers, while the other looks at her watch and says: 'He can't be hungry, he had a feed less than an hour and a half ago, he must be teething', and gives him a teething ring to chew. Two babies are moving their heads and making rooting noises; one mother picks up her baby and nurses him at once, and the other doesn't even realise because her baby was in his cot and the mother wasn't paying attention. Two babies say 'gaga'; one mother thinks: 'Oh no, he's already awake', and immediately begins to nurse him, and the other gazes at her baby and says: 'Ah, how sweet, he talked!'

A lot of Western mothers have heard people say: 'as he grows bigger, he'll be able to go for longer without feeding'. And the prediction is fulfilled; mothers who are convinced their child will be able 'to go longer', are increasingly less likely to hear their baby's demands to be fed, or more likely to misinterpret them (he's cold, he's hot, he's in pain, he's teething, he's bored… anything but hungry). And it is true that their children begin to nurse far less frequently, and within a year they stop nursing altogether. But it is also true that, when a mother ignores this myth, and really tries to breastfeed on demand, her baby carries on nursing as before. Yes, of course, there comes a time when the frequency of feeds diminishes; but this usually happens at a year and a half, not at three months.

The ten minutes every three hours rule has become so widespread in our society that almost all mothers, even those that wholeheartedly embrace breastfeeding, have undoubtedly tried, at one time or another, to make their baby 'go for longer' between feeds, or to make him nurse for longer when he releases the breast after two minutes. If they were left to their own devices, perhaps babies would nurse not ten but fifteen or twenty times a day, or more. Perhaps the period I described as the 'the final leg', when a child wants to nurse all the time, only goes on for a few weeks because the mother does her best to put a stop to it, and because the child, sensing his mother is upset, gives in; perhaps, if the mother were only too happy to oblige, the child would go on like that for months, or even years.

Perhaps we aren't so different from the !Kung after all. Given that they usually breastfeed for four years, perhaps when the anthropologists were counting the number of feeds, they observed fewer newborns than children of three and four. Perhaps !Kung newborns nurse less than six times an hour. Perhaps their mothers are so used to a child of two, three or four nursing more frequently, that when they have a new baby they find it strange that he nurses so little, and, unlike Western mothers, they try their best to nurse him more often. Or perhaps the desert heat is a factor, and !Kung babies need milk constantly.

Finally, it is worth remembering that 'on demand' doesn't only mean 'when the baby wants', but also 'when the mother wants'. Obviously, a newborn's needs always come first. But, as the baby grows older, the mother has more and more opportunities to intervene and decide when she breastfeeds and when she doesn't. Of course, a fixed schedule is undesirable for a baby of any age, and it is usually always best for him to decide when he nurses. This doesn't mean the mother can't bring forward or delay the odd feed.

For example, if your three-month-old wants to nurse in the middle of the street, you can either feed her immediately, or you can distract her for a while and feed her when you get home. With a five-month-old baby, the mother who breastfeeds according to a strict schedule can't go to the cinema at seven o'clock because at eight it is 'time for the baby's feed'. In contrast, the mother who breastfeeds on demand can feed her baby at six o'clock, try to feed him again at six-thirty, leave him with his grandmother and go off happily to the cinema. And if at eight-thirty the baby starts crying, his grandmother will do her best to distract him until his mother comes home half an hour later and breastfeeds him.

So, contrary to what a lot of people think, far from being a trap, breastfeeding on demand is a blessing for the mother. Most of the time her baby does what he wants, which means he is contented and doesn't complain, and his mother is also contented and doesn't complain. And, occasionally, she does what she wants, which isn't such a bad thing either. The real trap is breastfeeding by the clock. Having to pace up and down, fretting over a child that has been crying for fifteen minutes, or two hours, because 'it isn't time for his feed'. Trying to wake a child who is fast asleep because 'it's time for his feed'. Having to explain to the hairdresser 'I can't make 5.30. Can I come at 6.30 instead? I have to feed the baby at six.'

→ Konner, M. 'Nursing frequency and birth spacing in !Kung hunter-gatherers', *IPPF Med Bull* 1978;15:1-3

→ Manz, F., van't Hof, M.A., Haschke, F. 'The mother-infant relationship: Who controls breastfeeding frequency?' *Lancet* 1999;353:1152

Positioning: the key to success

A baby doesn't feed by creating a vacuum and sucking, the way you drink juice though a straw. He 'milks' the nipple, pressing with his tongue the lactiferous sinuses where, due to the oxytocin, the milk has accumulated.

So, in order for the baby to feed properly, these lactiferous sinuses must be inside his mouth, and his tongue must be underneath them.

Ultrasound images have been taken of a baby's mouth when he is nursing. *Figure 3* on page 56 shows the areola stretched out and, together with the nipple, completely filling the baby's mouth. The tip of the baby's tongue is placed over the gums and sometimes even over the lower lip underneath the areola. The baby's tongue moves up and back, squeezing the reserves of milk from the ducts. The tongue doesn't actually move, but a wave of pressure passes through it from tip to base, so that there is no friction between the tongue and the breast. As the pressure wave moves towards the nipple, the ducts empty, and the pressure inside them is reduced. Because the pressure in the breast acini is high (due to the oxytocin), the lactiferous sinuses fill up with milk again, and the tongue once more squeezes it out. After one or more movements of the tongue, enough milk accumulates in the baby's throat to trigger the deglutition reflex, and the baby swallows.

When the baby nurses, his mouth is wide open, the nipple thrust to the back of his throat, his top lip folded upward and his bottom lip folded downward. His nose is close to the breast. His chin usually touches the breast. Sometimes his cheeks press into the breast so that you can't see his lips at all. His cheeks aren't hollowed (as I said before, breastfeeding isn't like sucking through a straw, it is more like chewing), but rather they pump rhythmically. When the baby starts nursing, his lips usually move very fast, probably to stimulate the nipple to produce more oxytocin. But this rhythm soon changes, and the quick movements give way to a slower, more expansive movement of the jaw. You can see this from the way the angle of the baby's jaw moves in relation to his ear, and from the muscles tensing in his temples.

Consequences of incorrect positioning

When the baby is incorrectly positioned, instead of latching on to a large area of the breast he sucks at the nipple, which produces a whole host of symptoms:

1. Hollow cheeks

As the baby is unable to exert any pressure on the breast with his tongue, he is obliged to suck, creating a vacuum.

2. Sore or cracked nipples

The baby is exerting a great deal of force on a small surface area (the nipple), and therefore the pressure is far greater. The mother feels pain during the feed, and after a few days she may develop cracks.

3. Long feeds, staying latched on to the breast

Creating a vacuum is a very inefficient way of breastfeeding, and the baby will take much longer to nurse. A common complaint of mothers is: 'He nurses for thirty to forty-five minutes or more on each breast, and that's only because I take him off, otherwise he would take even longer'.

When the baby nurses properly, he automatically releases the breast when he has finished, which can be anywhere between two and twenty minutes. When a mother says: 'He falls asleep at the breast', normally what she means is that he releases the breast and then falls asleep. If a baby occasionally falls asleep still attached to the breast and has to be taken off it, well, these things happen. But if he does this nearly every time he nurses, it is almost always because he isn't nursing in the correct position (or because for some other reason, general weakness or problems with his tongue, he is unable to nurse properly).

4. He is still hungry

Despite nursing for over half an hour, he seems restless, annoyed, frustrated.

5. Frequent nursing

Because he is still hungry, he will soon want to nurse again. The mother complains that he is 'attached to her breast all day long'. It is normal for a baby to have the odd day, or certain hours during the day (usually in the afternoon) where he demands to nurse more than usual; it is also normal for him to nurse more frequently but for shorter periods of one or two minutes. But frequent nursing for periods of thirty to forty-five minutes, and then demanding to nurse again a few minutes later, usually suggests incorrect positioning.

6. Full breasts, breast engorgement, mastitis

In extreme cases, when a baby takes practically no milk at all, milk production begins to diminish and the breasts empty. However, if the baby is taking milk but nursing incorrectly, the breast is more likely to become too full. It seems the breast can differentiate between a baby who feeds correctly and little (when he is older and eating other foods), and one who is feeding little because he is feeding incorrectly. In the first case, the breast produces less milk. But in the second case, a safety mechanism is triggered; nature doesn't like children to starve to death, and it won't let a baby die because of the arbitrary positioning of his lips. When the breast *notices* that the baby isn't feeding properly, it begins to produce more *foremilk*, and the pituitary gland produces more oxytocin in order to eject this milk. Simplifying a lot, we could say that the *watery* foremilk is what comes out automatically, and the hindmilk, which is rich in fats, is the milk the baby gets when it feeds properly. When the baby can't get the milk out properly, the breasts serve the hindmilk to him on a plate. This safety mechanism allows the baby to survive, though not without difficulties. The combination of breasts producing too much milk and a baby who isn't feeding properly can lead to constantly, possibly painfully, full breasts and even mastitis.

7. Fast milk ejection reflex

I mentioned that mothers are usually able to feel the milk ejection reflex (the let-down) when the baby begins feeding, especially during the first few months (see page 25). But when the baby is feeding in the incorrect position, the mother often feels the let-down much more intensely and frequently while she is nursing. Her milk can sometimes literally spurt out. Rather than feeding, the baby is waiting for the milk, which, because of the oxytocin, is ejected automatically to fill his mouth. This is why he takes so long to feed. Some books, especially those published in America, talk about an excess of oxytocin as though it were a specific illness. Apparently, when the mother's pituitary gland produces an excess of oxytocin, her milk is ejected too fast, choking her baby, who becomes frustrated by this upsetting experience and soon refuses to breastfeed. The treatment they recommend is to express some of the milk by hand before the baby's feed, so that the first spurt doesn't shoot into his mouth, or to breastfeed lying on the bed, so that the milk has gravity to contend with. Some women may produce too much oxytocin, the same way others suffer from hyperthyroidism, but I am sure this is extremely rare, and that many of the problems attributed to an over-active pituitary gland are in fact caused by incorrect positioning. Placing the baby in the correct position will enable him to nurse properly, and the mother won't be forced to produce too much oxytocin.

8. Vomiting and regurgitation

All babies spit up, some more than others. This is normal, and it stops when the baby reaches about one year. But a baby who is nursing incorrectly is taking more of the diluted foremilk, and less of the more concentrated hindmilk. It could be that his stomach is overfull. He regurgitates the liquid and vomits copiously.

9. Diarrhoea

Because he is taking more foremilk, the baby is consuming less fat and more lactose than normal. This can lead to an overload of lactose. The baby isn't lactose intolerant; he is perfectly healthy and can digest a normal amount of lactose. But there is so much of it he can't digest it all. Undigested lactose reaches the large intestine where bacteria break it down, producing gases and lactic acid. The baby's stools will be even more watery than usual (all breastfed babies' stools are loose or runny) and more acidic, and this will irritate his little bottom if you don't change his nappy quickly.

10. Crying and colic

Our hero has many reasons to cry. He is hungry. He is tired. His mother frowns at him because her nipples hurt. He may be swallowing air when he feeds as he is unable to make a seal with his lips because they are incorrectly positioned. The bacteria turn the undigested lactose into gas, and he seems unhappy. His little bottom stings.

11. What about his weight?

That depends. If his mother tries to feed him for only ten minutes every four hours, obviously he will hardly gain any weight. But if his mother is breastfeeding on demand, morning, noon and night, and he is nursing all day long, he might gain the right amount of weight. He might even occasionally gain too much weight. Because he is not taking much fat, he doesn't feel full; in fact, even when he has taken enough calories he may still be hungry. Some babies put on lots of weight even though they are feeding in the incorrect position.

This is an important point. We can't just look at the baby's weight in order to evaluate whether he is nursing properly. We can't say: 'The baby is putting on weight so everything must be fine'. If, in order for the baby to gain weight, the mother has to nurse him day and night, putting up with painful cracked nipples and engorgement, and the baby spends all his time nursing, crying, and vomiting, then the baby is not nursing properly. It is safe to assume that breastfeeding is going well when, besides putting on weight, the baby and his mother are both contented.

Positioning at the breast isn't a black and white affair. There are many shades in between, ranging from the baby who is perfectly positioned through to the one who is completely incorrectly positioned. So, not all babies show all the symptoms described above, or they may be less acute. Almost invariably, feeds will be very long and the mother's nipples sore. She may have had cracks to begin with, but now her nipples are just sore. As the baby grows and his mouth gets bigger, he can fit more of the breast inside it, and this, together with experience, tends to ease the symptoms of incorrect positioning.

These many shades imply that there is no clear line between what is normal and what is abnormal. Chloe Fisher is a midwife based in Oxford, and perhaps the person who knows most about breastfeeding positions. She was asked how long a feed could last and still be considered normal (wouldn't it be great if everything was so clear cut, if we could say: 'Seventeen minutes is normal, eighteen minutes is too long!') and she replied: 'Normal is whatever is acceptable to the mother'. If the mother is enjoying breastfeeding, and the baby is too, if breastfeeding is the high point of her day, a moment of calm and relaxation, what does it matter if her baby nurses for eighteen minutes? On the other hand, another mother might find this situation uncomfortable. Perhaps her nipples are sore. Or the baby won't stop crying, or maybe she has other children, or other things she has to do, or she is spending so much time breastfeeding she feels 'tied down' and overwhelmed. In such cases, it is good to know that changing the baby's position when nursing can help.

How to achieve the correct position

We have seen that in order for the baby to nurse properly, a good bit of the breast has to be in his mouth, and his tongue should be underneath it. Years ago we used to tell mothers: 'The baby has to have the whole areola in his mouth, not just the nipple'. But there was a problem with this, because the mother can only see the breast from above and not what is going on below. When she tried to push the areola into the baby's mouth, the lower part of her breast slipped out. The nipple was too close to the baby's lower lip, and there was no room for his tongue, so he couldn't nurse properly. The idea, then, isn't to try to push the whole of the areola into the baby's mouth, but to make sure the baby takes a big mouthful of the breast and the nipple is in the upper part of his mouth. There has to be enough room for him to place his tongue between the nipple and the lower lip. (*Figure 3*).

In order to achieve this, it is a good idea to lift your baby to your breast so that your nipple is level with his nose. If your breast is level with his mouth, he may, of course, be able to nurse properly, but it could also happen that your nipple will remain in the middle or the lower part of his mouth, making it difficult for him to use his tongue.

On the other hand, if the nipple is level with the baby's nose, when he opens his mouth there will be enough room for his tongue (*Figure 4*).

The way the rest of the baby's body is positioned is of secondary importance. After a few months, the baby will be so skilled at nursing that he will be able to do it in almost any position. As

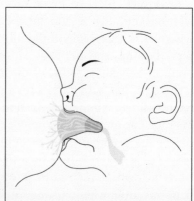

Figure 3: The baby takes a large part of the areola in his mouth (the area shaded in light grey) and 'milks' it with his tongue.

long as his mouth is correctly positioned, it doesn't matter where the rest of his body is. Having said this, there are, of course, positions from which it is more or less easy for the baby to latch on. Newborns may find it particularly difficult to nurse if their body isn't correctly positioned.

Ideally, the neck should be tilted back. Babies without a tongue-tie can usually also nurse with their neck in a straight line, but babies with a tongue-tie will need to have their neck clearly tilted back, so that their lower jaw comes closer to Mum. It is difficult for a baby to nurse with his neck in any other position, and in extreme instances it would make swallowing difficult. If you don't believe me, try drinking a glass of water with your neck bent forward (chin touching sternum) or twisted to the right or left (chin on shoulder), or bent over to the side (ear touching shoulder).

In most cases, holding the breast while the baby is nursing is unnecessary and even counterproductive; it is better to take the baby to the breast rather than taking the breast to the baby. Holding the breast can give rise to various problems: the mother's hand can get in the way, stopping the baby from latching on to the breast properly; the pressure from her fingers can pinch some of the ducts, stopping the milk from coming out, and she will no longer have a free hand.

In some cases, where the breast is very flaccid, it can be easier to cup it with one hand, but there is no need to use the thumb to hold it from above. The scissor position is a popular one, and it features in many old illustrations, showing that mothers have always used it. The scissor position has been much criticised by

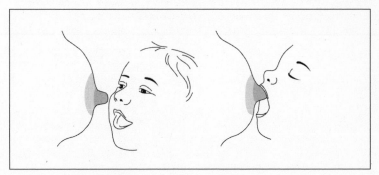

Figure 4: Place the baby so that his nose is level with your nipple; this way the nipple will remain in the upper part of his mouth.

experts, because when used incorrectly, with the fingers too close to the nipple, there is no room for the baby's mouth. When the fingers are far enough away from the nipple, the scissor position won't cause any problems, though it doesn't seem particularly effective. (*Figure 5*).

When the breast is very large, it is sometimes necessary to squeeze it so that the baby can latch on to the nipple more easily (*Figure 6*).

This is most often needed in the first weeks, when the baby's mouth is smaller. Once the baby is attached to the nipple, you can let go. Remember to squeeze the breast in the same direction as the baby's mouth. Wiessinger has demonstrated this perfectly with her analogy of a sandwich (*Figure 7*).

The baby's head should be positioned in such a way that the axis of his oral cavity and the axis of the breast are in alignment, and, depending on the shape of the breast, the baby's body should

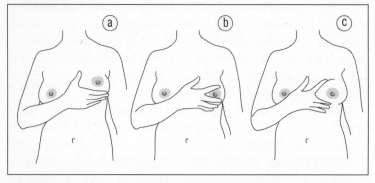

Figure 5: If it is necessary to hold the breast during nursing, it is best to cup it with the hand *(a)*. The scissor position often covers the nipple and makes it difficult for the baby to take the nipple *(b)*; the fingers must be widely spaced *(c)*.

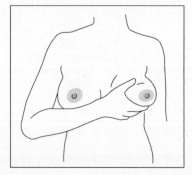

Figure 6: A large, voluminous breast can be squeezed so that the baby is able to latch on to the nipple more easily.

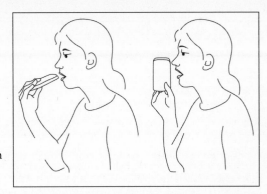

Figure 7: The thin part of the sandwich must be lined up with the mouth.

be turned completely on its side, or in a more or less diagonal position. (*Figure 8*).

If the baby's body is facing upwards, he will not be able to nurse comfortably. The baby's whole body should be touching that of his mother, curled around her like a belt. The baby in *Figure 9 (c)* is too far away from his mother, which means he has to stretch his neck too far. We sometimes use the expression 'navel to navel'. This isn't supposed to be taken literally (I have seen some mothers do precisely that, attempting to place the baby's navel level with their own). Stomach to stomach, or 'tummy to mummy' as it is sometimes called, is perfectly adequate.

Many books, especially those published in America, used to recommend holding the baby by placing a hand under his backside, so that his head is cradled in the crook of his mother's arm. But the elbow is to one side of the body, while the breast is in front of the body. Mothers who have no trouble breastfeeding

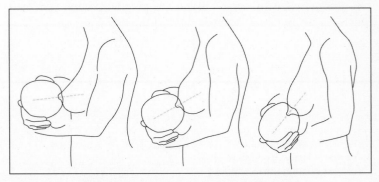

Figure 8: The baby's head must be pointing towards the breast.

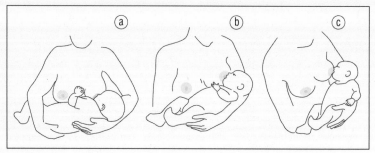

Figure 9: In order for the baby to nurse comfortably, his body must be pressed against the mother and facing her, *(a)*. Positions *(b)* and *(c)* are incorrect because the baby is forced to stretch his neck; in *(c)*, he is too far away from his mother and can't latch on to the breast properly.

their babies in this position usually have large, malleable breasts that can be easily stretched to the side, or else they move their arm inwards so their baby's head is aligned with their breast (quite an uncomfortable position that can put a strain on the shoulder). But if the mother's breast and arm remain in their usual places (*Figure 10*) the baby is forced to crane his neck to reach the breast. He will be uncomfortable, and will find it very difficult to latch on, managing only to take the nipple in his mouth.

It is better to support the baby by placing your hand on his back, so that his head is resting on your forearm. You can also hold the baby's head with your other hand (see *Figure 11*).

When the baby is in front of the breast, and his lip is brushing the nipple, he will begin to search for it, moving his head and his tongue. More than one novice mother, seeing her baby move his head from side to side, has exclaimed: 'He's saying no! He's doesn't want to nurse!' If you are pregnant when you read

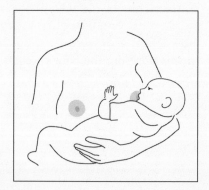

Figure 10: An incorrectly positioned baby. His head is cradled in his mother's arm, and he is forced to crane his neck to reach her breast.

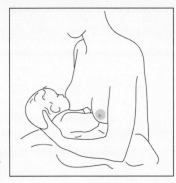

Figure 11: You can also hold the baby's head with your other hand.

this, or have been breastfeeding your baby for several weeks or months, you might think I am exaggerating. But believe me, after going through hours of exhausting labour, when you are unsure of yourself, and your hormones are raging, it is fairly easy for something like this to drag you down. Just remember, your baby isn't saying no; moving his head from side to side is instinctive, and is designed to help him find the breast. Our cousins the primates don't attach their babies to the breast, they simply hold them in their arms, and the babies do the rest.

Before starting to nurse, the baby has to be sure that it is the nipple he is taking. There is no sense in him sucking on his mother's arm or her tummy; apart from getting no milk he would give her a big bruise. And so he brings into play all his senses: he sees the nipple, he brushes it with the skin on his face, and then with his lips, he smells it, and licks it. When at last he is sure, he opens his mouth and goes for it. At that moment, to make sure he is firmly latched on, press him towards you with the same hand you are using to support his back. Don't push the back of his head as this might cause a reflex action, moving his head back.

Many babies nurse better if the mother is leaning back, like in a deckchair, with the baby lying face down on her front. When in this position, the baby's weight isn't resting on the mother's arm, but on her body; she can take her hand away and he won't fall. This position ensures their bodies are very close together – as they should be – with the mother's breast firmly in the baby's mouth.

Other positions

It is useful to know a few other nursing positions (*Figure 12*).

(a) With the baby's legs away from you (like holding a rugby ball). This is a particularly good way of nursing twins at the same time, and of preventing the baby's feet from touching your scar after a caesarean.

(b) Stretched out on the bed. This is essential at night, and more comfortable during the day. The best way is usually for you to lie on your back with your baby face down on top of you. Place his head between your breasts and wait for him to start searching for your nipple. You and the baby can also lie on your sides, facing one another; but you have to constantly press his back or he will fall away, and you cannot relax. In order to give him the second breast you can turn slightly further and nurse him from above, or clasp him to you and turn over with him onto your other side. If your breasts are very full and you are feeding on your side without turning over, it might be more comfortable to nurse from the upper breast first and then the lower.

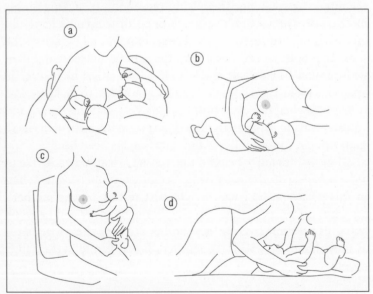

Figure 12: Other positions.

(c) Sitting. This is a very useful position for babies who have to nurse upright, for example if they have a cleft palate.

(d) The She-wolf (on all fours), and other resourceful positions. Believe it or not, they do sometimes work. For example, in the case of an obstruction or mastitis, it is necessary to find a position in which your baby's tongue is positioned just below the inflamed area. Don't forget to take a snapshot as a souvenir!

Why do babies nurse incorrectly?

Once the awful schedules have been put aside, and breastfeeding on demand has begun, most problems with nursing are due to incorrect positioning, tongue-tie or a combination of both.

How can so many babies be latching on incorrectly? After reading the lengthy and exhaustive explanation above, one is tempted to say, 'Well, because it's so difficult no one can explain it properly.' Yet it isn't that difficult. All mammals successfully nurse their young without anyone having to tell them what the correct position is, and the same was true of our ancestors for millions of years.

This subject made me worry. It took me years of reading books, watching videos and listening to experts to understand what the proper position was. So how did they manage in prehistoric times?

Post-partum interference

I found the answer in a piece of research carried out in Sweden in 1990 by Righard and Alade. They compared two groups of newborns: one group that had been in close physical contact with the mother from birth, and one group in which babies had been briefly separated from their mothers. Within each group there were mothers who had been given pethidine (a powerful pain-reliever) during labour, and others who hadn't. Almost all the babies who had been in constant physical contact with mothers who hadn't taken pethidine, sought out and found the breast of their own accord without any difficulty, and latched on perfectly. About twenty minutes after they were born, they began searching for the breast, and within forty to ninety minutes nearly all of them were nursing. Of the babies who had stayed close to their mothers, but were still affected by the pain-reliever, only half nursed in the proper position, and the same applied to the babies who hadn't been affected by the pain-reliever, but had been separated from their mothers. In other words, babies are born with a natural instinct to find their mother's breast and to nurse correctly, but if we intervene, by administering pethidine or by separating the newborn from his mother, this instinct fails. When both of these factors occurred together, the results were devastating; not one single baby was able to nurse properly, and the vast majority refused to nurse at all. Two hours after they were born, they had still not started feeding.

The most interesting detail (from a Spanish standpoint) was how the Swedes define being 'in contact with' and 'separated from' the mother. Immediately after delivery, before they were washed or had drops put in their eyes, the babies in the first group were placed on their naked mother's body for two hours. In the case of the babies in the 'separated' group, they were also immediately placed on their naked mother's body, but twenty minutes later they were taken from their mothers to be washed and weighed, and forty minutes after delivery were once again placed, still naked, on their mother's naked body for the remainder of the two hours. This twenty-minute separation, which wasn't immediate but occurred twenty minutes after delivery, was enough to interfere with the baby's ability to nurse. What of those newborns who aren't able to touch, or sometimes even to see, their mothers for three, six, twelve hours, or even longer? If only Spanish newborns had as much contact with their mothers as the Swedish newborns who are 'separated' from theirs!

Incidentally, this skin-to-skin contact between mother and baby isn't part of a new-age ritual or a return to nature. It has nothing to do with passing on good vibrations or earthly energy. It is about providing warmth in the literal sense. Various studies (among them those carried out in the Doce de Octubre Hospital in Madrid and Joan XXIII Hospital in Tarragona, pioneer centres in this field) show that babies who have skin-to-skin contact with their mothers maintain a normal temperature, or if they have caught cold their temperature returns to normal.

We mammals are warm-blooded creatures, and as such we need to maintain a stable body temperature. In order to ward off the cold we burn more sugar, by rallying our reserves and using more oxygen, which forces our lungs, heart and liver to work faster. This is a lot more difficult for a baby than for an adult, and makes them much more susceptible to hypothermia.

We adults wear warm clothes in order not to catch cold. But clothes don't provide warmth, they simply insulate. Our bodies produce heat effortlessly, and clothes stop it from dissipating. The same overcoat that keeps you warm can also stop a block of ice from melting. The problem newborns have is that they find it difficult to produce enough heat. They need an external source of heat. Inside the womb the baby obviously enjoys the same temperature as the mother's body, approximately 37°C (98.6°F). If a naked baby is placed on his mother's naked body, mother and baby will maintain the same temperature; this is a law of physics. A mother is the best, most efficient and most reliable source of heat for a baby because, even if the gas and electricity go off, she will go on giving off heat, and the baby will never be too hot in her arms. But if we place several layers of insulation between mother and baby, in the form of clothes, the baby will no longer receive the heat he needs.

→ Christensson, K., Siles, C., Moreno, L., Belaustequi, A., De La Fuente, P., Lagercrantz, H. et al. 'Temperature, metabolic adaptation and crying in healthy full-term newborns cared for skin-to-skin or in a cot', *Acta Pædiatr* 1992;81: 488.493

→ Gómez Papí, A., Baiges Nogues, M.T., Batiste Fernández, M.T., Marca Gutiérrez, M.M., Nieto Jurado, A., Closa Monasterolo, R. 'Método canguro en sala de partos en recién nacidos a término'. *An Esp Pediatr* 1998;48:631-3

→ Figueras Aloy, J., García Alix, A., Alomar Ribes, A., Blanco Bravo, D., Esqué Ruiz, M.T., Fernández Lorenzo. J.R. 'Recomendaciones de mínimos para la asistencia al recién nacido sano', *An Esp Pediatr* 2001;55:141-5

Nipple and teat confusion

Everybody knows that when babies get used to bottle feeding it can mean the end of lactation. A lot of mothers say: 'He wouldn't feed from me any more'. The most popular explanation is that 'the bottle is easier, the baby gets lazy and can't be bothered to breastfeed'.

But this is untrue. The bottle isn't easier. Various studies of premature babies, as well as those with serious heart malformations, show that their heart and respiratory rates and their oxygen levels are much more stable when they breastfeed than when they bottle feed. Babies are made to breastfeed; their muscles and reflexes are designed for it, whereas bottle feeding requires specific training.

The answer isn't that it is easier or more difficult, but that it is different. Apart from the few drops that come out by themselves, the milk has to be drawn from the mother's breast, and to do that the baby's tongue must push rhythmically backwards. Besides drawing the milk out, this gesture tends to pull the breast further into the baby's mouth, allowing him to feed more efficiently. In contrast, milk from a bottle comes out by itself; the baby has to stop it from coming out so that he can swallow the milk already in his mouth. When bottle feeding, the baby's tongue moves forward in a rhythmical movement, tending to push the bottle out of the baby's mouth. To prevent this from happening, teats and dummies are wider at the end, forming a kind of ball that acts as a stop. The rest of the teat is narrow, allowing the baby to feed from the bottle almost with his mouth closed; if he opened his mouth as wide as when he takes the breast, the ball would be useless and the bottle would fall from his mouth.

Slightly older babies will sometimes alternate between the breast and bottle (or the dummy) without any problem, adjusting the way they move their lips and tongues. However, during the first few weeks, a lot of babies get confused, and when they breastfeed they can't bottle feed, and vice versa. For the first few days, some mothers complain: 'He wants to nurse all the time, but he won't take the dummy' ('all the time' means 'before the three hours are up'), while others exclaim: 'I don't understand why he won't nurse, he sucks his dummy all the time', (and, of course, the oft-heard explanation: 'He won't nurse because you haven't got any milk', doesn't work, because a baby will happily keep sucking a dummy even though it won't provide even a drop of milk).

The first time a baby is given a bottle (for example by a nurse who wants to avoid waking the mother during the night), he will often refuse it. Besides the milk and the teat both tasting funny, and teat being hard and oddly shaped, when the baby tries feeding as he would from the breast, the milk shoots out so fast it chokes him. Spluttering and crying, the baby rejects the teat. The nice nurse will say: 'It's all right little one, be a good boy and take your milk', while the not-so-nice one says: 'We'll have none of that nonsense, who does he think he is,' but both nurses will persist. After a few moments, the baby realises that if he does this and not that with his tongue, he won't choke. 'Good boy, you see how easy it is?' says the nice nurse; 'I told you he was just being difficult,' says the other.

A few hours later, when they take the newborn back to his mother, he is 'thinking' what he will later say a hundred times: 'Look, see what I can do Mummy!' and he tries to do with the breast what he has just learned to do with the bottle, pushing his tongue forwards. Shock, horror, the breast slips out of his mouth. Because breasts don't have a ball on the end, they end *in a point*.

'He rejects my breast, crying,' the distraught mother says. Exhausted after hours of labour, her hormones raging, and suffering from post-natal blues (not as serious as post-natal depression, but far more widespread), what the mother is really saying is that she feels rejected by her own baby. Can things get any worse? 'Don't despair, he'll soon latch on,' says the nice nurse. 'Of course he does, you don't have any milk', says the not-so-nice nurse. And they take the baby away and give him another bottle. And that is the beginning of the end.

Because, of course, as every nurse knows (and every mother, grandmother, father and friend): you can always bottle feed a baby. If he refuses, you just have to be patient. You never hear anyone say: 'It's no use insisting, sometimes the bottle just doesn't work', or, 'my sister-in-law had the same problem, the baby refused to feed from the bottle and he almost starved to death, in the end she had to breastfeed him', or, 'you shouldn't get obsessed about bottle feeding, nowadays babies do just as well on breastmilk', or, 'I'm a great believer in bottle feeding, but sometimes you just have to accept that some women can't do it', or, 'it's better to breastfeed with love than to bottle feed with anger', or, 'you're only passing on your anxieties to your baby by trying to force him to bottle feed', or, 'there's no need to feel guilty, it isn't necessary to bottle feed your baby in order to be a good mother'...

If every mother was absolutely convinced that it was always

possible to breastfeed a baby, they would keep trying and nearly all babies would stop 'rejecting' the breast within minutes. And in the toughest cases, the nurse, equally convinced and with more experience, would help out. If every mother, nurse, grandmother, father and friend believed as much in the breast as in the bottle, I wouldn't have needed to write this book.

This refusal of the breast when the baby has become accustomed to the bottle is known as 'nipple confusion', or 'nipple and teat confusion'. In order to avoid it, mothers are advised not to bottle feed or give babies a dummy, at least during the first month. A lot of one-month-old babies will vigorously reject the bottle or the dummy; they are less easy to deceive than newborns. Others will bottle feed or use a dummy, and will no longer have this confusion, adjusting the movement of their tongue accordingly. But some babies (whatever age they are, even at six months), when they begin to use dummies or to bottle feed, will either refuse the breast, or nurse in a way that causes the mother pain.

A number of doctors insist there is no such thing as nipple confusion, and that giving newborns one or more bottles has no adverse effect on lactation. It is true that there is no experimental data to back this up, because that would require purposefully bottle feeding a random group of babies to see what happened. Those who see no harm in bottle feeding aren't interested in doing research, and those of us who do consider it unethical to carry out a study like that. 'What difference does it make if it exists or not?' the reader will be thinking; when in doubt don't bottle feed, and that's that. Well, it so happens that some of those who don't believe in nipple confusion recommend giving all babies a minimum of one bottle feed a week, to habituate them. Otherwise, they argue, when the mother goes back to work, or has to leave the house for any reason, the baby will reject the bottle. Well, at least they accept that the confusion works one way; that a baby who is 'habituated' to breastfeeding will refuse the bottle.

Lack of cultural models

Breastfeeding in the large primates isn't purely instinctive (see page 40). It requires learning through observation, which in the wild takes place naturally. However, a lot of women who give birth have never seen another mother breastfeeding. Some have never even held a baby. Many teenage girls have never seen a mother look after her baby, although some have worked as babysitters, looking after (and bottle feeding) a baby whose mother is absent.

On the other hand, it is relatively common to see a baby bottle feeding (in parks, films, magazines). This partly explains why, in many European countries, immigrant women breastfeed less than indigenous women. For example, Turkish women living in Sweden not only breastfeed less than their fellow countrywomen back in Turkey, they also breastfeed less than Swedish women. Sweden has one of the highest rates of breastfeeding but immigrant women don't see that. They can't read the local literature, they have no Swedish women friends to talk to, and all they see is pictures in magazines, from which they deduce that 'bottle feeding must be better, because that's what they do here'.

Also, because they have seen a lot of babies being bottle fed, either in pictures or in real life, a lot of mothers try to breastfeed their baby as if they were bottle feeding him, face up with his head in the crook of their arm. This position forces the baby to twist and crane his neck, and he has difficulty reaching the breast.

Art also provides some poor examples. Many paintings depict the baby Jesus nursing in a sitting position, his head twisted round. But if you look at the baby, he is usually several months old, and sometimes one or two years old. Newborns aren't very photogenic, it is true, and the painting looks nicer with a bigger baby. Older babies, as I mentioned before, can nurse in almost any position. And in some paintings the baby isn't even nursing, he is staring at the artist (no doubt the most interesting thing he has seen in his life), while pinching his mother's nipple hard.

Self-sacrifice

The myth of the self-sacrificing mother is partially responsible for many babies nursing incorrectly.

Why are nipples so sensitive? A pinch on the nipple is far more painful than a pinch anywhere else. Maybe they have to be that way in order to respond to stimuli and to trigger the oxytocin and prolactin receptors? Not necessarily. What we know as 'touch' is in fact several different senses, each with its own nerves and receptors. The nipple could still be very sensitive to pressure or contact without being sensitive to pain.

I think that the nipple's heightened sensitivity to pain is designed to make sure the baby is properly latched on to the breast when feeding. Why did cavewomen breastfeed? Why do animals breastfeed? Is it because the vet recommends it, or because they have heard that it is very nutritious and protects against infection? Obviously not. The main reason why both animal and human mothers breastfeed is quite simply to quieten their young. A baby's cry is extremely unpleasant, and compels the mother to do something to calm her baby. Nursing him, rocking him, cuddling him, singing to him, anything to make him shut up!

What happened in prehistoric times when a baby nursed incorrectly? 'The baby cries so I breastfeed him. It hurts so I take him off. He cries again, so I put him back on. It hurts so I take him off...' And so on, until they found the correct position: 'Oh, it doesn't hurt this time! He can nurse as long as he likes...' Pain is the body's way of warning the mother to change the baby's position. That way she can correct the problem before the cracks, mastitis, regurgitation and colic kick in.

Much more recently, breastfeeding acquired moral connotations. A 'good mother' goes on nursing her baby, even if it hurts. A 'good mother' is self-sacrificing and does her duty:

> Behold the suffering face of the mother nursing her child, despite the excruciating pain! See how she tries to blink back the tears, and how finally she cries out, tearing the baby from her breast!
> Dr José Muñoz 'Mother... Raise Your Child!!', 1941

A 'good mother' takes no notice of what her body is telling her, and carries on nursing incorrectly until she develops cracked nipples. And then, when the pain, anguish, and exhaustion are too much for her, and she gives in and starts bottle feeding, the same people who say to her face: 'Don't worry, babies do just as well on these new formulas', will comment behind her back: 'the problem with mothers nowadays is they can't put up with anything'.

In brief, for millions of years there can't have been many problems with positioning. After a natural delivery, when from the very first moment the baby was held in its mother's arms, where it stayed for months (where else could it go, to the cave-nursery?), when there were no dummies, no bottles and plenty of opportunities to observe other mothers with their babies, almost all babies breastfed properly. And if they didn't, the mother's pain instantly told her to correct the position. Nature had no way of knowing that in our society we would end up doing everything the wrong way round.

So why didn't nature invent a simpler way? If the oxytocin were a little more effective, and the milk came out in a stream without the baby having to do anything, he could feed regardless of being in a bad position, and since he wouldn't have to make any effort, there would be no pain and no cracks. It is an interesting idea, but it couldn't work. If the milk came out by itself, the baby would have no control. In order for the amount and composition of the milk to adapt to his needs, the baby has to nurse proactively. Milk doesn't come out of any mammal spontaneously; it has to be drawn out. That is why we have to milk cows, sheep and goats; we can't simply place a bucket under them and wait.

Incidentally, while we are on the subject of self-sacrificing mothers, I shall take the opportunity to give a homily against sacrifice. The word 'sacrifice' has many meanings, not all of them negative: 'An act of surrender or altruism inspired by intense affection'. But it can also mean: 'A gesture to which one submits with great reluctance', and this can lead to confusion.

Does a mountaineer sacrifice himself in order to reach the summit? Does a student sacrifice himself to become a lawyer, or a pianist? No. They aren't submitting reluctantly, they are doing what they want. I don't want to climb a mountain or become a lawyer, and so I don't do those things.

If you want to hold your baby, or breastfeed her, then go ahead. If you want to stop working for months or years in order to look after her, or pass up a wonderful opportunity to work abroad in order to be with your family, then go ahead. But only if this is what you want. If it isn't what you want then don't do it. Saying: 'I sacrificed my career to be with my child' is as absurd as saying: 'I sacrificed my child for my career'. These aren't sacrifices, they are choices. To live is to choose. There are only twenty-four hours in a day, and when we do one thing we can't do another. Choose what you consider best at every moment. When we do what we want, we aren't renouncing anything, we are achieving something: we aren't making a sacrifice, we are triumphing.

This is an important nuance, because someone who is making (or believes he is making or wants people to believe he is making) a sacrifice does so, by definition, with great reluctance. He doesn't consider himself fortunate, but feels he is owed something. There will come a time when you clash with your children. When that happens, those of you who consider you have made a sacrifice will think (or, worse still, will say): 'You ungrateful brat, after all I've done for you' or 'if it weren't for you, I could have…' You can't take words back once they have been said. On the other hand, those of you who are conscious of having done what you wanted, are more likely to think (or, better still, to say): 'What a pity that after all the years of happiness you've brought me we should quarrel like this' or 'thanks to you, I've had the good fortune to be a parent'.

Chapter 3
PREGNANCY

A few decades ago, there was a revival of interest in breastfeeding, and people thought up various ways of preparing the nipples during pregnancy. These involved rubbing, stretching, twisting, and smearing them with creams, ointments and other concoctions. Occasionally the advice was contradictory: some women would 'soften' their nipples with ointments, while others 'hardened' or 'toughened' them with alcohol.

The collapse of lactation was so widespread in the West, with so few women breastfeeding, and for such short periods, that there was a desperate rush everywhere to find solutions. Many believed the problems started prior to delivery; we now know that they begin afterwards. The solution wasn't for mothers to do more (prepare their nipples, follow a special diet, eat certain herbs...), but rather for us professionals to do less (stop separating mother and baby, stop handing out free samples, stop recommending feeding schedules, and so on).

Preparing the nipples for breastfeeding is like preparing the feet for walking or the nose for breathing. These things are specially designed: the nose is made for breathing, the feet for walking and the breast for feeding. A less hands-on version suggests exposing the nipples to the air and the sun, not wearing a bra so that clothes rub against them, arguing that breasts would receive this natural preparation if they weren't always covered up. The idea seems logical, especially when a few decades ago we compared the failure of breastfeeding in Europe with its growth in Africa. And yet, up until the beginning of the twentieth century, European women, who were equally if not more covered up than the women of today, breastfed without any problem. And Eskimo mothers breastfeed, too. If you prefer not wearing a bra, or you like topless sunbathing (be careful, breasts get sunburnt) go ahead, but obviously it isn't obligatory in order to be able to breastfeed your baby.

Yet this supposed obligation poses the greatest danger. Generally speaking, preparing the nipples is physically innocuous. Theoretically, over-stimulating the nipples can cause contractions and even premature labour, but obviously any woman noticing such contractions would immediately stop rubbing her nipples. Theoretically, too much pulling and twisting could damage the nipple ducts, but if that has ever happened, it must be extremely rare.

However, it is quite common for some women to feel obliged to do things they find bothersome, painful or uncomfortable because they have been told that 'if they don't prepare, they won't be able to breastfeed'. In some extreme cases, women decide against breastfeeding to avoid having to go through this 'preparation'. Others who develop cracked or painful nipples after they give birth, instead of asking for help, stay at home feeling guilty: 'If only I'd prepared my nipples like they told me. Now I'll just have to put up and shut up…'.

So there is no need for women to prepare their nipples for breastfeeding. If you have decided to bottle feed, and then, for whatever reason, you change your mind the day you give birth, there is nothing to stop you breastfeeding. On the other hand, if you have the time and are willing, there is one sort of preparation for breastfeeding you might find beneficial: learning.

Find another woman who can teach you. Perhaps your mother (or mother-in-law, or one of your grandmothers) breastfed. But bear in mind that a few decades ago women were subjected to intense brainwashing. They were told that everything they had done in their day had been misguided. The mothers or grandmothers who breastfed their children for two years are often the ones who now say: 'Only feed him every three hours', or, 'this baby is still hungry', or, 'your milk isn't good enough'. They are probably only repeating what they have subsequently been told. Say to your grandmother: 'So, granny, are you telling me you only fed mum every three hours? That during those two years when you were breastfeeding, you were constantly looking at the clock?' 'Well, no, because in those days we didn't know what we were doing. Imagine, I even breastfed her in bed! But when your mother had you, the doctor explained about feeding schedules. What a shame her milk dried up after two weeks, she was doing so well to start with…'

So, if you are lucky enough to have a woman in your family who breastfed successfully, ask her. And if you have a friend or relative who is currently breastfeeding, go and watch how she does it (but no criticising, please! You'll soon see how annoying it is if they do it to you…).

Breastfeeding support groups

There are many support groups for nursing mothers in the UK, the US and around the world. These may be run by breastfeeding organisations (La Leche League, NCT, ABM, BfN), or the NHS in the UK (often through the network of Children's Centres or social enterprises). Groups often have weekly meetings, offer help over the phone and publish pamphlets. They offer information, support, companionship and the chance to see how other mothers breastfeed.

Try to get in touch with a mothers' group and attend some meetings. Going to these when you are pregnant is very useful, because although the idea is to keep going after you give birth, it isn't always easy to get out when you have a baby. Your midwife or health visitor should be able to give you information about local groups.

→ La Leche League www.laleche.org.uk (UK), www.llli.org (USA)

→ Association of Breastfeeding Mothers (UK) abm.me.uk

→ National Childbirth Trust (UK) www.nct.org.uk

→ Breastfeeding Network (UK) www.breastfeedingnetwork.org.uk

→ National Health Service (UK) www.nhs.uk/Conditions/pregnancy-and-baby/pages/breastfeeding-help-support.aspx

→ Australian Breastfeeding Association (Australia) www.breastfeeding.asn.au

Chapter 4
GIVING BIRTH

Anaesthesia

There is much debate over whether using anaesthesia during delivery affects the ability to breastfeed.

The use of general anaesthetic during delivery is extremely rare nowadays. One study showed that mothers who had a caesarean delivery using an epidural anaesthesia breastfed (on average) for the same length of time as those who had given birth normally. In contrast, a caesarean delivery using general anaesthetic often led to premature weaning. Clearly the anaesthetic itself doesn't directly affect milk production, but it can trigger a series of minor problems that gradually snowball: the first feed is delayed, the baby is drowsy and doesn't feed properly, the mother gets cracked nipples, the baby loses a lot of weight and is given supplements… In one study where all the mothers were helped by a nurse specialised in breastfeeding, those who had received anaesthesia or pain relief during labour breastfed the same as the others. Unfortunately, not all mothers receive this level of help, and a bad start will probably lead to premature weaning.

The effects of epidural anaesthesia are controversial. Some studies have found that the babies' behaviour changes for several days (imperceptible changes that only show up on neurological tests), and that at one month old mothers who had given birth without an epidural considered their babies easier to look after, and they breastfed them more frequently. (Those who have no children could be forgiven for thinking that the baby who demands to be breastfed *less* is 'easier to look after', but the mothers saw it the other way round. It is possible the babies were less drowsy, and therefore demanded to be fed more often, or perhaps it wasn't that they demanded to be breastfed more, but that the mothers responded to their babies more because they looked 'more cute'. The mother-baby relationship is an exquisite choreography, in which it is difficult to separate nurture and nature.) Other studies found none of these effects in cases where a low dose of epidural was used (the current trend is towards lower doses, but some anaesthetists may continue using higher ones).

In any event, one thing is clear: anaesthesia, whether general or epidural, doesn't harm the baby via his mother's milk. If the newborn is a little drowsy, it isn't because of the miniscule amount of the drug that might have transferred to his mother's milk, but rather to the huge amount he received via the placenta. It is nonsense to delay the baby's first feed 'so that the mother has time to eliminate the drug'; on the contrary, she must breastfeed as soon and as often as possible so that despite the anaesthetic, lactation gets off to a good start.

For the treatment of afterpains it is usual to administer simple painkillers, which don't interfere in any way with breastfeeding. In fact, in one study, mothers who were given some pain relief tended to breastfeed more frequently, perhaps because it is easier to attend to your baby if you aren't in pain. There are some drugs (rarely used) that can affect breastfeeding, but the doctors at the hospital where you give birth will know what these are. So if anyone says to you: 'You mustn't breastfeed because we've prescribed a very strong painkiller', you can simply reply: 'Well, prescribe a different one, because I intend to go on breastfeeding'.

Don't use iodine

The iodine contained in antiseptics such as Betadine® or Topionic® is absorbed by the skin and the mucous membranes (for example, the vagina) and transfers to the baby via the placenta. In older children or adults, this is harmless. In fact, the occasional application of iodine to cuts may have prevented cases of iodine deficiency in people who don't eat iodised salt. But the amount of iodine absorbed from the antiseptic is enormous, hundreds of times above the recommended daily intake.

Foetuses and newborns are extremely sensitive to this overload of iodine, and it can block their thyroid glands and cause transitory hyperthyroidism. A few of the 'scares' that result from an early diagnosis of metabolic disorders (the neonatal heel-prick test) are caused by iodine: the test result is abnormal and needs to be double-checked urgently. A second test proves negative. False alarms cause enough problems, only this isn't a false alarm because the iodine has actually caused hypothyroidism, although fortunately it is only transitory. However, it isn't good for a baby to suffer from hypothyroidism, even if only for a few days.

For this reason, iodine should never be applied to pregnant women or to newborns during their first few months. Pregnant women shouldn't be treated with it even for the tiniest cut, and it shouldn't be applied to their abdomen prior to a caesarean, or to their arm before being given a drip or to their vagina before an episiotomy, or to the baby's belly button. The hospital will know which antiseptic to use; when at home use soap and water. (Mercurochrome isn't recommended either because it contains mercury).

On the other hand, pregnant women and nursing mothers should take iodine supplements (see page 170.) The amount of iodine contained in the supplement is hundreds of times lower than in an antiseptic, and is therefore harmless.

→ Arena Ansotegui, J., Emparanza Knörr, J.I. 'Los antisépticos yodados no son inocuos', *An Esp Pediatr* 2000;53:25-9 http://db.doyma.es/cgibin/wdbcgi.exe/doyma/mrevista. fulltext?pident=1104

Clamping the umbilical cord

For many decades now it has been customary to clamp the umbilical cord only a few seconds after the baby has emerged. This is done for fear that blood from the placenta may transfer to the baby. And, indeed, too much blood in the baby (policythemia) can cause serious problems, such as blood clots or breathing difficulties. I imagine this fear has some foundation in reality: perhaps a century ago it occurred to someone to hold the placenta up, like a drip, or even to squeeze it to make sure the baby was nice and full with blood, with disastrous results, and doctors at the time decided it was necessary to clamp the umbilical cord.

However, modern research has found that clamping the cord too soon can also cause problems. When the baby is placed on his mother's chest (which is where he should be placed as soon as he is born) for three minutes before clamping the umbilical cord, he receives 30 per cent more blood: it has been observed that a) this modest increase doesn't harm the baby, as it doesn't produce blood clots or affect the baby's circulation, and b) the baby's iron reserves increase and this reduces the risk of anaemia a few months later. These results have been observed both in babies born at term and those born prematurely.

So you see, much of the anaemia blamed on the mother's milk not containing sufficient iron (and on the mother herself for insisting on breastfeeding her baby) are in fact the 'fault' of clamping the umbilical cord too soon. Breastmilk contains sufficient iron, but nature didn't foresee the invention of clamps and scissors. Obviously, animals in the wild don't clamp the umbilical cord; they simply wait a few minutes for it to close of its own accord and then sever it with their teeth.

Discuss this during your pregnancy with your midwife or your obstetrician, and print out some of the articles referenced below to show them (you can find them easily on www.pubmed. gov, under the names of their authors).

→ Pisacane, A. 'Neonatal prevention of iron deficiency', *Br Med J* 1996;312:136-7 http://bmj.com/cgi/content/full/312/7024/136

→ Nelle, M., Zilow, E.P., Kraus, M., Bastert, G., Linderkamp, O. 'The effect of Leboyer delivery on blood viscosity and other hemorheologic parameters in term neo-nates', *Am J Obstet Gynecol*. 1993;169:189-93.

→ McDonnell, M., Henderson-Smart, D.J. 'Delayed umbilical cord clamping in preterm infants: a feasibility study', *J Paediatr Child Health* 1997;33:308-10.

→ Ibrahim, H.M., Krouskop, R.W., Lewis, D.F., Dhanireddy, R. 'Placental transfusion: umbilical cord clamping and preterm infants', *J Perinatol* 2000;20:351-4.

→ Rabe, H., Wacker, A., Hulskamp, G., Hornig-Franz, I., Schulze-Everding, A., Harms, E. et al. 'A randomised controlled trial of delayed cord clamping in very low birth weight preterm infants', *Eur J Pediatr* 2000;159:775-7.

→ Mercer, J.S. 'Current best evidence: a review of the literature on umbilical cord clamping', *J Midwifery Womens Health* 2001;46:402-14.

→ Grajeda, R., Perez-Escamilla, R., Dewey, K.G. 'Delayed clamping of the umbilical cord improves hematologic status of Guatemalan infants at 2 mo of age', *Am J Clin Nutr* 1997;65:425-31.

→ Gupta, R., Ramji, S. 'Effect of delayed cord clamping on iron stores in infants born to anemic mothers: a randomized controlled trial', *Indian Pediatr* 2002;39:130-5 www.indianpediatrics.net/feb2002/feb-130-135.htm

Chapter 5
INITIATING BREASTFEEDING

Baby-friendly hospitals

In 1989, WHO and UNICEF published a joint statement entitled 'Protecting, Promoting and Supporting Breastfeeding: The Special Role of Maternity Services', in which, for the first time, ten steps to successful breastfeeding were presented.

Every facility providing maternity services and care for newborn infants should:

1. Have a written breastfeeding policy that is routinely communicated to all health care staff.
2. Train all health care staff in skills necessary to implement this policy.
3. Inform all pregnant women about the benefits and management of breastfeeding.
4. Help mothers initiate breastfeeding within half an hour of birth.
5. Show mothers how to breastfeed, and how to maintain lactation even if they should be separated from their infants.
6. Give newborn infants no food or drink other than breast milk, unless medically indicated.
7. Practise rooming-in – that is, allow mothers and infants to remain together – 24 hours a day.
8. Encourage breastfeeding on demand.
9. Give no artificial teats or pacifiers (also called dummies or soothers) to breastfeeding infants.
10. Foster the establishment of breastfeeding support groups and refer mothers to them on discharge from the hospital or clinic.

Later on, in 1991, WHO and UNICEF launched The Baby-Friendly Health Initiative (BFHI), the aim of which was to have every hospital in the world implement these ten steps. Each country sets up its own committee to oversee the initiative. The Spanish committee is made up of representatives from UNICEF, from the Department of Health, midwives' organisations, paediatric nurses, gynaecologists, hospital managers and paediatricians, mothers' groups and breastfeeding support groups.

Hospitals that sign up voluntarily are very strictly assessed, and if they fulfil the ten steps are awarded the title 'Baby-Friendly Hospital'. In 2013 there were ninety-two UK hospitals with full Baby-Friendly accreditation, 165 in the US and sixty-six in Australia.

If there is a baby-friendly hospital in your area, you should try to give birth there. If there isn't, don't despair. Fulfilling all ten steps and being awarded the title is no easy feat, and fortunately there are a lot of other hospitals which might not be perfect, but come very close.

Ask your obstetrician or your midwife, ask your women friends and acquaintances who have given birth recently, and don't hesitate to visit the hospitals in person and find out.

What you want to know is how they manage the birth: whether you are 'allowed' to walk during dilation, and squat or adopt any other posture you like during labour, whether your husband or a birth partner is allowed to be present, whether they habitually shave, use enemas or do episiotomies. Discussing in detail how a normal birth should take place would be beyond the scope of this book. You will find useful information on the internet (see below).

→ WHO: www.who.int/reproductivehealth/publications/maternal_perinatal_health/MSM_96_24_/en/

→ The Royal College of Midwives: www.rcm.org.uk/college/campaigns-events/campaign-for-normal-birth/

→ The Royal College of Obstetricians and Gynaecologists: www.rcog.org.uk/womens-health/clinical-guidance/making-normal-birth-reality

→ National Childbirth Trust: www.nct.org.uk/professional/research/pregnancy-birth-and-postnatal-care/birth/normal-birth

In her book *Becoming a mother* Dr Gro Nylander gives a very interesting description of maternity care in Norway.

Finding out the number of caesarean sections your hospital performs is also important. Clearly there are cases where a caesarean is vital, and it can save the mother's or baby's life or both. However, a lot of caesareans are performed unnecessarily. In Spain the national average is just below 20 per cent. You would expect there to be fewer caesareans in small hospitals, where they don't deal with high-risk deliveries, than in the referral hospitals, where women with high-risk pregnancies are usually admitted. And yet, in some of Spain's general hospitals fewer than 15 per cent of deliveries are caesareans, compared to more than 35 per cent in some private clinics. Don't be afraid to ask your hospital the percentage of caesareans they performed last year; they can easily provide you with that information. In the UK www.birthchoiceuk.com gives easy access to information about hospitals in your area.

But let us return to our subject: breastfeeding. Find out how many of the hospitals in your area fulfil the abovementioned ten steps. Of particular interest is whether they place the baby on your breast in the birthing room, and whether you are allowed to keep your baby with you in your room day and night. Ask other mothers, and find out whether they really do what they have said, or whether they are paying lip-service to it. Find out, too, whether the staff are friendly, whether they support breastfeeding or not, and whether they usually find ways of solving the various minor problems mothers have.

If you have no choice but to give birth in a hospital where mothers are separated from their babies for several hours, or where babies are taken away at night (some hospitals may still take the baby away during the day, and only bring it every three hours to breastfeed), or where they give water or glucose to all newborns, it isn't too late to try to change things. You still have a few months to go before you give birth; fight for your health and that of your baby.

You have two powerful weapons at your disposal: reason, and the recommendations of the RCM (Royal College of Midwives) and RCOG (Royal College of Obstetricians and Gynaecologists), whose websites you can consult. If necessary you can print out the ten steps, and show them to those concerned. They are only recommendations, so doctors aren't legally bound to follow them, but at least they won't be able to say: 'This is nonsense concocted by breastfeeding fanatics'. They will have to listen to you, and they may take what you say on board. At the very least they will be forced to come up with a counter-argument.

If the problem is that mother and baby have to remain under observation for two hours after the birth (or however long), then ask them if they can at least observe you and the baby together. This should be easier for the hospital, because they won't need to have a nurse watching the baby while a midwife takes care of the mother; one person can watch over both. If they say: 'that's how we've always done things', or 'those are the rules', then find out who has the authority to make an exception. At this moment, you aren't asking them to change the rules; you aren't suggesting they put all babies and mothers together. You only want them to put *your* baby in with *you*. Hasn't the head of paediatrics or the medical director the authority to do this? Go as high up as you need. If you come up against a lot of resistance, but in the end they agree, ask them to make a note on your medical file. Don't give the impression you don't trust them, of course you do! But what if you give birth on a Sunday, and the doctors on the weekend shift don't know about the director giving authorisation? If you have had to beg them to let you keep your baby with you all night, try to get someone (your husband or your mother) to stay with you overnight to help look after the baby. Because you can imagine what they will say if after making such a 'fuss' you have to 'bother' them for something in the middle of the night.

More than ten years ago, I heard about a clinic where they would only allow the baby to stay in the room with the mother if she signed a document stating that the hospital was absolved of all responsibility in the event that her baby died in the night. As though newborns were in the habit of dying all the time! This was nothing short of an underhand way of controlling the mothers by terrifying them. Naturally, such a document has no legal worth; the hospital is still obliged to attend to your baby's needs should a problem arise. Besides, hospital nurseries aren't like intensive care units, and babies usually spend the night alone, with a nurse checking up on them occasionally from a distance. I also knew of a private clinic where, in the end, the problem was about money. A separate fee was charged for the 'nursery' service, and provided the mother agreed to pay it, she was allowed keep her baby with her in her room. I would like to think such practices no longer exist.

When your milk comes in

Around the third day, the mother's breasts usually feel fuller than usual. This is because the milk is 'coming in'.

A few decades ago, when babies weren't placed on their mother's breast until twenty-four to forty-eight hours (or more) after delivery, (and even then according to a strict schedule), the milk coming in was spectacular. Our mothers' – or grandmothers' – breasts grew as hard as bullets. They even ran a temperature (milk fever). This wasn't due to an infection, but was an inflammation caused by the accumulation of milk, which burst the ducts and acted as a foreign body. Some grandmothers speak of this with the same excitement as old men recounting their war experiences, and this can cause some mothers to feel discouraged or worried. Things are done differently nowadays – even in hospitals that aren't perfect. Mothers are encouraged to breastfeed soon after delivery, babies are placed with their mothers during the day, if not at night, and the schedule, even if not on demand, is at least flexible. And as the baby is emptying the breast, milk is no longer able to accumulate. Those bullet-hard breasts are now considered an illness (mammary ingurgitation, see page 140); most mothers only notice a very slight, or moderate increase in breast size, and some don't notice any. More than one mother has complained to me, two to three weeks after delivery, that her milk hasn't come in yet. If her baby were losing weight, I would believe it, but when the baby is growing nice and plump and he isn't being bottle fed, he has to be getting his nourishment from somewhere.

Occasionally there are two episodes of milk coming in. If, for example, a newborn isn't properly latched on, or is in the incorrect position and fails to gain weight, and then one or two weeks later he begins to nurse properly (or the mother begins to express her milk), within two or three days the mother's breasts may suddenly begin to feel very full. It is important to know this, because some mothers get into a panic and turn up in casualty. If they smile and say: 'Don't worry Madam, it's your milk coming in', she will simply have wasted her time. But in at least one case I know of, a mother was told she had mastitis (first mistake, she didn't), prescribed amoxicillin (second mistake, amoxicillin is almost useless for treating mastitis) and ordered to stop breastfeeding (third mistake, when you have mastitis there is no need to stop breastfeeding).

Some mothers have also noticed a second episode of milk coming in when their child of a few months or years suddenly increases his number of feeds, as in the case of the little girl of two who was on holiday, and didn't like any of the food in the hotel buffet.

Weight loss

All newborns lose weight, and a few days later they put it back on. This is perfectly normal.

It is common for babies to lose between 4 and 6 per cent of their body weight at birth, and then put it back on within a week. Some may lose a little more, or may take longer to put it back on, but this is also considered normal. How much (and how long) is normal? I am not aware of any scientific data that allows us to set limits. Nearly all paediatricians accept that a newborn can lose up to 10–12 per cent of his bodyweight. Babies who weigh more at birth may lose up to 14 or 15 per cent. High weights at birth can be due to water retention, and the excess weight is got rid of through the urine; these babies lose more weight and take longer to put it back on. When a mother has been on an intravenous drip during labour, her baby is sometimes born 'bloated', and will lose a lot of weight in a few hours, which is excess liquid. How do you know whether the baby is losing liquid or fat? Because it takes days, not hours, to lose fat.

There is even less data available concerning time limits for regaining weight lost after birth. Some authors say two weeks, others three, the majority don't say anything. Clearly these are arbitrary, approximate figures. In my experience, I have seen two baby girls take twenty-two days to regain their birth weight.

What you mustn't do is sit back and wait for your baby to put on weight by herself. Many of those babies who lose 8–10 per cent of their body weight will undoubtedly put it back on automatically, whatever the mother does. But some babies go on losing weight until they develop serious problems. There comes a time when a baby is too weak to cry, so she sleeps all the time and appears calm, and even if, despite not crying, she is breastfed, she scarcely feeds at all because she is too weak. There are cases of babies who have been taken into intensive care units having lost 30 per cent of their body weight. Some have even died. I do not say this in order to alarm pregnant women; it rarely happens, and above all it is preventable. A baby doesn't lose 30 per cent of her body weight all at once. First she loses 10, then 15, then 20 per cent. It takes several days. During that time, an experienced person will notice that the baby isn't feeding properly, that she isn't behaving normally and is unusually drowsy.

Breast compression

Breast compression is a very useful technique for when a baby isn't nursing properly. This can happen for a number of reasons: because she is very drowsy, or has lost weight and is weak, or because her mother hasn't managed to position her correctly, or she isn't using her tongue properly, or is unwell or premature and tires easily when feeding… It is also useful for shortening the feed if the mother has cracked or painful nipples.

The baby will normally feed properly (or at least passably well) for the first few minutes, but after that she will keep the breast in her mouth without suckling. She won't let go of the breast, but she won't feed either. She might stay on each breast for 30–45 minutes, but most of the time she isn't feeding. If the baby isn't feeding, there is no point in keeping the breast in her mouth; it is better to compress the breast, and if that doesn't work then to express milk.

During those first few minutes when the baby is actively feeding, leave her alone. When she stops, take care not to let the breast fall out of her mouth, and compress the base of your breast (touching your ribcage) between your thumb and forefinger. Give it a good squeeze, taking care not to hurt yourself. Don't pump your breast, by squeezing repeatedly, but instead squeeze and do not release. As you compress the breast, a jet of milk will usually spurt out, and the baby, who has stopped nursing, will get a nice surprise and begin nursing again. As long as you can see that she is still feeding, carry on squeezing. When she stops again (or has almost stopped) release your breast (sometimes when you do this another spurt will come out and she will begin feeding again). When she stops feeding again, squeeze until she stops again and then release your breast, and so on. You can alternate, compressing above and below, side to side, above and below, and so on. Repeat the manoeuvre until your baby stops responding when you compress your breast, because there is no milk coming out. Now is the time to switch her over to the other breast and begin the procedure all over again. This may seem like an exception to the rule of breastfeeding on demand – i.e. letting your baby feed until she is sated. But it isn't: one thing is 'letting her nurse' and another 'letting her keep the breast in her mouth without nursing'. It is better to give your baby a short feed and then feed her again in an hour's time, than to keep her on your breast for hours when she isn't nursing. Giving her frequent, shorter feeds will enable you to rest, and even to express your milk, if necessary, and you feel like it and have the time.

Supplements

In some cases, when a baby has lost too much weight, or is taking too long to put it back on, and all of the above has failed, he must be given a formula supplement. Of course, it would better to give him breastmilk; but sometimes the mother can't express enough milk, and there comes a moment when it is impossible to wait any longer.

There is no fixed rule about this. You can't say: 'The baby needs a supplement if he loses more than 12 per cent of his body weight'. Some babies will need one before that. In each case it is the doctor who must decide. It depends on the baby's general state, and how things develop. For example, a baby who loses 100 grams one day and 20 grams the next is considered to be 'still losing weight'. But a baby who loses 20 grams one day and 100 grams the next is a different matter; in the first case it is possible to wait and see whether the baby continues to improve, in the second the baby needs a supplement immediately.

Both the American Academy of Paediatrics and ESPGHAN (European Society for Paediatric Gastroenterology, Hepatology and Nutrition) recommend that babies with allergies in the family should be given a supplement made with hydrolyzed milk (not with one of these 'hypoallergenic' milks, which are completely useless, but with an 'extensively hydrolyzed formula' designed especially for babies who are allergic to milk). This is because babies who are always bottle fed normally develop an immunological tolerance to cow's milk. But nursing babies who are given artificial milk for only a few days don't have time to build up a tolerance, and can easily develop an allergy to cow's milk. Many paediatricians don't know about this recommendation; you may want to pass on the scientific article mentioned below to them.

To begin with, try to give your baby the supplement in a cup or a dropper, or with a breastmilk supplementer (also known as a Supplementary Nursing System, or SNS). You can either buy these ready made, or you can make one with a syringe and a butterfly needle, by removing the needle (see *Figure 13*). However, if your baby has lost a lot of weight, and none of the above methods are working, don't hesitate to bottle feed him. It isn't the end of the world; you will be able to wean him off the bottle later.

When it becomes necessary to give your baby a milk supplement, it is important not to stint on the amount. When the baby requires a supplement, it is because the situation is serious, and 30ml a day won't be enough to solve the problem. A baby who only needs 30ml probably doesn't need a supplement at all. You don't want the situation to drag on, so that the baby spends two to three weeks gaining 30–40 grams per week. You want her to gain weight quickly, and to become strong and healthy. Then

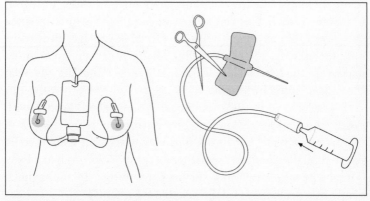

Figure 13: A breastmilk supplementer and how to make one yourself.

she will nurse better, more milk will come out and you can stop giving her the supplement. So, try to give her around 30–60 ml every three hours, always just after she nurses. And if she takes it all, and seems to want more, give her another 30ml.

An important warning: because we are always saying how wonderful mother's milk is, there are those who seem to think artificial milk is bad. I have come across parents determined to give their baby everything except artificial milk (milk formula). They prefer giving him soymilk, almond milk, rice milk, goat's milk…

This is a serious mistake. There is a soy formula adapted for babies, but many experts recommend not using it unless advised by a doctor. Soy contains natural phytoestrogens, which should be consumed in moderation. However, normal soymilk for adults sold in health food shops is completely different from the soy formula adapted for babies and mustn't be given to children under one year old. Almond milk, rice milk and oat milk are even worse. They have nothing in common with breastmilk, and if a newborn were fed this and nothing else, he would die. These 'milks' usually contain very little protein, almost no fat and a lot of sugar, and as far as vitamins, minerals and other nutrients are concerned, well, the less said the better. They are only referred to as 'milks' because they are pale and watery, but all similarity to milk ends there. It would be more correct to call them 'drinks'. Goat's milk is very like cow's milk, and nothing like breastmilk. In Germany there is a brand of infant formula based on goat's milk. In other words, they take out a lot of things, and add a lot of other things, like they do with cow's milk, in order to turn it into something babies can take. You can buy this milk in some shops or on the internet. It has no special advantages over cow's milk formula. In any event, before giving your baby goat's milk, make sure the label states clearly that it is formula that has been specially adapted for infants.

I implore you, don't endanger your baby's health with exotic concoctions. Manufacturers have been researching and improving artificial baby milk for many years, and there is strict international legislation regulating its composition. When a baby is unable to take breastmilk, the next best thing is infant formula, a milk that has been specially adapted for infants.

→ Zeiger, R.S. 'Food Allergen Avoidance in the Prevention of Food Allergy in Infants and Children', Pediatrics 2003;111:1662-71 pediatrics.aappublications.org/cgi/reprint/111/6/S2/1662

→ American Academy of Pediatrics Committee on Nutrition, 'Soy protein-based formulas: recommendations for use in infant feeding', Pediatrics 1998;101:148- 153 aappolicy.aappublications. org/cgi/content/full/pediatrics;101/1/148

→ New Zealand Ministry of Health, 'Soy-based infant formula' Wellington 1998 www.soyonlineservice.co.nz/downloads/ mohsoy.pdf

Chapter 6
A FEW INTERESTING FACTS ABOUT BABIES

Babies' breasts

Both male and female newborns often have swollen breasts as a result of the female hormones they have received through the placenta. They can even produce drops of milk – so-called 'witch's milk'. This is perfectly normal, even in male babies. There is no need to do anything. Don't squeeze or otherwise try to get the milk out, as manipulation can cause mastitis. This has absolutely nothing to do with whether babies are breast or bottle fed, and of course you can continue breastfeeding normally.

In female babies under two years, one or both breasts may grow. This is known as 'isolated premature thelarche'. The size varies from case to case, and the same baby girl's breasts may grow and then shrink again. There are no other signs of puberty, such as pubic hair or underarm hair, and this condition shouldn't be confused with precocious puberty. When in doubt, your paediatrician may perform some tests. In cases of precocious puberty there is early bone maturation, and increased levels of LH (luteinizing hormone), whereas in isolated premature thelarche both these indicators are normal. Between the ages of three and five the breasts usually go down again, but in some children they may remain swollen until puberty takes over. I repeat: this is perfectly normal and has nothing to do with breastfeeding, which can carry on as before.

The belly button and bathing

On average, your baby's umbilical stump will dry out and drop off between five and ten days after birth, but it is quite common for this to take two to three weeks, or even as long as a month and a half. Applying alcohol and other antiseptics to the stump will only delay the process. Iodine or Mercurochrome (which contains mercury) should not be applied (see page 77).

The newborn's belly button can be the point of entry for lethal infections, which explains this habit of applying antiseptics. However, a study of various products showed that none has the advantage over simple hygiene: keeping the belly button clean and dry.

Up until a few years ago, babies were washed moments after birth, and then not bathed again until after the umbilical stump dropped off. Interestingly, both these recommendations have since proved mistaken. It is best not to bath newborns for the first twenty-four hours (or more), even in warm water, mainly because of the risk of hypothermia (catching cold). During the brief interval between the baby getting wet and being dried off, water will evaporate on his skin, rapidly lowering his body temperature. Nowadays, newborns are wiped with a warm towel, placed skin-to-skin with their mother, and both mother and baby are covered with a blanket.

During the days that follow, there is normally no need to bath the baby because he won't get very soiled. You can rub him down with a damp sponge. But if he does a copious, watery poo, don't hesitate to wash him in warm water and dry him very quickly. (Wash him very quickly, too, because you don't want him soaking in water soiled with poo.)

Incidentally, while we are on the subject of bathing, we have a curious obsession in our society with bathing babies. Before they begin crawling, babies don't get much dirt on them (besides poo). They say babies like being bathed, it relaxes them, and you should bath them before putting them down for the night. But the fact is some babies enjoy it while others protest vigorously, some appear relaxed while others get overexcited with all the splashing, so you can bath your baby any time of the day, whenever it suits you best.

If your baby doesn't like being bathed, twice a week is ample. If he really hates being in water, you can also wash him with a damp sponge.

There is no need to clean your baby's eyes with gauze or anything else (except to gently wipe away the sleep). Don't clean his ears with cotton buds. They are dangerous because they can easily damage the eardrums, and they also compress the wax, which can lead to blocked ears. Ears should be left alone for the wax to come out of its own accord. If necessary, clean the outer ear, but never the ear canal itself.

Don't pull back the foreskin of male babies in order to clean it. The foreskin in almost all newborns is stuck to the head of the penis, meaning that you can't pull it back. The foreskin will come loose of its own accord in a few years (*years* not months), or never. This is normal and doesn't lead to any problems. Early attempts to pull it back can produce lesions, which when they heal can make the foreskin tighter and lead to phimosis. So, I insist: don't touch your baby's foreskin, even if the doctor tells you to, and don't allow the doctor to try to pull it back either (there are many cases of bleeding foreskins as a result of these absurd attempts).

Poo

A newborn's first poo is black and sticky, like paint, and it is called meconium. Then come the so-called transitional stools, which are a grey-green colour and very runny and last a few days. And finally come the typical stools of a breastfed baby: semi-liquid and lumpy (containing lumps, or strings of mucous), and pleasant-smelling (in so far as stools can smell pleasant). These are frequently yellowy, but also come in a brownish or greenish colour.

These changes in the baby's poo reflect the changes in her diet. While she is in the womb, she eats nothing (and drinks a lot of amniotic fluid). The meconium comes from digesting cells from her own intestinal mucosa, which have been desquamating for months (a diet consisting exclusively of human flesh). For the first few days after the baby is born, she eats very little (not because there isn't enough milk, but because she isn't supposed to feed much) and her poo is almost like water. The normal poo of breastfed babies indicates that they are drinking substantial amounts of breastmilk, and it differs from that of bottle fed babies (which is usually darker and stronger-smelling, and occasionally hard, like pellets, which don't soil the nappy).

If after five days the baby still isn't producing normal stools – yellow, lumpy and with the consistency of purée – she may not be getting enough milk. You can check this by weighing her; if she is gaining weight normally, then her stools are probably normal and there is nothing to worry about. When a baby (or an adult for that matter) isn't eating enough for some reason, she may go back to getting those very runny grey-green stools, known as 'hunger' or 'starvation stools'. This explains why many children suffering from an ear infection, a cold or a sore throat have diarrhoea at the same time. They don't really have diarrhoea; their stools are loose because being unwell has made them lose their appetite. This is why we no longer reduce the food intake of children (or adults) when they have diarrhoea. Not eating, or eating very little, makes diarrhoea worse. By eating normally, you get rid of diarrhoea more quickly.

For the first few weeks, babies poo frequently, usually each time they feed (as if their tiny bodies haven't enough room for both, and putting one in forces the other out). Some babies won't poo as much, perhaps 'only' four or five times a day. Others will poo more often between feeds, sometimes more than twenty times a day. This is all completely normal. The baby doesn't have diarrhoea and you don't have to do anything: you don't need to stop breastfeeding, or to give the baby water, or any other liquids, or drugs. It is unusual for a baby who is exclusively breastfeeding to have diarrhoea, although of course it can happen. Diarrhoea can be detected in sudden changes in the baby's stools: for example, if they are much runnier or more copious than the day before, or if there is blood in them, or if the baby is running a temperature. Many mild cases of diarrhoea in young babies no doubt go undetected: what difference can it make if they poo six or eight times a day?

Later on, between the age of six weeks and six months (sometimes a bit before, sometimes a bit after, though the average is between three and five months) there is usually a period when babies who are fed *exclusively* on breastmilk virtually stop passing stools altogether (this doesn't apply to mixed-fed babies: it only takes a small amount of formula to change a baby's stools). A few decades ago, it was rare for a Spanish baby to still be breastfeeding (not to mention exclusively) at three months, so many older mothers and grandmothers, and doctors and nurses, don't know that this is normal. But now that an increasing number of women breastfeed their babies exclusively for six months, we can see how unusual it is for a baby to pass stools every day. Most do a poo every two to three days, and some every five or seven days. If you join a breastfeeding group, you will probably meet babies that haven't done a poo for ten or twelve days. I know of a baby who went for twenty-three days without doing one, and Dr Jack

Newman (a breastfeeding specialist in Toronto who treats rare cases) has seen babies who haven't done one for more than thirty days.

When the baby eventually does a poo, it is perfectly normal, semi-liquid or sticky as before, and very copious. Whatever you do, don't weigh your baby before and after he does a poo, because you will be in for a big shock. All this is perfectly normal, and your baby isn't constipated. If he were constipated, his poo would be round and hard. Constipation is a condition where the stools are hard and dry. If your stools are like billiard balls, you can thank heaven if you only go once a week, because if you went three times a day you would be no less constipated, and you would suffer a lot more. On the other hand, if your stools are soft you aren't constipated, even if you only go once a month. A number of doctors still don't know that this is normal, and will insist on treating your baby as if she were constipated. A few of your female relatives or friends may voice the same opinion. Don't listen to them. You mustn't give your baby any of the following: water, orange juice (or any other type of juice), herbal teas, herbal, homeopathic or Chinese remedies, laxatives (or other drugs) or prune water. Don't give your baby enemas, or insert suppositories, rectal thermometers, or the tip of a clean little finger, into her bottom. Do absolutely nothing.

Some mothers maintain that their baby is uncomfortable and cries a lot when he hasn't done a poo for a few days, and that as soon as he does one he is fine. Most, however, say their baby is as right as rain. It is risky to doubt what mothers say, because more often than not they are right; but I find it hard to believe that this soft, sometimes runny poo can cause a baby any real pain or discomfort. Genuine constipation is no doubt uncomfortable: passing a hard pellet hurts, and it can even cause pain as it travels through the intestine, but surely not a soft poo? I suspect that, rather like with teething, not doing a poo is blamed for things that are purely coincidental. When a baby of two to six months cries, screams or won't go to sleep, it is more than likely that she hasn't done a poo for several days, and when a child of six to eighteen months cries or screams, it is more than likely he is teething. When the child who cries is two, they blame it on 'the terrible twos', and from the age of three onwards any problem is blamed on pre-adolescence.

If your baby doesn't go through this phase, but carries on doing several poos a day during the whole time she is nursing, this is also normal.

If, on the other hand, during the first four to six weeks she *doesn't* poo several times a day, this could also be normal, but check her weight anyway. Some babies who don't poo very much at that age are nursing incorrectly. If you see that she is gaining weight normally, then there is no need to worry.

If, from day one, your baby does a poo every few days, but doesn't go through the stage (long or short) of doing several poos a day, consult your doctor. This could be perfectly normal, but it could be a sign that she has a digestive problem. Try to see whether she at least passes wind; this is a healthy sign.

Pee

Small babies usually pee at least six to eight times a day, except during the first few days, when they are losing weight, when they don't pee as often.

This doesn't mean they need six to eight nappies. Disposable nappies are highly absorbent and you can sometimes get away with using only four or five (if the baby hasn't done a poo). When you are changing the nappy of a baby who has done a poo, it isn't always easy to know if he has done a pee as well (it is more obvious with an older baby, but very small babies do small amounts each time, and the mother might be less experienced).

If a baby pees very little it can mean that he isn't taking much milk. You can check this by weighing him. The same applies if he doesn't poo very much during the first month, or if his poo is a grey-green colour and very runny. These are merely pointers telling us to check the baby's weight. Provided he is gaining weight normally, and is contented, then it doesn't really matter how much he poos or pees.

It would matter if we were able to measure the exact amount, of course. A baby who pees very little hasn't had enough liquid, which means not enough milk. But our only method is to count soiled nappies. A baby who pees ten times and produces 30ml each time has peed less than a baby who pees five times and produces 80ml each time.

In addition, the fact that a baby pees a lot is no guarantee that he is getting enough liquids. Nursing babies don't need water. They get all the water they need and more from the milk. If they took a little less milk they would still pee a lot. They have to be taking very little milk indeed for their pee to decrease.

This is why counting soiled nappies doesn't give us a very good idea of how well a baby is nursing. But since the idea first appeared in a few books, under the heading: 'How to find out if my baby is getting enough milk', it has been passed on by word of mouth, and has achieved the status of dogma, no doubt to the surprise of the authors of these books. Some mothers spend months obsessively counting nappies, when it is obvious from their baby's happy face that he is getting all the milk he needs (and if there is any doubt he can be weighed). What is worse, when everything points to the baby having a problem, the mother can look at his nappy for false (and dangerous) reassurances ('My baby only gained 250 grams between the first and second month.' 'Does he wet many nappies?' 'Yes, he pees a lot.' 'In that case don't worry.') I recently came across the opposite case: a healthy, chubby five-month-old baby, who was nursing perfectly well and gaining weight normally, but whose mother was fretting ('I'm sure I don't have enough milk, because he pees very little and has done since he was born; but he absolutely refuses to take the bottle'). A five-month-old baby who has genuinely peed very little since he was born would be in hospital.

Forget about urine, please. If your baby is happy and active, and looks healthy and nurses as much as she wants, then everything is fine. If she is gaining weight normally, then everything is fine. If everything is fine, but she isn't soiling many nappies, this just means she is retaining her urine for longer and peeing more each time. If your three-month-old baby suddenly needs to feed more, it won't be her nappies that tell you this, she will tell you herself by wanting to nurse more (and when you breastfeed her, she will stop being hungry, and there will be no more problem).

Urine can be more important during the first few weeks, when babies are often very drowsy, and it is harder to tell from their faces how healthy they are. If you suspect your baby isn't nursing well (because she takes a long time and your nipples hurt, or because she isn't latched on properly), and is still hungry (because she cries all day) or is weak (because she sleeps all day) it might be a good idea to check on her urine while you are taking her to be weighed. But in any event, whether her nappy is dry or soiled you must still have her weighed.

Sleep

Should I wake my baby in order to nurse him?

Generally speaking, no.

Babies usually feed a lot just after they are born, after which they become very drowsy for eight, ten or twelve hours and hardly nurse at all. This is normal. And whilst they should be given every opportunity to nurse (by being placed close to their mother, preferably skin-to-skin, and offered the breast when they seem more awake, before they start to cry), this should not extend to waking them up. They will nurse in good time.

But, of course, they have to start nursing at some point. After about ten or twelve hours, begin insisting a little more, and if after several more hours your baby still won't feed, it is a good idea for the doctor to take a look at him to make sure there is nothing wrong, and also for you to express some of your milk and try to feed it to him with a dropper or a syringe. If you let him go for too long without feeding and don't try to give him milk, he will go on sleeping because he is too weak to feed, and will lose more and more weight.

As I re-read the last paragraph, I think to myself: 'This is going to alarm pregnant women'. Well, please don't be alarmed. In the vast majority of cases, newborns nurse vigorously and with gusto, and there isn't the slightest need for concern. But you will understand that it is precisely the exceptions that pose a risk, and it is my duty in a book like this to point them out. We don't want a mother turning up with a five-day-old baby and saying: 'I breastfeed him on demand, but he hasn't demanded yet so I haven't fed him.'

Once breastfeeding is underway, when the baby has been nursing for a few days without any problem, and he looks contented and is gaining weight normally, there is no need to wake him up to feed him. If one day he sleeps for eight hours, use the opportunity to have a rest, because at four months he probably won't sleep for that long (once again, it is a matter of common sense: if your baby sleeps a lot longer than usual, watch him, make sure he is breathing properly, check his forehead to see if he has a temperature, etc.)

However, if he is losing, or gaining very little weight, and in addition he is sleeping a lot, it is a good idea to try to wake him up to feed him. It can be quite difficult to rouse a baby from a deep sleep, so rather than wake him, be alert to when he begins moving or is *almost* awake, and lift him to your breast. This means having him beside you at all times. A baby who doesn't cry much because he has a quiet nature, or because he is too weak due to illness or weight loss, will miss a lot of feeds if he sleeps out of sight of his mother. He will half wake up, move his head from side to side, whimper, and no one will notice, so he will go back to sleep. And it will be said afterwards: 'He slept for six hours in one go.'

During the first few days, all babies lose weight, and so you need to be attentive in order to try to breastfeed your baby as often as you can. There is no strict rule that says at exactly what hourly intervals. You have to use your common sense. A baby who nurses several times in the morning (and nurses well, so that you can see her jaw working and hear her swallowing) and then sleeps for five hours in the afternoon, isn't the same as a baby who sleeps for five hours, and then another five hours, and another, and between naps scarcely latches on to the breast, struggles to nurse, and only feeds for two minutes or less, or stays attached to it for half an hour, but without nursing.

When will she start sleeping through the night?

Various methods claiming 'to teach children how to sleep' have recently come into fashion. This is nonsense; all children know how to sleep. Foetuses already sleep before they are born, and newborns usually sleep for more than fifteen hours a day (and some much more than that). A baby who didn't sleep would die within a few days, the same as an adult.

In fact, what children 'learn' with time is not how to sleep, but how to stay awake. They have to pass from the fifteen or twenty hours of sleep of a newborn to the seven or eight hours of sleep of an adult, so obviously they have to sleep less and less. However, this isn't really something they learn (i.e. something they have to be taught), but rather it is part of the maturing process, like sitting and walking: all children will do all these things when they are ready, without their parents having to do anything in particular (just loving and caring for them in the usual way), and no amount of intensive or early stimulation will make them do these things any earlier or better.

One of the milestones in this maturing process takes place at about four months old, when the baby starts waking up frequently during the night. This takes many mothers by surprise, and they worry or even get alarmed, because they have been told their baby will start sleeping longer and longer (Really? if he slept any longer he would be in a coma!). But now you are forewarned: at two or three months, your baby may sleep for six hours in one go, possibly even eight; but when he reaches about four or five months he will probably begin to wake up several times in the night, roughly every hour and a half to two hours. Remember, this is a normal part of the maturing process. There is no need for you to teach him this by waking him up every two hours, he will do it all by himself. Apparently, some babies don't start waking up, but carry on sleeping right through the night. If your baby happens to be one of these don't worry, he is also normal.

After this, we begin moving into uncharted territory: there is very little information about the natural evolution of sleep patterns in children. It is certainly very varied, and every child is different. It seems that around the age of two children wake up quite a lot less, and when they are about three they begin to sleep through the night (the majority, anyway – those who haven't suffered any trauma from being left alone at night against their will). Also around three years old, many children who have been sleeping with their parents will accept sleeping in a different room, provided someone stays with them until they fall asleep. Children of about seven can go to sleep on their own (meaning, you can kiss them goodnight and leave the room, and they will stay in bed without crying, protesting or calling out.)

Gas

Both children and adults can have gas in their stomachs or intestines (mainly in the large intestine). But these are two quite different things.

Gas in the stomach is just air that that has been swallowed (doctors refer to this as aerophagia, 'eating air'). Babies swallow air when they eat, when they cry, or even when they suck their thumb or dummy.

The gas found in the intestine is different. You can tell from the smell. It contains nitrogen from the swallowed air (the oxygen has been absorbed through the digestive tract) and other gases the intestine produces when digesting certain foods, which account for its particular odour.

When a baby swallows too much air, he may get rid of it by passing wind, but he will more likely expel it through his mouth in the form of burps. An excess of gas in the intestine probably comes from his digestion rather than from swallowed air. When a baby isn't feeding properly because he is in the incorrect position, or for any other reason, he may be getting too much lactose and not enough fat, and the relative overload of lactose is producing the excess of gas (see page 54). In addition, if he is not latched on properly, he is more likely to swallow air while he is nursing. However, incorrect positioning isn't the main cause of gas, and gas isn't the main symptom of incorrect positioning.

An excess of gas in the intestine can only be expelled by passing wind. Fortunately it isn't able to travel in the other direction and come out of the mouth.

It is easier to expel gas from the stomach in an upright position than it is lying down. As our ancestors spent most of the time more or less upright in their mothers' arms, they probably didn't have much of a problem. During the last hundred years, bottle feeding and cots have become widespread. A baby can swallow a lot of air while bottle feeding, and then have difficulty expelling it in his cot; this is why it seemed important to burp the baby before putting him down.

However, it appears that babies aren't all that bothered by gas, except perhaps in some extreme cases. A lot of people think the main reason why small babies cry is because of gas. And many of the old treatments for baby colic supposedly helped expel gas (this is the meaning of the word 'carminative'), or prevent the formation of air bubbles (I've never understood the reason, but it is true that some drops for treating colic contain anti-foaming agents).

Not everybody agrees about what causes colic (I will explain my pet theory further on), but nobody, it seems, seriously defends the theory that it is caused by gas. Years ago, before it became known that too much radiation was a bad thing, people were given X-rays for the most ridiculous reasons, and it occurred to someone to X-ray crying babies (gas is clearly visible, and comes out as a big black spot on an X-ray). It showed that babies have very little gas when they start crying, and lots more gas after they have been crying for a while. The fact is, when they cry they swallow air, and because they can't cry and burp at the same time, the air builds up until they stop crying. The mother usually explains it thus: 'Poor little thing, he was crying because he had a lot of gas. I picked him up, patted his back a few times and after he had burped he was all right'. A more likely interpretation is: 'Poor little thing, he was crying because he missed me. When I picked him up and stroked his back, he calmed down, and all the air he'd swallowed came out in a big burp'.

I think this explains the importance given to burping in the previous century. When the mother tried to place the baby in his cot straight after a feed, the baby cried inconsolably. If, however, she held him in her arms and rocked him and stroked him before leaving him in his cot, the baby was more likely to calm down and fall asleep. While he was still in his mother's arms, the baby, of course, burped. And, as no one wanted to admit that it was good for a mother to hold her baby (Good? Nonsense, it is bad, it spoils the child, turns him into a cry-baby!), they preferred to think that it was burping and not the mother's presence that explained the miracle.

The fact is that many of today's mothers still believe burping is terribly important, essential to their baby's health and happiness. He has to burp, come what may. But when babies nurse correctly, they swallow almost no air at all (their lips form a seal around the breast, so the air can't get in, and, unlike the bottle, the breast contains no air). Babies often don't burp after they nurse. However, when they are incorrectly positioned, it is possible for them to swallow air (their lips make a smacking sound) because there is a gap between breast and lips.

Occasionally, a mother will tell me that her baby has 'difficulty burping', and that she has to pat his back for an hour, during which he cries all the time because he is so uncomfortable, until finally he expels the trapped gas. Poor little thing, he doesn't need to burp, he is crying because his mother keeps patting his back and shaking him, until finally he expels the air he swallowed while he was crying.

Don't become too fixated on burping. After your baby nurses, it is a good idea to hold him for a while. He likes this. If while you are holding him he burps, fine. If he doesn't, then he probably hasn't any gas. Don't pat his back or give him camomile tea, or aniseed, or water, or any herbal, artificial, or homemade 'remedy', whether from a chemist or a health food shop.

Colic

It is common in the West for babies to cry a lot during the first few months. This is known as infant or baby colic. Colic is a spontaneous, painful spasm in a hollow viscera. You can have colic of the kidneys, bladder and intestine. But since a baby isn't 'a hollow viscera', the expression 'baby colic' seems rather inappropriate. The word colic was used because it was thought that the baby's stomach hurt, although this is impossible to verify. Pain can't be seen; the patient has to describe it. When you ask babies: 'Why are you crying?' they refuse to answer, and when you ask them again years later they say they can't remember. So nobody knows whether it is their stomach, head or back that hurts, or whether they have an itchy foot, or the noise bothers them, or they are simply upset by something they heard on the radio. That is why books today avoid the word 'colic' and prefer to talk about 'excessive infant crying'. It is reasonable to suppose that babies don't all cry for the same reason; one might have a stomach-ache, while another is hungry, or cold, or hot, and another simply wants to be cuddled (probably the most common reason).

Crying usually takes place in the evening, between six and ten o'clock – 'the witching hour'. Sometimes it is from eight until midnight, or from midnight until four in the morning, and some babies seem to be on permanent crying watch. It usually starts after two or three weeks, and improves around three months (though not always).

When a mother is breastfeeding, and her baby cries in the evening, some thoughtful person will always say: 'Obviously, your milk dries up in the evening!' But in that case, why do babies who are bottle fed suffer from colic? (Colic appears to be evenly distributed among breastfed and bottle fed babies.) Perhaps some mothers prepare the morning bottle with 150ml and the evening one with 90ml just to annoy the baby and make him cry? Of course not! Both bottles contain exactly the same amount, and yet the baby who was sleeping more or less peacefully in the morning won't stop crying in the evening. Hunger isn't the cause.

'So why is my baby attached to my breast the whole afternoon, and why are my breasts empty?' There are several things a mother who bottle feeds can do when her baby cries: she can pick him up, rock him, sing to him, caress him, give him a dummy, give him a bottle, leave him to cry (I am not suggesting leaving him to cry is a good idea, I am simply listing it as one of the things the mother can do). The mother who is breastfeeding can do all those things (including giving him a bottle and leaving him to cry), but there is one other thing she can do: she can put him to her breast. Most mothers discover that putting the baby to the breast is the quickest and easiest way to calm him (at home we called it 'the anaesthesia'), and so this is what she does repeatedly as the evening wears on. And of course in the end, her breasts become flaccid, not because her milk has dried up, but because all the milk is inside her baby's stomach. The baby is no longer hungry; on the contrary, he is full of milk.

If the mother is happy for her baby to be attached to her breast all the time, and her nipples don't hurt (if the baby wants to nurse all the time, and the mother's nipples *do* hurt, the baby is most likely incorrectly positioned or has a tongue-tie), and if this calms the baby down, then this is fine. She can put him on her breast as often and for as long as she wants. She can lie down and rest while her baby is nursing. But if the mother is exhausted, at her wits' end, tired of constantly breastfeeding, and if her baby is gaining weight normally, there is no reason for her not to say to the baby's father, or grandmother, or the first volunteer she can find: 'Take this baby away, take him into the other room, or go out for a stroll and don't bring him back for a couple of hours'. Because we can be reasonably sure of one thing: if a baby who is breastfeeding correctly, and gaining weight normally, nurses five times in two hours and still won't stop crying, he isn't hungry (a baby who is gaining very little weight, or who was gaining little or no weight up until two days ago, and is now making up for it is a different matter: he may need frequent, consecutive feeds). If you manage to find someone to take the baby out for a stroll, make sure you use the opportunity to rest, and if possible to have some sleep. Don't start washing up, or catching up with the ironing, otherwise you will be back to square one.

The mother is sometimes at her wits' end after alternately breastfeeding and holding her baby for two hours. She greets her husband as if he were the cavalry arriving: 'Please, do something with this baby, I'm going crazy'. The father takes the baby (not without some anxiety, given the circumstances), the baby lays her head on his shoulder and, hey presto!, she falls asleep. There are several possible explanations for this phenomenon. Perhaps it is that we men have broader shoulders, which are more conducive to sleep. Because the baby has been active for two hours, and it is only normal that she is tired. Perhaps all she needed was a change of scene, to be held by someone different (it often happens the other way round: the father is at his wits' end and the mother manages to calm the baby in a few seconds).

My feeling is (and I have no evidence to back this up, it is simply a theory) that, in some cases, the baby is also tired of nursing. She isn't hungry, but she can't lay her head on her mother's shoulder and fall asleep. It is as though nursing is the only relationship she has with her mother. Perhaps she feels the way we do when after a big meal someone offers us a helping of our favourite dessert. We can't refuse, and afterwards we suffer from indigestion for the rest of the afternoon. When the baby is in her mother's arms she is constantly torn between wanting and not wanting to nurse, whereas with her father there is no choice: he has no breasts, so she can go to sleep.

My theory evidently has many weaknesses. To begin with, most of the babies in the world spend all day in their mother's arms (or on her back), and generally speaking they are calm and hardly ever cry. But perhaps these babies do have a different way of relating to their mother, apart from nursing. In our culture we insist on leaving babies in their cots for several hours a day. Perhaps, by doing this, we convey the idea that they can only be with their mother if they are nursing.

Because the truth is, baby colic appears to be exclusive to our culture. Some see it as a malaise of our civilisation, the result of our not giving children as much physical contact as they need. In other societies, the concept of 'colic' is unknown. Dr Lee didn't discover a single case of colic among 160 babies in Korea. One-month-old babies in Korea spend only two hours alone every day, compared to sixteen hours in America. Korean babies were held twice as much as American babies, and their mothers responded almost unfailingly to their cries. American mothers purposefully ignore their children's cries almost fifty per cent of the time.

In Canada, Hunziker and Barr showed that it is possible to prevent baby colic by advising mothers to carry their babies for several hours a day. Carrying your baby in a sling, the way the majority of the mothers in the world do, is an excellent idea. There are lots of different baby-slings and carriers available on the market, all of which are very comfortable for carrying your baby around in, both inside and outside the house. Don't rush to put your baby in his cot as soon as he falls asleep; babies like being close to their mothers even while they are sleeping. And don't wait until your two or three-week-old baby starts to cry before picking her up; it may be too late by then, and even picking her up won't calm her. From the moment they are born, babies need a lot of physical contact, a lot of holding. It isn't good for them to be separated from their mothers, much less left alone in a separate room. If during the day you put her in her cot to sleep for a while, it is better for the cot to be in the sitting room; this way both mother and baby will feel reassured, and more able to relax.

In our society we find it extremely difficult to accept that babies need holding, that they need physical contact and affection; that they need their mothers. Any other explanation is preferable: maybe an immature digestive system, maybe the nervous system. We prefer to think the baby is ill, that she needs drugs. A few decades ago, Spanish chemists used to sell a remedy for colic that contained barbiturate: 'miraculously' the baby fell fast asleep. Others turn to herbal remedies or teas, homeopathy, massage. All the treatments I know of have one thing in common; in order to administer them you are obliged to hold the baby. The baby is crying in his cot, his mother picks him up, gives him some camomile tea, the baby stops crying. He would have stopped crying without the camomile tea, if she had put him to her breast, or simply held him. Imagine a robot that administers camomile tea and is activated by the baby's crying. A micro-camera watches the baby's cot, a computer discovers the baby's mouth, and a syringe aims a spurt of camomile tea into it: do you think the baby will stop crying? It isn't the camomile tea or the homeopathic remedy that calms him; it is his mother's arms that cure his colic!

An American paediatrician by the name of Taubman demonstrated that a few simple instructions for the mother (see *Table 1*) made her baby's colic disappear within two weeks. Babies whose mothers paid attention to them went from an average of 2.6 hours crying per day to only 0.8 hours per day. Babies in the control group, that were left to cry, went from an average of 3.1 hours crying to 3.8 hours. In other words, babies don't cry because they want to, they cry because something is happening. If they are left to cry they cry more, and if they are consoled they cry less. It is so simple! Why do so many people try to convince us of the opposite?

---

1. Try to never let your baby cry.
2. In attempting to discover why your infant is crying, consider these possibilities:
   a) The baby is hungry and wants to be fed.
   b) The baby wants to suck, although he is not hungry.
   c) The baby wants to be held.
   d) The baby is bored and wants stimulation.
   e) The baby is tired and wants to sleep.
3. If the crying continues for more than five minutes with one response, then try another.
4. Decide on your own in what order to explore the above possibilities.
5. Don't be concerned about overfeeding your baby. This will not happen.
6. Don't be concerned about spoiling your baby. This also will not happen.

Table 1: Instructions for Treating Colic According to Taubman (*Pediatrics 1984;74;998*)

In the control group the instructions were: when your baby cries and you don't know why, leave her where she is (in her cot) and leave the room. If after thirty minutes she is still crying, go back in, check (briefly) that she is all right, and leave the room again. If after thirty minutes she is still crying, go back in and so on. If after three hours she is still crying, feed her, and begin again.

The last two instructions on Dr Taubman's list seem to me particularly important: it is impossible to overfeed your baby by offering her too much food (ask any mother who tries to feed solids to a child who doesn't want to eat); and it is impossible to spoil a child by giving her too much attention. The only way you can 'spoil' a child is by inflicting on her beatings, insults, and ridicule, and by ignoring her when she cries. On the contrary, it has always been true that the way to nurture a child is by giving her attention, cuddling her, caressing her, consoling her, talking to her, kissing her, and smiling at her.

There is no such thing as a mental illness caused by *too much* affection, cuddling, or caresses. No one in prison or in a mental hospital is there as a result of his parents cuddling or singing to him *too much*, or letting him sleep in their bed. In contrast, there are people in prison or in the mental hospital because they had no parents, or because their parents abused or abandoned them. And yet, society's biggest concern seems to be to prevent this completely imaginary form of mental illness: 'chronic child-spoiling'. If in doubt, dear reader, try to remember and compare how many people have warned you since you got pregnant about the importance of buying child-proof plugs, keeping your house chemical-free, using a car seat, or vaccinating your baby against tetanus, and how many have warned you not to pick up your baby, not to have her in your bed, and not to 'spoil' her.

→ Lee, K. 'The crying pattern of Korean infants and related factors', *Dev Med Child Neurol* 1994;36:601-7

→ Hunziker, U.A., Barr, R.G. 'Increased carrying reduces infant crying: a randomized controlled trial', *Pediatrics* 1986;77:641-8

→ Taubman, B. 'Clinical trial of the treatment of colic by modification of parent-infant interaction', *Pediatrics* 1984;74:998-1003

Clarifications

Somebody will no doubt say that thanks to Dr González (and Dr Taubman – they are two of a kind!), mothers everywhere will now be enslaved, poor things, their attention completely taken up by their child. This isn't true. I am not the one who tells the poor baby to cry, he cries all by himself. Some will say that if your child cries all you can do is to go out of the room and leave him to cry. And that you must keep doing this, again and again, day after day, regardless of whether it works or not. And what does a mother do while her baby is crying? Do you think she reads a book, or has a rest or does the ironing? Anyone who has a heard a baby crying inconsolably (especially their own baby!) knows that the mother will be incapable of doing anything. The noise a baby makes when it cries is one of the most disagreeable sounds in the world (it is specially designed to cause a response in adults, to leave nobody indifferent). All the poor mother can do is grit her teeth, and watch the clock, waiting for the thirty minutes to pass. On the other hand, the mother who has been told to attend to her baby has five options (and if she can think up a sixth, even better). She can decide which one she tries first, and if that doesn't work and her baby goes on crying, she can try another. Incidentally, one of these options, 'the baby is tired and wants to sleep', could be understood to mean: 'put him in his cot and leave the room', except that, if this doesn't work, the mother isn't forced to wait another thirty minutes before picking him up.

It is the mother who is forced to leave her baby to cry who is enslaved, while the mother who is allowed to do what *she* thinks will best calm her baby is liberated. And in addition, she will see that her baby cries less and less.

So, if I leave my baby to cry, will he be traumatised for the rest of his life? No, I am not saying that. I am not talking about lasting damage, only about baby colic. If you leave your baby to cry, he will simply go on crying.

All babies cry. This is normal. Inevitable. Korean babies cry, African babies cry, they all cry. Even if you hold them twenty-four hours a day, they will still cry. But they will cry less. I am not suggesting that as soon as your baby starts crying, you must drop everything and rush to pick her up. Of course you will sometimes be in the shower, or in the kitchen trying not to burn the dinner, or doing something else. If so, at least try speaking to him, looking at him, smiling at him. It isn't the end of the world if a baby occasionally has to wait for a few minutes before someone goes to him. The problem is leaving the baby to cry on purpose and frequently. And doing it because someone who claims to know better than you (a relative, friend, a doctor, the author of a book…) has told you that crying is the best thing for your child, and that if you pick him up you will 'spoil' him.

We adults also cry, when there is a reason for it. So do babies. They don't cry 'for no reason', but their reasons are different from ours, and often we don't know why they are crying. Imagine you are the one crying: somebody very close to you has been in a terrible accident, and you are crying all alone at home. Isn't it sad to suffer when there is nobody to support you, to console you? Now imagine that you aren't alone, but that your husband is in the room, reading. You are crying, and he doesn't even glance up from his book. Or he screams at you: 'Shut up, will you, I'm trying to read!' Isn't that even worse than crying all alone? Besides your grief, you now feel abandoned and humiliated. You feel your husband no longer loves you. When a loved one cries, we go to them.

Of course, a two-month-old baby doesn't know whether his mother only went to him after ten minutes because she was busy, or because she was purposefully leaving him to cry ('Let him wait for a while, he has to learn he can't always get his own way'). He doesn't know, but you do. We do what we think is right, regardless of whether anyone else realises it.

Teething

A while ago, a mother told me that her six-week-old baby girl was teething. It is rare, though not impossible, for a six-week-old to begin teething, and so I examined the baby's mouth with interest. 'Well, I can't see anything.' 'There's nothing to see, yet.' 'So, how do you know she's teething?' 'Because she's restless, she cries and chews her fists…' 'Ah! But that's normal, all babies cry and chew their fists, it doesn't mean they're teething.' Month after month she said the same thing, the baby was 'teething', and I stopped arguing with her. After six months of this, a tooth finally emerged, as happens with all babies. 'You see, doctor? I told you she was teething!'

A comprehensive study found that teething was associated with only mild symptoms, which only affected some babies for a few days: drooling, chewing, pimples on the face (probably caused by drooling), crankiness, a slightly raised temperature when the teeth actually appeared (only detected because the researchers took each baby's temperature twice a day). The majority of babies showed no symptoms at all, and none of the symptoms increased more than 20 per cent during the teething phase. Moreover, no one symptom or combination of symptoms enabled them to predict when the baby's tooth would emerge. Teething didn't produce fever, diarrhoea, a runny nose, vomiting, a sore bottom or night-time waking.

However, we don't need a study to tell us that teething doesn't cause any serious symptoms. Babies aren't the only ones who cut teeth. At six years old, children begin cutting their permanent teeth, not all of which replace milk teeth (in case anyone argues that the cavity was already there), because there are no molars among milk teeth. Eight and ten-year-olds don't cry or chew their fists, or gnaw on teething rings when they are cutting teeth. Nobody rubs ointments on their gums. Thanks to the tooth fairy, we all remember when as children our first tooth fell out, but we don't remember the exact day when a new one began to emerge. Usually, you don't even notice. One day you look in the mirror and, surprise, surprise, you have a new tooth! (Wisdom teeth are different; some people's gums haven't enough space for them, and this can cause considerable discomfort).

And yet, many people are convinced that teething causes serious problems in babies, so many that they require treatment. They buy ointments from the chemist containing local anaesthetic (!), 'natural', herbal or homeopathic folk remedies, teething rings made of plastic, rubber and other materials (not so long ago, babies were given cuttlebone). The latest fashion is amber necklaces (not for the baby to chew on, it seems, but to put round his neck!). Some mothers believe in these 'cures': 'I gave him X for his teeth and it worked really well'. I have always wondered what that means. If it weren't for 'X', would their children have no teeth, or would they have died of teething?

Given that babies cut twenty teeth in the space of a few months, it is always possible to blame any problem on a tooth that is 'about to come in' or 'has just come in'. I think in part that, as with baby colic, this is another manifestation of our society's fear of the mother-child relationship. If a baby cries we can't accept that it is because he needs his mother. We prefer to think he must be ill, frightened, suffering from colic or teething…

While we are on the subject of supposed reasons why babies cry, for a while I was mildly concerned that my own children didn't cry when their nappies were soiled. Everybody says they cry. Even in films, when a baby cries they always check his nappy. But my children's nappies could be heavily soiled and they didn't make a sound, and I only realised because of the smell. I felt vindicated when I read somewhere (I don't remember where) about an experiment on this very subject carried out a few decades ago. Half the babies were given a clean nappy, and the other half were given the soiled nappy they had just been wearing. They calmed down just the same! The babies weren't crying because of soiled nappies; this was mere coincidence. They calmed down because, during an era when babies were left for hours alone in their cots, their mothers picked them up, carried them to the nappy-changing table, touched them, rubbed them (with a sponge), looked into their eyes, and probably said loving things to them.

I suspect that the famous effect of the relaxing bath before bed belongs to the same category of myth. What your baby needs in order to relax and fall asleep is contact, attention, holding.

→ Macknin, M.L., Piedmonte, M., Jacobs, J., Skibinski, C. 'Symptoms associated with infant teething: a prospective study', *Pediatrics* 2000;105:747-52

Hunger

The big question! 'Is he hungry?' often contains the implicit question: 'Is my milk no good, will I have to bottle feed him?' When a baby is tired, there is no problem, he sleeps; but when he is hungry, many a mother will turn pale, as though she were to blame.

The problem is that when we use the word 'hunger' we are referring to two very different things. On the one hand hunger is a lack of food, undernourishment. There is hunger in the world, children who die of hunger. Our parents and grandparents experienced hunger in times of war. How lucky we are not to have gone through that! On the other hand, hunger is an unpleasant sensation that makes us want to eat. I know what hunger feels like: I get hungry several times a day, which is why I eat. If I never felt hungry I would never eat. This is the irony: a child (or adult) who never felt hunger would die of hunger.

'My baby already wants to nurse after an hour and a half. Is this because he's hungry?' Of course he is hungry! That is why he wants his mother's breast! But if you breastfeed him on demand, he will stop being hungry. If you only feed him every three hours he will still be hungry. Don't let your baby suffer hunger. Let him nurse when he is hungry.

Growth spurts

A great many books on breastfeeding talk about babies going though periods of needing to nurse more frequently (so-called 'growth spurts' or 'frequency days'). Typically, from one day to the next, a baby who has been more or less happy with a steady pattern of breastfeeding will suddenly want to nurse all the time. If his mother panics ('My milk has dried up!') and starts him on bottles, the baby will bottle feed more and more, and will soon stop breastfeeding altogether. If, instead of starting him on bottles, his mother breastfeeds on demand, she will produce more milk, and in two or three days, his increased demands to nurse will stop. Supposedly these are periods when babies grow more quickly, and therefore need more milk, and some claim they occur at specific times – at two weeks, six weeks, three months and so on.

The theory appears plausible, because some authors have found that babies can go for several weeks without growing at all, and then grow one or two centimetres in a few days. And yet, to my knowledge, nobody has been able to show that these 'frequency days' actually coincide with periods of sudden growth, or that they occur at two or six weeks, and not at three or five weeks. Let us just say that they can occur any time, and we don't know the cause. But we do know the solution: breastfeeding on demand, and no bottles.

The three-month crisis

The three-month crisis (I invented this term, so you won't find it in any other books) concerns the mother, not the baby. The baby is fine; there is nothing wrong with him. But his mother panics, and thinks that her milk has dried up. This usually occurs somewhere between the second and fourth month, but this can vary.

There are several factors that work together to trigger the crisis. The mother's breasts, which, when lactation started, swelled up and then emptied noticeably with each feed, now always seem to look the same (empty!). The milk that used to leak from the other breast, sometimes all day, has stopped leaking. The baby, who used to need fifteen or twenty minutes on each breast, now nurses in five minutes, and sometimes only two or less. And on top of all that, he doesn't poo! (See page 94).

All of these changes are normal. Swollen breasts and leaking milk don't mean plenty of milk. They are more like little hiccups at the start of the lactation process, which stop when the breast is fully functioning. Otherwise you would be using breast pads for two years! The baby is growing stronger and more skilful, and he nurses more and more quickly. His weight gain shows us there is no problem. Well, those of us, that is, who know that each month babies gain less weight than the month before (apparently some people don't know this, and they alarm mothers unnecessarily). A mother who is expecting her baby to gain exactly the same amount of weight each month will have one more thing to worry about: 'this month he gained less weight'.

So, the solution to the 'three-month crisis' is in the mother's own hands. It is simple: stop worrying, keep breastfeeding on demand (which also means letting the baby stop nursing when he wants) and no bottles.

Breast refusal

Babies can refuse the breast for many reasons. If you find out the cause, you will quickly discover the solution.

'False' refusal

Newborns usually nurse without any problem for the first two hours after delivery. But for the following eight to ten hours they are often a bit drowsy, and almost stop nursing. You should give your baby every opportunity to feed by maintaining skin-to-skin contact with her, and putting her to your breast whenever possible, but don't become overly concerned. If as the hours go by she still hasn't nursed, you will need to make more of an effort to wake her, and if that doesn't work then you will have to express some of your milk and feed it to her using a dropper or a small cup.

When babies are near their mother's breast they move their heads from side to side, in a searching movement. Some mothers will think this means their baby is refusing to nurse. But newborns don't know how to shake their heads, they are simply searching for their mother's breast.

When you try to direct the baby to your breast, exert pressure on her back, not on her crown, otherwise she will instinctively jerk her head back. This is a reflex.

When something brushes against a baby's mouth, cheek, upper lip or chin, she will automatically move towards whatever has touched her. Under normal circumstances, this reflex helps her to find the nipple. But if what brushes her cheek is a finger, or clothing, she will move away from the nipple.

As I mentioned above, when babies get older, they nurse much more quickly. They release the nipple and refuse to go on feeding. Don't insist. The most common cause of breast 'refusal' is in fact that the baby isn't hungry.

Infant pain or illness

A lot of babies suffer bruising to the head or a fractured collarbone during delivery. Both these things can be painful, and it is necessary to find a position in which he is able to nurse comfortably. The same may apply later on when he is vaccinated. Try not to press on the sore area.

When a baby's nose runs, he finds it hard to breathe and nurse at the same time. And, naturally, he prefers to breathe. You can put him on his back and place a few drops (not a spurt) of physiological saline solution in each nostril (chemists sell small bottles). The dry mucus will soften, and a few moments later the baby will sneeze, expelling all the mucus. When using a nose-sucker, be careful not to insert it into the baby's nostril, as it may damage the mucosa (the old-fashioned ones were pointed, nowadays they are rounded), and remember to suck, not blow, otherwise you will push the mucus further inside.

Babies who suffer from a congenital heart defect sometimes refuse to nurse because they are too weak.

If a baby has an ear or throat infection, and it hurts when he swallows, he won't have much desire to nurse.

If he is restless and has been crying for a while, he may refuse to latch on to the breast. Calm him first by cradling him in your arms, and after a while try putting him to your breast again.

He may have had an unpleasant experience during a previous feed: for example, if he was given an injection while nursing, or if he bit you by accident and you screamed.

He may have an allergy to something the mother has eaten: 'As soon as he swallows my milk, he starts crying'. It is important not to confuse this with the 'three-month-crisis' (see page 115). In the latter, the baby is happy nursing and when he releases the breast, and only starts protesting when the mother tries to make him nurse more. When there is an allergy, the baby will cry while he is nursing even though no one is forcing him. He will go on crying when he releases the breast because the allergy is irritating his stomach. But he will soon want to nurse again because he is still hungry, and when he does he will start crying again. He doesn't know what he wants, and struggles while nursing.

Problems of technique

If the baby has become used to feeding from a bottle or to having a dummy in her mouth, she will try to latch onto the breast as if it were a bottle, and, of course, the breast will slip out of her mouth (see page 65).

When the baby is incorrectly positioned, it can produce an excess of oxytocin: the milk comes out in a spurt, choking the baby (see page 53).

Nipple creams may also cause the baby's mouth to slip off the breast. Sometimes it is necessary to apply creams to treat a specific problem such as cracked nipples, or a fungal or other infection; if you don't have any problem don't use any 'preventative' creams.

If your breast is very full, it is hard for the baby to get a grip on it. Try expressing some of your milk before feeding her (see page 52).

Changes that upset the baby

Some of the all-too-common practices in the delivery room (probes, aspirations, teats, a finger being placed in the baby's mouth) are unpleasant experiences, and can cause the baby to develop an oral aversion. The baby refuses to have anything else put in his mouth. It will take a lot of patience and gentle cajoling.

When the mother has been out (for example, if she has gone back to work), when she returns the baby may respond by being 'clingy', or he may push her away, or both. This is normal. Your baby will need lots of attention and affection to overcome this.

Babies sometimes refuse the breast if they notice their mother isn't paying attention to them because she is distracted by a family discussion, problems at work, preparations for a party, renovations to the house, or because someone has dropped by unexpectedly.

Some babies refuse the breast when the mother is pregnant or has her period; it seems the taste of her milk changes.

A baby may be put off by the taste of something the mother has eaten (see page 162), or the salt on her skin when she has been sweating, or by the taste or smell of the soap, perfume, cream or deodorant she uses.

Many older babies are distracted by their surroundings. For a while you may have to find somewhere quiet to breastfeed your baby.

If a loud noise or an abrupt movement frightens your baby while he is nursing, he may refuse to nurse the next time.

Refusal of one breast

It is perfectly normal for a baby to nurse from a single breast at each feed. Sometimes she will want the second breast, sometimes she won't. However, when a baby always wants to nurse from the same breast, and completely rejects the other, this is a different thing.

It may be more difficult for her to latch on to one of the mother's breasts, because the nipple is very flat, or too big, and won't fit into her mouth.

She may be uncomfortable nursing from one of the breasts, because she has earache, or a sore collarbone, or one of her buttocks is painful after being vaccinated, or because her mother is less skilled at holding her with one arm than with the other. In cases like these, try breastfeeding in a different position, with her feet facing the other way, or holding her with the other arm.

When the mother is suffering from mastitis, there is a build-up of sodium in her infected breast. Her milk has a salty taste, and some babies will refuse it. Sodium builds up when milk production goes down, and milk production goes down when the baby doesn't nurse, creating a vicious circle.

Start off trying to make your baby accept the other breast by patiently experimenting with different positions. In the meantime, you should express your milk in order to prevent engorgement, maintain milk production, and prevent a build-up of sodium in your milk. If your baby is gaining weight normally, don't feed her the expressed milk (you can freeze it and keep it for when you go back to work), because if she is full and you keep offering her more milk, she will have even less desire to nurse.

If after several days your baby still refuses the other breast, it is probably better to stop trying, gradually to stop expressing the milk, and to carry on breastfeeding from one breast, which is perfectly possible. One breast will produce enough milk for the baby, and milk secretion in the other breast will stop completely. The only problem is aesthetic: if the difference in breast size is noticeable, you can pad out the other bra cup.

In a few very rare cases, months after a baby rejects one of the mother's breasts, it is found to have a tumour. This may affect the taste of the milk. As I said, it is extremely rare, and there is usually another cause (or no apparent cause). If your baby has been happily nursing from both breasts and she suddenly starts refusing one, and if all attempts to make her feed from it fail, wait a few days and then examine your breast for lumps (I say wait a few days because while the breast is still producing milk which the baby isn't taking, it will of course be lumpy). And then a few months later examine it again.

→ Healow, L.K., Hugh, R.S. 'Oral aversion in the breastfed neonate', *Breastfeeding Abstracts* 2000;20:3-4 www.llli.org/ba/Aug00. html

→ Saber, A., Dardik, H., Ibrahim, I.M., Wolodiger, F. 'The milk rejection sign: a natural tumor marker', *Am Surg* 1996;62:998-9

How to overcome breast refusal

You have to have a lot of patience. Try to cajole your baby into taking your breast without forcing her to latch on to it, hold her a lot, and give her lots of cuddles. Experiment with different positions. It can be very helpful to lie on your back (either on a bed, or leaning back in an armchair) with your baby face down on top of you. Place her close to your breast, and let her look for it herself.

If she continues to refuse, you will need to express your milk and feed it to her from a cup. Some babies refuse a cup from their mother, and someone else has to do it. Don't feel hurt. Imagine how bad your baby must be feeling in order to behave like this. Don't try to make her yield by starving her. She will probably nurse even worse if she is hungry. It is better if you first feed her the expressed milk from a cup, and try to get her to nurse when she isn't hungry or upset. Try using skin-to-skin contact (see page 63).

Don't try to make her to latch on to your breast, or force her mouth open, or press her to your breast. This is usually counter-productive, as it can result in both mother and baby getting upset, and the unpleasant experience helps perpetuate the refusal.

Weight

How much a baby weighs is the source of a great deal of unnecessary anxiety. Some doctors stipulate a certain weight and alarm parents unnecessarily. Others, possibly as reaction against this, go to the other extreme: 'So long as he is nursing his weight doesn't matter'. Of course it matters! A baby who only gains 200 grams between the first and second month has a serious problem. An experienced person often doesn't need to weigh a baby to see that he is perfectly healthy or severely undernourished. However, where there is any doubt, the baby's weight must be carefully compared with a baby growth chart, and this is when serious mistakes can arise.

Growth curves aren't straight

If they were, babies would gain the same amount of weight each month. The reason they curve is precisely because each month babies usually gain less weight than the month before. The same baby who for the first two or three months gained 500 grams, 1,000 grams or even 1,500 grams, may only gain 200 grams in the fourth month, or may not gain any weight between the ninth and the twelfth month. Sometimes, the babies who gained the most weight to begin with seem to gain less weight in subsequent months, as if they had gained all their weight in one go instead of in instalments.

→ Mei, Z., Grummer-Strawn, L.M., Thompson, D., Dietz, W.H. 'Shifts in percentiles of growth during early childhood: analysis of longitudinal data from the California Child Health and Development Study', *Pediatrics* 2004;113:e617-27 pediatrics. aappublications.org/cgi/content/full/113/6/e617

Half of all babies are below the average

This is why it is called 'the average'. Babies who weigh below the average are as normal as those who weigh above the average. A baby who weighs below the average isn't 'underweight', he is completely normal. In fact, if all babies weighed above the average, the Department of Health would issue a health alert warning about the biggest epidemic of child obesity in the history of the world.

Three per cent of babies are below the third percentile (the lowest line on the chart). Not three per cent of all babies, three per cent of those weighed in order to make up the charts. By definition, the participants were all normal healthy babies, who weren't premature, weren't in hospital, and didn't have congenital heart conditions. This means that in real life, more than three per cent of babies are below the third percentile. Possibly four to five per cent. The doctor's job is to distinguish between the three who are healthy and the fourth or fifth, who might be ill.

In the UK around 700,000 babies are born each year; this means that 21,000 healthy babies weigh less than the third percentile. Plus another 21,000 one-year-olds, 21,000 two-year-olds, 21,000 three-year-olds…

Children don't grow strictly along growth chart lines

The lines on a baby growth chart are artistic representations (they are designed to look nice) of mathematical functions. They bear no relation to a baby's growth in the real world. It is perfectly normal for a baby to cross one or two lines on the chart (obviously over several months, not in one go) in either direction, in weight as well as size. It is perfectly normal for a baby to go up one percentile in weight and down one percentile in size, and vice versa.

If your baby really isn't gaining weight...

When a baby's weight is genuinely low, lower than 'normal', or he is gaining weight too slowly, this can be for a multitude of reasons:

1. The baby is very small or skinny, but perfectly healthy. A particular case could be a case of constitutional growth delay (CGD) (see page 125).
2. The baby has an illness that primarily affects growth (growth hormone deficiency, Down's syndrome...).
3. The baby is malnourished, which may be the result of:

   a) Malnutrition secondary to an illness that interferes with the absorption of food (diarrhoea, coeliac disease, cystic fibrosis) or the metabolism (diabetes), or increases the use of energy (a fever...), or causes a loss of nutrients (nephrotic syndrome, parasitosis...), or of appetite (tuberculosis, urinary tract infection, tracheomalacia, repeated viral infections or otitis...).

   b) Primary malnutrition (not enough food). In this case, and if the baby is exclusively breastfed, we can have

   - A tongue-tie that makes breastfeeding difficult
   - Inadequate breastfeeding technique (insufficient length or frequency of feeds, interference from dummies, water or other liquids; incorrect positioning, suppression of night feedings...). Most babies who gain little weight when exclusively breastfeeding don't need to be bottle fed, they need to be breastfed more.
   - Primary hypogalactia; that is, insufficient secretion of milk by the mammary gland, which doesn't respond to the usual interventions (increasing the number of feeds, good positioning). Hypogalactia can be treatable, like hypothyroidism, or untreatable (at present), like breast agenesis.

Only in the highly unlikely case of untreatable primary hypogalactia, the solution would be mixed feeding. There is no available data on the relative frequency of the different causes of low weight in babies, but experience shows that in Spain the most frequent causes are: a) the baby is small, but healthy, b) the baby has an intercurrent illness (usually mild) and c) poor breastfeeding techniques (imposed feeding schedule, feeding the baby water from a bottle). Fortunately this is less and less common.

And yet, many doctors will automatically tell mothers to bottle feed their baby if he doesn't gain enough weight: without looking any further, or considering any other options. First the baby is weaned off the breast, and if he still doesn't gain weight after he is weaned, the problem is taken seriously, and the necessary tests carried out, only to discover he has a urinary infection, coeliac disease or cystic fibrosis. The sad truth is that some mothers feel obliged to lie, and tell their doctor they aren't breastfeeding in order for their baby to be properly examined.

New growth charts for nursing babies

The growth charts in common usage till recent times were compiled using babies who were generally breastfed very little or not at all. The WHO has published a new set of charts, based only on the growth of babies who are fed normally (that is, who are breastfed for over a year, and who are exclusively breastfed for the first six months). You can see them at www.who.int/childgrowth. This isn't about using two different charts, one for children who are breastfed and one for children who are bottle fed. The same chart should be used for all babies. Artificial feeding aims to achieve the same growth rates for bottle fed as for breastfed babies. Seventy years ago, babies who were bottle fed didn't gain as much weight. Now, it would seem, after the age of six months they gain more. More research needs doing before they come up with a type of artificial milk that doesn't cause obesity.

When comparing the WHO growth charts with those recently used in Spain (from the Fundación Orbegozo), you see that they are almost identical up until six months. But after five or six months, on the WHO chart each of the lines (the average, the third percentile, the ninety-seventh percentile) is lower by several hundred grams than its Spanish counterpart. This means that an eight-month-old baby, who on the Spanish chart is 'below the norm', on the WHO chart is probably 'within the norm'. However, the difference is very slight and affects only a few children. In many more cases, the problem isn't with the chart, but with how the chart is interpreted. Those who claim that a baby is underweight if he weighs below the average, or is losing weight if he goes down a percentile, will carry on interpreting the new charts in the same way and alarming parents unnecessarily.

The 1990 UK reference charts were also very similar to the new WHO charts for the bigger babies, but percentile lines 3 to 50 are lower in the WHO charts (so a baby who was below the line in the British charts can be OK in the WHO ones). Also, to follow the WHO chart, a baby has to put weight on more quickly in the first two months, and then more slowly for the rest of the year.

As for the American CDC 2000 growth charts, they were lower than the WHO charts for the first four to six months. So a baby who is gaining enough weight for CDC may not be gaining enough by WHO standards.[*]

There is no point in weighing your baby every week

A baby's weight goes up after she feeds and goes down after she does a pee or a poo. Accidental variations in weight over such a short period can be enormous in relation to expected weight gains, and it is impossible to assess the result accurately. With the exception of special cases requiring strict observation (for example during the baby's first few days, before she regains her birth weight, or in the case of serious illness) weighing a baby more than once a month (or once every two months for babies of between six and twelve months) is not only pointless, but can give rise to serious errors.

No amount of weighing will make your baby grow bigger. He grows bigger because you breastfeed him.

---

[*] See Scientific Advisory Committee on Nutrition. The Royal College of Paediatrics and Child Health. Application of WHO Growth Standards in the UK. August 2007 http://www.sacn.gov.uk/pdfs/report_growth_standards_2007_08_10.pdf and Onis M, Garza C, Onyango AW, Borghi E. Comparison of the WHO Child Growth Standards and the CDC 2000 Growth Charts. *J. Nutr.* 137: 144–148, 2007. http://nutrition.highwire.org/content/137/1/144.full.pdf

Constitutional growth delay

When a baby doesn't gain weight because he isn't eating enough, his weight is low, but to begin with his size is normal. In the long run, malnutrition will also affect his size. His weight/size ratio is below average.

But when a baby neither gains weight nor grows, his weight/size ratio is normal and the problem is different, and he may need to undergo tests in order to rule out diseases such as growth hormone deficiency. Bear in mind, however, that there are two normal variations, which aren't diseases, but which can cause undue concern if they aren't taken into consideration.

The first is very obvious: familial short stature. The father is small, the mother is small, and when the baby grows up he will be small.

Constitutional growth delay (CGD) is less well known, and causes more concern. Yet it is the most frequent cause of smallness and delayed puberty. At around three to six months, the growth rate (weight and size) decreases. The baby is on the third percentile (or lower) in terms of weight and size, and his weight is proportionate to his size. The baby's bone age is delayed, but is in accordance with his size. From the age of two or three onwards, the child's growth speed will pick up again, and he will grow in the lower part of the curve, or below the third percentile, but in a parallel way. The puberty growth spurt is delayed, so that for a few years he will slip even further off the chart, but will also have more time to grow. Finally puberty arrives, and his adult size will be normal. This often runs in families. It is very reassuring to ask the grandmother; frequently one or both parents or other family member 'was always tiny', or 'was a puny girl' or 'the family doctor used to prescribe vitamins for him', and in the end they all grew to a normal size.

CGD is completely normal and requires no treatment. Unfortunately, a lot of babies who grow more slowly in the second trimester are 'treated' (needless to say, in vain) with supplementary bottle feeding, early introduction of solids, or forced weaning.

On the subject of bone maturation: I have seen many parents in distress after being told their baby has delayed bone maturation. Firstly, bone age doesn't coincide exactly with chronological age; one year more or less is perfectly normal, and only differences of two or three years are considered clinically significant. If you are told your baby has 'a nine-month delay', you can shrug it off. Secondly, it is advanced bone maturation, not delayed bone maturation that is bad. If a child is small and his bone age is normal, or still worse, his bone age is advanced, this means he will stop growing at the same age as other children, and will probably remain small. On the other hand, if his bone age is delayed by three years, it means he will go on growing for another three years, and will have time to catch up a bit.

→ Clark, P.A. 'Constitutional growth delay', 2003. emedicine. medscape.com/article/919677-overview

→ Rodríguez Rodríguez, I. 'Diagnóstico de la talla 4baja idiopática' www.comtf.es/pediatria/Congreso_AEP_2000/Ponencias-htm/ Ilde_Rguez.htm

Chapter 7
BREAST PROBLEMS

Inverted nipples

Years ago, we paediatricians considered inverted nipples a substantial impediment to breastfeeding. We tried to persuade obstetricians to examine pregnant women's nipples. We had to draw them out before the baby was born! In order to do this, two types of treatment were proposed: breast shells (see page 140) and the Hoffman technique.

Fortunately, obstetricians weren't convinced, and we were spared the embarrassing task of having to retract our advice. In the past few years, we have learned two important facts: treatments for inverted nipples don't work (and so early diagnosis is futile); and (the good news) mothers with inverted nipples have no problem breastfeeding.

In the late 1980s, an English midwife, a Ms Alexander, asked herself which of the two treatments (breast shells or Hoffman technique) would work better. She did what most people would do in this situation: she looked for research papers on the subject. She looked and looked but found nothing. Only one article about the Hoffman method had been published, written by Dr Hoffman himself, explaining how beneficial his exercises had been for two mothers. She found nothing on breast shells.

And so Ms Alexander decided to carry out a study herself. She divided a hundred pregnant women with inverted nipples randomly into four groups. One group used the breast shells during pregnancy, a second carried out the Hoffman technique exercises, a third group did both, and a fourth group did nothing at all.

The results couldn't have been more surprising: in all four groups, 60 per cent of previously inverted nipples were normal at the time of delivery (in fact, the percentage was slightly higher in the group that received no treatment, though not enough to be statistically significant). In other words, they 'corrected' themselves, no thanks to the treatment. At six weeks, the percentage of mothers still breastfeeding was lowest in the group that had used only breast shells; some found the contraption so uncomfortable that they decided to stop breastfeeding.

This is a clear example of the importance of rigorous scientific studies. A control group is necessary in order to be able to evaluate the results of the treatment as compared with the random results. For years, many mothers (60 per cent, to be precise) testified to the success of these treatments, and many doctors and midwives would say: 'I always recommend breast shells (or exercises), and in most cases they work very well'. It is equally essential for the study to measure a really important result (how successful breastfeeding was), and not simply an intermediary outcome (the shape of the nipple). Let us imagine that mothers who used the breast shells breastfed their babies for longer, despite the percentage of nipples that 'corrected' themselves being the same. This would suggest that the breast shells were useful, and should be recommended, only we wouldn't know why. Or, on the contrary, it could be that the breast shells were very useful for changing the shape of the nipple, but when it came to it, the mothers who used them breastfed for exactly the same length of time as the other mothers, in which case what are the benefits of having nipples that stick out?

The Alexander study went down like a lead balloon. It was very difficult to accept that these two treatments, which had been 'seen' to work for so many years, were in fact ineffective. And so another similar study was undertaken, only on a much larger scale, and involving more pregnant women from different hospitals. The results were very similar: at six weeks, the percentage of mothers still breastfeeding was exactly the same in all four groups. At least this time the breast shells didn't prove to be counterproductive, just ineffective.

Some maintain that certain brands of breast shell were used when carrying out these studies, and that there are other brands on the market that may be effective. To my knowledge, no studies have been done using these other brands of breast shell, and therefore no one has been able to prove that they are any more effective.

Suddenly, without a leg to stand on, we realised that inverted nipples weren't as problematic as we had supposed, and that women who had them were able to breastfeed after all. In a sense this was logical; it was one of those things that makes us exclaim: 'Of course! Why didn't I see that before!' The baby nurses from the breast, not the nipple. It is the areola the baby latches on to, it is the areola she has to squeeze with her tongue. While the baby is nursing, she is unable to tell the difference between an inverted nipple and a 'normal' nipple. A friend and midwife, Lourdes Martínez, once met a mother who breastfed for months despite having only one nipple. The other had been removed when she was little due to a skin infection.

The nipple itself isn't meant for nursing, only to show the baby where to feed, like the flag on a putting green that shows golfers where the hole is from a distance. If the breast were completely smooth, like a ball, the baby wouldn't know where the milk came out. She would try to feed from all sides. This happened to my wife one night: the baby got confused and gave her a huge love bite. In order to prevent confusion, nature has provided a complex system of detection, using four of the senses: smell, sight, touch, and taste. The baby smells the nipple (in one study they washed one breast with soap during delivery, and the newborn was placed between the two breasts; most latched on to the unwashed one); she sees the areola (which is like the target surrounding a bull's eye, and which becomes darker when lactation begins and the baby has to learn to feed); she touches the nipple with her cheeks and lips, and licks it to make sure it tastes of nipple. When all four senses correspond, the baby knows she has found the treasure! If the breast is completely smooth, and she can't use her sense of touch, the other three senses will still guide her.

For thousands of years, these three senses were probably enough to guide our ancestors, and nearly all babies were able to nurse properly even if their mothers had flat nipples. As I explained above (see page 63), things are slightly more complicated nowadays, due to the use of anaesthesia during delivery, babies being separated from their mothers in the first few minutes, and mothers not having the opportunity to learn how to breastfeed by watching other mothers. But if the midwife or nurse helps the mother to position her baby correctly, the baby will nurse however inverted her nipples are.

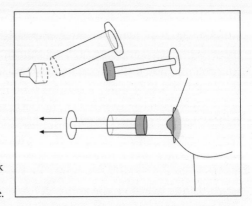

Figure 14: In exceptional cases it is possible to suck the inverted nipple out using an inverted syringe.

After a few days of the baby nursing, the mother's nipples usually begin to stick out. This is because the power of a baby, applied to them for more than two hours a day (divided up into several feeds) is equal to anything. Sometimes, this change can be permanent; but many mothers discover to their surprise that their nipples go back to being inverted after weaning, until their next baby draws them out again. After the experience of a first child, they need less help with the second.

So inverted nipples are only an impediment to breastfeeding when the mother has no assistance. But if nurses and midwives know how to help her, inverted nipples can almost be an advantage. This is because with a nipple that sticks out, the baby can nurse correctly or incorrectly, and nursing incorrectly will end up causing cracked nipples and other problems. Whereas when the nipple is inverted, the baby either nurses correctly or he doesn't nurse at all. Staff offer special help to mothers with inverted nipples, and so breastfeeding goes smoothly from the beginning.

Other ways of drawing out inverted nipples, using suction devices such as the Niplette®, have been invented. But generally speaking, I don't think any of them are particularly effective or necessary: you don't need them in order to breastfeed. In some exceptional cases it is possible to use a syringe that has been cut in half and inverted (see *Figure 14*).

→ Alexander, J.M., Grant, A.M., Campbell, M.J. 'Randomised controlled trial of breast shells and Hoffman's exercises for inverted and non-protractile nipples', *Br Med J* 1990;304:1030

Nipple pain

Breastfeeding shouldn't be painful. Many people think that pain is an unavoidable part of breastfeeding, and that mothers must grin and bear it. This isn't true. Breastfeeding shouldn't be painful. At most, it may cause slight discomfort for the first few days, due to lack of practice. But it shouldn't *hurt*. Pain is a sign that something is wrong. The most frequent cause (and in the first few days almost the only cause) is incorrect positioning, tongue-tie or a combination of both.

Cracked nipples

It is the incorrect positioning of the baby when nursing that causes cracked nipples. The baby's mouth is too closed, he is only latched on to the teat, and he is too far away from the breast. Instead of pressing with his tongue, he tries to suck and his cheeks become hollow. He spends a long time at the breast, and nurses frequently. The mother will often misinterpret this and think it means her baby is feeding well, for a long time and vigorously, when in fact he is doing it all wrong.

The nipple is especially sensitive to pain, in order to alert us to a problem. If it hurts when your baby is nursing, you can either remove your breast from his mouth (first opening his mouth gently with your finger to break the seal), and start again, or you can try to find the correct position while the baby is still nursing. You can usually do this by holding him closer to you, and shifting him slightly in the direction of his own feet, so that his neck is stretched back. On page 56, I explained in a wealth of detail how to achieve the correct position. It is far easier to prevent cracks than to cure them, so don't wait until you have an open wound, do something the moment you feel any pain. Besides, when a baby has been nursing incorrectly for months, it can be difficult to make him change.

It isn't always easy to achieve the perfect position. And, obviously, the baby will end up getting distressed if you keep taking him off the nipple and putting him back on every five minutes. Sometimes, after the third or fourth attempt it is best to stick with a position which may not be perfect, but is clearly an improvement on the first, and wait for the next feed before trying to find the ideal position.

Once the position has been corrected, the pain will immediately disappear. Or at least it will subside to the point where the mother won't notice it anymore. It is wonderful to see the expression of relief and surprise on the face of a mother who has just achieved a pain-free feed after days or weeks (or sometimes months) of torment. Of course, the crack is still there, at the base or tip of the nipple. But it no longer hurts, because in the correct position, the baby's gums are pressing much further out from the nipple.

From this point on, the crack will heal in a matter of days, the same as a slight scratch. The only reason it didn't heal before was because the baby was pressing on it every few hours when nursing. When correct positioning doesn't lead to a rapid recovery, the crack may not be the problem, or it could be infected (see below).

If the pain is intense, or takes time to ease, breast compression (see page 87) may prove useful for a few days, to shorten the feeds and ease the pressure on the nipple. Some mothers will express milk for a few hours or days, and feed it to their baby from a cup to avoid the baby sucking on their nipple. This may help in a few extreme cases, but generally speaking it isn't necessary, and may even be self-defeating, because on the one hand the baby won't be able to practice nursing correctly, and on the other hand breast pumps can be more painful than the baby suckling.

There are no ointments for treating or preventing normal (uninfected) cracks. If the baby is nursing incorrectly, ointments won't stop the pain or prevent cracks. If he is nursing correctly, there is no need to apply any ointments or moisturisers. By the same token, once a crack appears, it won't heal with or without ointment until the baby's position is corrected.

Nipple shields have long been recommended to avoid the pain of cracks. Whilst they might help in some special cases, I wouldn't recommend them for general use. The old models (made of rubber, or rubber and glass) made suction very difficult, and the baby wasn't able to get all the milk he needed. Recent models (made of fine silicone) also reduce milk consumption slightly. The baby will have difficulty learning to nurse properly if he can't feed from a naked breast (the nipple shield stops the breast and nipple from stretching and adapting to the baby's mouth). In some cases, the surface of the nipple shield rubs against the crack, increasing rather than diminishing the pain. And, if the nipple shield isn't dispensed with after a few days, breastfeeding usually becomes impossible: nursing with a nipple shield is tricky, and although I have known a couple of cases where women have nursed with nipple shields for months, it is much more common for breastfeeding to go badly, and for mothers to end up abandoning it after a few days. So, if the pain is unbearable enough for you to decide to try using a nipple shield, there are two important things to keep in mind:

1. Stop using the nipple shield if there is no immediate improvement. The only reason for using it is to protect the wound while the baby is nursing, and to avoid pain. If it hurts as much or more when using the nipple shield, there is no point in persisting. It won't work any better on day two than on day one.

2. If you notice some improvement, only use it for a few days. Stop using it as soon as the fissure gets better.

Cracked nipples usually appear during the first few days of breastfeeding. If the problem isn't solved, breastfeeding will cease, because very few mothers are able to put up with the pain for weeks and months on end. As the baby gets bigger, he usually latches on to the breast better, because he is more practised, he has a bigger mouth, and the mother usually manages to find a better nursing position. It is not unusual to come across cases of partial healing, in mothers who, after two or three months, explain that they had cracks, which healed, but which still hurt each time their baby feeds. In cases like this, correcting the baby's nursing position can be difficult; if he has been moving his tongue and jaw in a certain way for months, he may not want or be able to change. Because the most important thing is the way the baby moves his tongue, he may still nurse incorrectly even once his mouth is correctly on the breast.

Once a baby learns to nurse correctly, he will usually continue to do so until he is weaned. If, after a few weeks or months of problem-free breastfeeding, you suddenly start to feel pain in your nipples when your baby is nursing, could this be because you have been giving him bottles or dummies? Many babies are able to alternate between breast and bottle without any problem (when their mother goes back to work, for example), whereas others, no matter what age they are, get confused and start nursing incorrectly.

Tongue-tie

Some babies can't feed properly because they have a short lingual frenulum, or tongue-tie. When the baby is nursing, he normally places his tongue above his gums and upper lip. Sometimes you can even see the tip of the baby's tongue poking out while he is nursing. If the baby's frenulum is too short for his tongue to reach over his gum and upper lip, it is more difficult for him to draw out the milk (which is why it takes him so long to nurse), and moreover, his gum bites down directly on the nipple. I came across one mother who had discovered and diagnosed the problem herself. She had been putting up with the pain for a few weeks, and had noticed his frenulum was so short that his tongue was almost stuck to the floor of his mouth, and the tip made a heart shape. It so happened that her sister had given birth to a baby boy at almost the same time, and they tried switching babies for one feed: when she nursed her nephew her nipples didn't hurt at all, whereas her sister was in agony. Unfortunately, a lot of doctors don't believe a short frenulum causes any problems, and they prefer to leave it alone. At most they think that, in some rare cases, it may lead to speech problems, so before cutting it you have to wait until your child learns to talk to see whether he has a speech problem or not. The woman I knew had to see several ear, nose and throat specialists before one of them agreed to cut her son's frenulum.

Sometimes the tip of the baby's tongue does poke out, but only in a downward direction (the baby can't raise his tongue as if to touch the tip of his nose). Sometimes the back of the baby's tongue is too inflexible for him to press correctly on the breast. This type of tongue-tie is known as submucosal, or posterior, and isn't visible, but you can feel it with your fingers, or identify it through the effect it has, because the back of the tongue doesn't lift up.

When breastfeeding is painful, or the baby isn't gaining weight, despite being positioned correctly, it is essential to have someone experienced check your baby for tongue-tie.

Cutting the frenulum is a simple, quick procedure and no more painful than an injection. There seems to be an interaction between the tongue-tie and the position at the breast. Babies with a very mobile tongue can nurse quite well in a bad position; babies with a mild case of tongue-tie can nurse with little or no problem if the position is very good. Severe cases of tongue-tie will improve a little (but will still have problems) even with a very, very good position.

It's important not only to cut the frenulum, but also to improve positioning and to stimulate milk production with breast compression (see page 87) and/or pumping.

Babies feed with their lips folded outwards. In a few rare cases, the labial frenulum (upper or lower) can cause problems when nursing, because the lip remains stuck to the gum and won't fold outwards. This is sometimes known as lip-tie.

→ Ballard, J.L., Auer, C.E., Khoury, J.C. 'Ankyloglossia: assessment, incidence, and effect of frenuloplasty on the breastfeeding dyad', *Pediatrics* 2002;110:e63 pediatrics.aappublications.org/cgi/content/full/110/5/e63

Nipple Candidiasis

Candida is a microscopic fungus commonly found on people's skin (and in many other places). It is harmless, until it starts to grow and becomes invasive.

Candida infections (candidiasis) can occur after taking antibiotics for another illness. Besides killing off the bacteria that cause the other illness, antibiotics also kill many of the good bacteria that live in our digestive tract, on our skin and elsewhere. This leaves room for other microbes to flourish, among them candida.

In adult women, candida usually causes vaginitis (vaginal discharge, itching and soreness) and in men it can cause balanitis (inflammation of the penis gland). It can also cause skin lesions, especially in humid places (armpits, groin, beneath voluminous breasts).

Babies can get candidiasis in their mouths and on their bottoms, and less frequently in their skin folds. In the mouth it produces thrush, white patches on the tongue, gums, inside the lips and cheeks, and on the roof of the mouth. Traces of coagulated milk can be mistaken for thrush, but milk can be easily scraped away with a wooden stick or spoon, whereas thrush is firmly rooted in the mucosa.

The type of lesion it presents on the bottom is different from a simple nappy rash. It is a red, raised patch, redder towards the edges than in the centre, and is clearly delineated, unlike nappy rash, which is more diffuse. There are often 'satellite lesions', tiny red circles like paint spots, near the main lesion.

For years it was thought that candidiasis was a frequent cause of nipple pain. Recent research suggests that other bacteria cause most nipple pain attributed to candidiasis. Apparently nipple candidiasis is extremely rare. Before we discovered this fact, many such infections were treated with anti-fungal creams. Some cleared up over time (few infections last forever, even if untreated), some because the anti-candida creams also happened to eradicate other bacteria, and some because they were in fact candida infections. When the infection didn't go away, we said: 'what a nasty resilient bacteria candida is.'

Nipple infections

When pain and cracks persist despite correcting the baby's nursing position, this can be due to a bacterial infection in the nipple. Many species of bacteria can cause the infection, like *Staphylococcus epidermis*, which make up part of the human skin flora (the millions of harmless bacteria we carry around with us). Occasionally there is redness, soreness or discharge around the nipple area, but often there is nothing to see, because the bacteria are inside the lactiferous ducts. Local treatment with antibacterial creams often doesn't work, and an oral antibiotic is necessary.

Often (though not always) the pain from cracked nipples and from bacterial infections differs. Pain from cracks can be intense, but superficial – i.e. the breast hurts on the outside, not on the inside. The pain from a crack starts when the baby latches on and begins nursing ('the first bite'), then usually diminishes slightly throughout the feed, the mother giving a sigh of relief when the baby finally finishes nursing.

The pain caused by infection (normally caused by bacteria, sometimes candidiasis) is much worse. The first bite doesn't hurt. The pain starts while the baby is nursing, and continues to intensify. But there is no use gritting your teeth until it is over, because when the baby releases the breast, it hurts even more, and goes on hurting for quite a while. It is a sharp, throbbing pain, like a pin being stuck in your nipple (some mothers have said it feels like having liquid fire injected into their nipple).

This is a new field of study, and many changes will doubtless occur in the next few years. It would be ideal to be able to grow a skin culture in suspect cases, in order to discover which bacteria is the infection and how best to treat it. More and more professionals perform cultures, and in the future, when we have more information about the most common sources of infection, perhaps skin cultures can be reserved for cases that are more resistant to treatment. If you have scabs or pus, wash your nipple several times a day with soap and water.

A word on the naming of things: mastitis is traditionally defined by the presence of an inflammation (a mass, or lump) in the breast. I stick to this criterion, and therefore any infections where there is no mass I refer to as 'nipple infections'. I think this distinction is useful for the reader: on the one hand, problems where the main symptom is nipple pain, and on the other, problems where the main symptom is a mass. However, what I have referred to as nipple infection, other authors refer to as 'mastitis', claiming that in most cases of mastitis there is no lump or mass. Let it be clear that this is simply a difference in name, and that we are in fact referring to the same thing.

→ Delgado, S., Arroyo, R., Jiménez, E., Fernández, L., Rodríguez, J.M. 'Mastitis infecciosas durante la lactancia: un problema infravalorado (I)', *Acta Pediatr Esp* 2009;67:77. www.gastroinf. com/SecciNutri/Febrero_09.pdf

→ Jiménez, E., Delgado, S., Arroyo, R., Fernández, L., Rodríguez, J.M. 'Mastitis infecciosas durante la lactancia: un problema infravalorado (II)', *Acta Pediatr Esp* 2009;67:125. www.gastroinf. com/SecciNutri/Marzo_09.pdf

Raynaud's of the nipple

Raynaud's syndrome is a circulatory disorder in what doctors refer to as 'acral parts' – i.e. the parts of the body that are tapered (fingers, toes, earlobes… and nipples). It affects many more women than men, and apparently one in five women between the ages of twenty and fifty has suffered from it at one time or another. Sometimes the disease has already affected other parts of the mother's body, and sometimes the nipple is the first area to be affected.

Incorrect positioning can trigger Raynaud's, or a lingual frenulum that has damaged the nipple tissue. The problem can flare up at any moment, and unlike in the case of cracks or infections, the pain doesn't only come on during or after nursing, but also between feeds. The blood vessels in the nipple contract, and the supply of blood and oxygen to the nipple is cut off. The pain is very intense (remember that a lack of oxygen to the heart is what causes angina). The nipple turns completely white, and a few moments later turns blue. Sometimes there is a third phase where it turns red. Blisters, cracks and ulcers may appear, which take a very long time to heal (partly because of the original problem of incorrect positioning, but also because of the lack of blood supply).

Episodes can be triggered by cold, and when they happen while the baby is nursing, it is more likely to be because the breast is exposed to the air, than because of the baby's suckling. Some mothers describe a searing pain when they go out in the cold, or open the fridge door, or walk down the frozen food aisles at the supermarket. Smoking exacerbates the problem.

Treatment is based on correcting the baby's nursing position, avoiding the cold, and giving up smoking (and that includes everyone in the house). Direct heat should be applied in the form of a hot water bottle or an electric blanket – not burning hot, of course – as soon as the baby has finished nursing. If there is no improvement, your doctor will give you a prescription for something like nifedipine. Some mothers need to take nifedipine for several months.

→ Lawlor-Smith, L., Lawlor-Smith, C. 'Vasospasm of the nipple – a manifestation of Raynaud's phenomenon: case reports', *Br Med J* 1997;314:644-645 bmj.bmjjournals.com/cgi/content/full/314/7081/644

→ Anderson, J.E., Held, N., Wright, K. 'Raynaud's phenomenon of the nipple: a treatable cause of painful breastfeeding', *Pediatrics* 2004;113:e360-4 pediatrics.aappublications.org/cgi/content/full/113/4/e360

Nipple Eczema

As well as problems relating to lactation, the breast can suffer from the same skin disorders as any other part of the body.

In eczema the skin becomes raised, inflamed and scaly (dandruff is a form of eczema). There may be vesicles (small deep blisters) and lesions caused by scratching.

There is another type of eczema known as atopic eczema, which is sometimes caused by an allergy. A mother who develops nipple eczema may already have had eczema on other parts of her body.

First make sure the eczema isn't an allergic reaction to something that has come into contact with your skin. Stop using any creams or ointments, including moisturisers and stretch-mark creams – unless they are being used to treat a serious problem, such as an infection, in which case consult whoever prescribed it. Have you recently changed your soap, deodorant, or washing powder? Have you left a wet breast pad in your bra for too long?

If after taking these simple steps there is no improvement, your doctor will probably prescribe a corticosteroid cream. Rub the cream in to your nipple after the feed. There is no need to wash it off before the next feed.

If after a few days there is no improvement, return to your doctor. The vast majority of nipple eczemas are simple eczemas. However, there is a rare type of nipple cancer that resembles eczema, called Paget's disease of the breast. It makes up about 1 to 2 per cent of all breast cancers, and usually occurs in women around the age of fifty, but it can occur earlier and coincide with lactation. In 50 per cent of cases, there is no tumour in the breast, only lesions on the nipple. Persistent nipple eczema should be given serious attention.

Milk blisters

These are also known as nipple blisters or blebs. These are smooth and shiny, and the size of a pinhead. They hurt when the baby nurses, and can swell up. Sometimes they are associated with a blocked duct. Treatment consists of bursting with a sterile needle, preferably after a feed when the blister is larger. Milk blisters tend to recur. It is advisable, after bursting them, to massage the area. Sometimes a thick white substance, like coagulated milk, will come out.

Breast shells and nipple shields

The nipple shield is worn during the feed, and the breast shell is worn between feeds. Breast shells have been recommended during pregnancy in theory as a way of correcting inverted nipples, but they don't work (see page 127).

Modern nipple shields are made from fine silicone, and are apparently useful in some cases, for example to help small premature newborns begin nursing. They can also help mothers suffering from cracked nipples (see page 132).

Another possible use for nipple shields is to correct inverted nipples: once again there is no evidence to suggest that they work, and they are usually unnecessary and sometimes counterproductive. They should only be used as a last resort.

In some hospitals they overuse nipple shields, recommending them to a third of mothers (or more). Some hospital nurses consider them very useful in helping mothers to cope for the first few days. Many community nurses loathe them, precisely because they see the consequences a few days later: inefficient suction, nipple confusion, low weight gain, and an early end to breastfeeding. In some parts of Spain, wax nipple shields are all the rage and are used between feeds to treat cracks. I don't know of any studies as to their effectiveness, and in other parts of the country mothers seem to manage perfectly well without them.

Breast inflammation

Almost all doctors-to-be learn four Latin words when they begin their studies: *calor*, *rubor*, *dolor*, and *tumor* – the definition of inflammation given by Celsus, who was a contemporary of Christ. If your ankle is swollen, red, hot, and painful, you have an inflamed ankle.

There are several different types of breast inflammation. The most frequent are engorgement (which usually affects both breasts in their entirety), blocked ducts and mastitis (these two usually affect only part of one breast).

Engorgement

Sometimes breasts get too full and become enormous, swollen and painful. This usually occurs in the first week, and is caused by a combination of factors. Approximately three days after labour, the mother's milk comes in. This isn't a sudden increase in milk production, which is gradual. The thing that happens suddenly, allowing the mother to say: 'My milk came in last night' is a change in the breast, which becomes inflamed. When the breast wakes up from its long sleep, it shows proper signs of inflammation: the secreting cells multiply and swell up, the blood vessels expand and dilate in order to transport more water, nutrients and oxygen to them, the leucocytes leave the blood and regroup among the secretor cells in order to produce the immunoglobulin in the milk, the water filters through the blood capillaries and into the breast tissue.

When the baby nurses properly, the breast doesn't swell up much, sometimes hardly at all. Some mothers are convinced their milk hasn't come in, even when their baby is already two or three weeks old and is clearly gaining weight. But when the baby doesn't feed enough (because they don't let him, or because he is incorrectly positioned), the milk accumulates, and, in addition to the usual inflammation, produces painful swelling or engorgement. In extreme cases this can result in a vicious circle: the pressure of the accumulated milk bursts some of the acini and the milk ducts, and the milk spills into the interstitial tissue. Because the milk isn't supposed to be there, it is treated as a foreign body, which causes further inflammation. It is like being bitten by an insect, or having a reaction to an injection. It may produce common symptoms of inflammation such as general malaise, and sometimes fever (see page 51).

The treatment for engorgement is to empty the breast. Increase the baby's feeds, making sure she is correctly positioned, and try to express the remaining milk, either by hand or with a pump.

Sometimes, the breast is so swollen the baby has trouble latching on, and you have to express some of your milk to soften the breast so it will go into the baby's mouth.

'If I empty my breast won't I just produce more milk?' Well, yes. But if your breasts hurt and you don't empty them, they will hurt even more. You aren't strictly emptying your breasts (which is impossible), only extracting enough milk to stop them from hurting. And if you produce more milk, you extract it again.

Bear in mind that engorgement has two components: milk retention and inflammation. Milk can be extracted from the breast, but the inflammation can't. If you try to extract milk from an inflamed breast when there is no more milk to extract, you will end up hurting yourself (and exacerbating the inflammation). If your breasts are very full, try expressing your milk, but if this fails, leave it until later.

The inflammation around the areola can sometimes constrict the milk ducts, preventing the milk from being ejected. The area becomes swollen due to liquid retention (oedema), and when you press it, your finger leaves an indentation. It is difficult to express the milk either by hand or using a pump, or for the baby to nurse, because the ducts are almost completely closed up. When this happens, using a breast pump can be counterproductive, because the pressure of the vacuum concentrates the oedema in the area of the nipple, which becomes even more swollen. What you need to do is clear the area from the outside in, not from the inside out. Press the area firmly inwards, with your thumb and forefinger, or with the tips of all five fingers, until it begins to soften (this may take between twenty and thirty minutes); afterwards, you can either let the baby nurse or try expressing your milk by hand. This is known as 'reverse pressure softening'.

'What do I do with the milk I express?' This depends on whether your baby has nursed enough or not. When the problem is too much milk, your baby may not need to nurse more. In this case she will be gaining weight, peeing and pooing, and more or less contented. Conversely, when the problem is due to inflammation, or when the engorgement is due to your baby nursing incorrectly, you must feed her the expressed milk with a dropper or from a small cup (not from a bottle). When in doubt (it may be too early to tell whether the baby is gaining weight or not, or perhaps as a first-time mother you aren't sure whether your newborn is 'normal' or 'weak') try feeding her the milk. If she takes it, fine, if not it is probably because she doesn't need it.

A word of warning about the word 'probably': when a baby of several weeks or months who is gaining weight and clearly healthy and happy, refuses milk, we can be sure it is because she has had enough. But in the case of newborns, we can't be so sure: they are already fairly docile, and may be weak from weight loss or drowsy from an anaesthetic administered during labour. It could be that your baby is too weak to nurse, rather than not hungry, and you have to keep trying. If you are in any doubt, if your baby seems weak or 'not quite right', or she nurses very little and sleeps a lot, consult someone who has more experience of babies (such as your mother, or another mother), and don't hesitate to ask to see your midwife, doctor or nurse as often as you need. That is what they are there for.

So, this is the basic treatment: getting your baby to nurse, expressing the remaining milk, and waiting. If your breasts are very painful, you can take an analgesic or anti-inflammatory, such as ibuprofen (yes, it is perfectly compatible with breastfeeding; the amount of ibuprofen a baby ingests in one day while nursing is 500 times lower than what you would give the same baby if she were running a temperature).

Other treatments may ease the symptoms. For example, applying heat or cold. Both have their advocates: a fairly common recommendation for reducing the pain is to apply dry cold to the inflamed area between feeds (a bag of frozen vegetables, or ice cubes wrapped in a towel). Alternatively, applying wet heat before nursing or expressing milk helps the flow of milk (a flannel soaked in hot water, dipping the breast in a basin, taking a hot shower or bath). However, because these treatments only deal with the symptoms, they are only worth doing if they bring relief. If applying cold doesn't relieve the symptoms, then don't apply cold. If on the other hand applying heat seems to bring you some relief, then apply heat as often as you want.

In some countries, cabbage leaves in the bra are highly recommended. Take them cold from the fridge, wash them and make a hole in the middle for the nipple, and crumple them up to break the veins (the ones in the leaves, not in the breast!). If you find this method helps, by all means use it, although I don't know of any studies showing that cabbage leaves work better than simple ice.

An important warning: two treatments you mustn't try are stopping drinking water, and bandaging your breasts. Tightly bandaging the breasts doesn't reduce the engorgement, it only increases the pain. Stopping drinking water is pointless (you would have to be seriously dehydrated for the engorgement to go down), disagreeable (when you are thirsty, water deprivation is a form of torture) and dangerous (if you substantially reduce your liquid intake you risk becoming dehydrated).

Blocked ducts

This looks straightforward, doesn't it? As the title suggests, one of the milk ducts in the breast becomes blocked. And yet it isn't as simple as that (why are things never as simple as they look?). In fact, our knowledge is so limited... The fact is that sometimes a red, hot, painful lump forms in one sector of the breast (I use the word 'sector' in the geometrical sense, to denote the section of a circle between two radii, like a cheese triangle). This type of inflammation doesn't affect the whole gland, only one (or several) of its lobules.

The usual explanation for this is that the duct is blocked, causing milk to build up. To start with, this only causes a slight swelling, but when there is a big build-up of milk, the acini can burst and the milk spills out and causes an inflammation. Sometimes, after lengthy massaging and squeezing of the affected area, a thin white tube, like a plug, will emerge from the nipple. However, there is an alternative explanation: there is a build-up of milk, the water from the milk is reabsorbed and the solids remain, drying up to produce the plug. But which comes first, the plug or the build-up of milk? Perhaps it is a combination of both, or a vicious circle, or perhaps in some cases it begins with the plug, and in others it begins with the build-up of milk.

A few decades ago, Dr Yamanouchi, from Okayama in Japan, analysed some of these plugs and discovered they were largely made up of saturated fats. Unsaturated fats, such as vegetable oils, are liquid at room temperature; saturated fats, such as butter, are solid. Most of the fats in breastmilk are unsaturated. Unsaturated fats are converted into saturated fats using hydrogen. This is how they turn vegetable oils into margarines (and explains why on the label it says: 'made with partially hydrogenated vegetable oils'). Dr Yamanouchi thought that the milk ducts became plugged when the mother ate too much animal fat, meat and butter, and he recommended returning to a traditional Japanese diet of vegetables and fish (with unsaturated fat). However, apart from his analysis of the plugs, he found no evidence that eating butter leads to blocked ducts or that eating fish can prevent blocked ducts. The opposite theory is equally plausible: fat in the milk is normal (predominantly unsaturated), but as the milk builds up and becomes more concentrated, it is somehow converted into saturated fat, which solidifies, producing the plug.

If the initial problem is a build-up of milk, we don't know what causes it. In some cases the culprit may be a tight-fitting bra: never wear a bra that isn't comfortable or leaves marks. Babies nurse using their tongues, and the part of the breast that comes into contact with the tongue empties more easily. Blocked ducts usually occur in the part of the breast that is furthest from the tongue, towards the armpit (furthermore, breasts aren't symmetrical, and there is a bigger concentration of glandular tissue towards the armpit than in other areas of the breast).

The treatment is more or less the same as with engorgement: massage the breast, try to empty it by frequent nursing, apply a cold compress between feeds if it eases the pain, and apply heat before breastfeeding to get the milk flowing. Try to find a nursing position where the baby's tongue is pressing on the area of the breast with the blocked duct. This can take a lot of ingenuity, and a measure of contortionism. You can nurse your baby at any angle if he is on his back on a big bed and you dangle over him on all fours.

Besides continuing to breastfeed, it is a good idea to express more milk, either by hand or with a pump. Some mothers find the pump more painful than the baby nursing; if this is the case, you can express the milk from the healthy breast and discard it, and let your baby nurse exclusively from the painful breast.

One mother told me a trick her grandmother taught her: tearing the baby abruptly off the breast while he is nursing – i.e. without breaking the seal. Her breast instantly unblocked.

Mastitis

Mastitis is an infection of the mammary gland (although some make a distinction between 'infectious' and 'non-infectious mastitis', which for the purposes of this book I have referred to as 'blocked ducts').

A blocked duct left untreated can become infected and turn into mastitis, and no doubt some cases of mastitis are due to this.

Mastitis usually produces fever and a feeling of general malaise, what doctors call 'flu-like syndrome' (tiredness, feeling unwell, muscle ache). There is an old maxim: 'Flu in the nursing mother is mastitis unless proven otherwise'. And it is true that the mother can experience such pain in her legs and back, and feel so unwell, that no one notices the inflamed mass in her breast. However, although this is rare, the engorgement resulting from a blocked duct can also produce fever and flu-like symptoms due to a simple inflammation, without any infection being present.

Therefore, it isn't strictly possible to tell the difference between a simple blockage and mastitis only by looking at the symptoms. Doctors should do a milk culture, but this isn't usual practice in Spain, and diagnosis is based on a physical exam.

It has been shown that half of all cases of mastitis (genuine mastitis, which has been diagnosed by culturing the milk) get better without any need for antibiotics, simply by following the above-mentioned treatment for blocked ducts and engorgement: frequent feeding, and expressing backed-up milk. For this reason, unless the mother's condition is acute, many doctors prefer not to prescribe an antibiotic straight away, and they recommend emptying the breast, and waiting for twenty-four hours. If the mother's temperature goes down to normal, it means she is better. If she still has a temperature, they prescribe antibiotics (although half of cases clear up on their own, the other half don't). Some doctors, depending on the circumstances, or habit, may prescribe antibiotics from the start.

The antibiotic prescribed has to be effective against staphylococcus (the most common germ, which is resistant to both penicillin and amoxicillin). The fever and flu-like symptoms will normally disappear two or three days after starting the antibiotic, but it is essential to finish the course as prescribed, even if you start to feel better. It is easy to have a relapse if the treatment is interrupted. If, on the other hand, after three days of taking the antibiotic you still have a temperature, go back to the doctor. You may have a resistant strain of bacteria, and need to be prescribed a different antibiotic. This time your milk should be cultured to make certain.

You can still nurse from both breasts when you have mastitis. There is no danger of infecting your baby. And the antibiotics you are taking won't harm him either. Anyone who tells you that you have to stop breastfeeding completely, or for a few days, or that you should only nurse from the healthy breast, is mistaken. In addition, if the breast isn't emptied, the mastitis can get worse and turn into an abscess. Not only *can* you carry on breastfeeding, this is the only case where *it is essential* that you go on breastfeeding. And if you were already planning to wean your baby, don't. Wait until the mastitis has completely cleared up.

Conversely, the baby may reject the sick breast. Mastitis causes an increase in the milk's sodium content. This won't harm your baby, but your milk will taste salty and some babies don't like this. If so, continue to offer him both breasts, without forcing him, and don't worry if he only accepts the healthy one: milk production in this breast will quickly increase, and your baby won't go hungry. But you will still need to empty the sick breast several times a day. Firstly, to prevent an abscess from forming, secondly, so that the breast continues producing milk, and thirdly, so that the taste of the milk goes back to normal. The sodium content also goes up when a breast doesn't produce much milk. Some mothers don't take the precaution of expressing their milk, and get caught in a vicious circle: their baby refuses the sick breast because of the mastitis, and when it is cured they continue to refuse it, because the small amount of milk that comes out of it tastes funny. These mothers have to go on nursing from the other breast. This won't harm mother or baby, of course, but it can look a bit odd (see page 118).

→ Departmento de Salud y Desarrollo del Niño y del Adolescente, 'Mastitis. Causas y manejo', Ginebra: Organización Mundial de la Salud, 2000. Doc. WHO/FCH/ CAH/00.13

Breast abscesses

When mastitis isn't properly treated (by frequent feeding and expressing milk), pus can accumulate in the breast, forming an abscess. This is usually drained with a needle and syringe, although sometimes a small incision is made, and a draining tube inserted. Despite all this, the baby can carry on nursing from both breasts, provided the drainage incision is far enough away from the mother's nipple. In order to prevent the baby's face coming into contact with any pus, cover the wound with a piece of gauze.

If the drainage incision is too close to the nipple, the baby will have to nurse from the other breast for a few days, and in the meantime you will have to express milk from the sick breast.

A breast too many?

Many people have an extra breast. Usually this takes the form of an atrophied nipple, located somewhere between the armpit and the groin, which the lucky owner believes is a mole or a wart.

Underneath this supernumerary nipple, there is sometimes actual breast tissue, which swells up and secretes milk after delivery. If the breast is properly formed, the milk can come out. There are documented cases of mothers who nurse from all three breasts (or rather from two and a quarter, as the third tends to be very small). If you don't want to walk around with an extra breast, it is best not to try to squeeze out the milk, or let your baby nurse from it. In other cases, the third breast is atrophied, so the milk can't come out. For the first few days it will feel a little sore. Try applying a cold pack (if this helps), don't express milk, and wait patiently. Milk secretion will soon stop, and the swelling will go down.

Some women may have excess breast tissue (usually in the armpit), which isn't connected to the nipple and so can't be emptied. Similarly, use a cold pack to ease the pain, and wait a few days for it to stop secreting, while continuing to breastfeed normally.

Chapter 8

DEFICIENT MILK SECRETION (HYPOGALACTIA)

Do all women have milk? Of course not! Just as there are women who don't produce insulin, or who can't walk, there are women who don't have milk. The mammary gland is one more organ, which, like the heart or kidneys, can go wrong or stop functioning altogether.

What can't be true is that there are as many women who don't have milk as some suppose. Few mothers stop breastfeeding voluntarily. Most do so because their milk has 'dried up', because their baby 'is still hungry', or because their milk 'isn't good enough'. It isn't possible that half or three-quarters of women don't have milk, or that their breasts don't work. If this were true, we would be facing the biggest epidemic the world has ever known.

On the face of it, hypogalactia (insufficient secretion of milk) must be as rare as any other illness, for example diabetes or high blood pressure. Actually, if we look a bit closer, we find it must be even more rare. For one thing, natural selection doesn't work against high blood pressure. A woman with high blood pressure can give birth to as many healthy children as a woman with normal blood pressure. On the other hand, natural selection is implacable in the case of hypogalactia: if the mother has no milk, her offspring will die, unless they are adopted and nursed by another female (which is almost unknown in the wild). It is only in the last hundred years that babies have begun to survive without a mother's milk.

Anyone can have diabetes: a little girl, an old woman, or a woman with serious birth defects. But none of these women can suffer from hypogalactia. In order to find out that you have no milk, you must first give birth to a child. You must be a fertile woman (in theory between the ages of twelve and fifty-five, but almost always between the ages of eighteen and forty, the best years), who is sufficiently healthy in body and mind to become pregnant and to give birth, i.e. a woman in the best of health. What bad luck if the one thing that doesn't work is this woman's breasts. Of course this can happen, but it is extremely rare. So rare, in fact, that it is worth ruling out all other possibilities first.

The problem in our society is that we have lost faith in lactation. We have come to believe that the 'norm' is not to have milk, and if some women do, it is only by the most extraordinary coincidence. When you ask a pregnant woman how long she is going to breastfeed, she will rarely give a specific answer: 'Three months' or 'A year and a half'. She is much more likely to say: 'As long as I can', or 'As long as I have milk'. She doesn't believe she has any say in the matter; that she can make a choice and stick to it. She sees herself simply as a plaything of destiny. When my wife was breastfeeding, her friends didn't say to her: 'How do you manage it? Tell me what to do, I want to breastfeed my daughter, too'. On the contrary, they said: 'How lucky you are to have milk! I wish I'd had milk, I would have liked to breastfeed my daughter.'

The anxiety is so great that, nine times out of ten, the mother believes she has no milk. If her breasts are empty it is because 'she has no milk', and if they are full it is because 'the baby won't nurse', because, understandably, her milk 'must be bad'. If her baby constantly wants to nurse, it is because he 'isn't getting enough milk', and if he sleeps a lot it is because, 'well, my milk has dried up'. If he doesn't gain enough weight it is because he 'needs a bottle', and if he does then 'such a big baby won't be satisfied with just the breast'. Small breasts are 'no good', but neither are large ones. If a mother was bottle fed she will say, 'The women in my family don't have milk'; and if her grandmother or great-grandmother breastfed seven children she will say: 'I wish I had as much milk as my grandmother, who after nursing seven children, took in an orphan during the war and nursed him too, but, of course, women today don't have milk'. In short, under no circumstance will a mother say: 'I have plenty of milk!'

In the vast majority of cases, when the mother thinks she has no milk, there in fact is no problem. Statistically, she has more chance of winning the rollover Christmas lottery than of suffering from hypogalactia. Sagging breasts, a baby who wakes up in the night, who is said not to have gained enough weight when in fact he has, who 'can't go three hours without nursing', aren't signs of decreased milk secretion. In order for anyone to think there may be a genuine deficiency, it is necessary to fulfil the following three criteria:

1. The baby really (truly!) isn't gaining enough weight.
2. After days of trying to increase her milk supply, using the proper techniques several times a day, the mother is unable to make more milk.
3. The baby is given supplements and gains more weight than before.

If the baby is gaining weight normally, it means he is getting enough milk, and that is that. However, if the mother does have milk, and the baby refuses to nurse and isn't gaining weight, then the baby might be sick, but the mother doesn't have hypogalactia.

A few causes of genuine hypogalactia

Hypothyroidism

A woman with untreated hypothyroidism will normally be unable to get pregnant. However, some mothers with undiagnosed mild hypothyroidism are able to give birth, though they may have trouble nursing. The thyroid hormone is essential for milk secretion. If she receives hormone substitution therapy she will be able to breastfeed.

Some cases of hypogalactia have also been associated with hyperthyroidism, although the causal mechanism is unknown. Both hypo and hyperthyroidism are fairly common during pregnancy and after childbirth, so this possibility should be taken into consideration when a genuine case of hypogalactia is suspected. Thyroid problems are due to the chronic iodine deficiency many children suffered in infancy. The thyroid glands were obliged to hypertrophy in order to utilise the small amounts of iodine available, and the added stress of pregnancy produces an imbalance. This is why mothers are advised to take iodine supplements (see page 170), so that their children won't suffer from the same problem.

→ Shomon, M. 'Breastfeeding and thyroid disease, questions and answers', www.thyroid-info.com/articles/breastfeeding.htm

Placental retention

The oestrogens and gestagens produced by the placenta inhibit milk secretion, so that a partial retention may present hypogalactia as an initial symptom. Interestingly, the opposite effect has also been observed: galactorrhea (excess of milk) due to placental retention.

→ Neifert, M.R., McDonough, S.L., Neville, M.C. 'Failure of lactogenesis associated with placental retention', *Am J Obstet Gynecol* 1981;140:477-8

→ Byrne, E. 'Breastmilk oversupply despite retained placental fragment', *J Hum Lact* 1992;8:152-3

Agenesis of mammary tissue

The breasts haven't developed normally (they probably haven't grown during pregnancy), prolactin levels are normal, but milk production is very low, despite every effort to increase it. This is a very rare problem. The first three cases were identified in America in 1985, and all three mothers were able to breastfeed (with supplements) for more than a year, because even a little milk is better than none.

→ Neifert, M.R., Seacat, J.M., Jobe, W.E. 'Lactation failure due to inadequate glandular development of the breast', *Pediatrics* 1985;76:823-8

Surgery

If you have had a silicone implant, you can breastfeed without any problem (unless you had a real agenesis of the breasts before the surgery). The operation doesn't damage the mammary gland, and silicone isn't harmful for babies (some dummies are made of silicone!)

If you have had a breast reduction then it depends on the type of operation. One technique involves removing the nipple completely from the breast, cutting away the necessary tissue, and replacing the nipple in the centre, to achieve the 'perfect' look. After this type of operation, breastfeeding is almost impossible, although occasionally (due to nature's stubbornness!) a few ducts manage to reconnect, and some milk may come out. Occasionally, women will notice that with their first baby almost no milk comes out, but with their second, milk production increases; it is thought that the area of the breast where the ducts don't reconnect atrophies, while the small area which is able to secrete milk grows in size.

There is another breast reduction technique which keeps the nipple attached to the breast, its milk ducts, and nerves at all times, and after which breastfeeding is possible. A few of the milk ducts may be severed by accident, in which case for the first few days a painful lump will appear, because the milk won't be able to come out of one of the lobules. Apply a cold pack, be patient and after a few days the lobule will stop secreting milk and the problem will go away.

If you have had surgery for breast cancer, or undergone radiotherapy, you can nurse from the healthy breast. And even sometimes from the unhealthy one, where breast-conserving surgery has been performed.

→ Hughes, V., Owen, J. 'Is breastfeeding possible after breast surgery?' *Am J Matern Child Nurs* 1993;18:213-7

→ Marshall, D.R., Callan, P.P., Nicholson, W. 'Breastfeeding after reduction mammaplasty', *Br J Plast Surg* 1994;47:167-9

→ Berlin, C.M. 'Silicone breast implants and breastfeeding', *Pediatrics* 1994;94:547-9 Jordan, M.E., Blum, R.W. 'Should breastfeeding by women with silicone implants be recommended?' *Arch Pediatr Adolesc Med* 1996;150:880-1

→ Higgins, S.; Haffty, B.G. 'Pregnancy and lactation after breast-conserving therapy for early stage breast cancer', *Cancer* 1994;73:2175-80

Sheehan's syndrome

Sheehan's syndrome is a necrosis of the pituitary gland due to a lack of blood supply during delivery because of severe haemorrhage. In the absence of prolactin and oxytocin, there is no milk production. Later on other problems occur, because the pituitary gland is responsible for secreting several different hormones. This is a very serious illness.

Women rarely present with the complete syndrome, but post-partum haemorrhage has also associated been with an occasional reduction in milk secretion (the baby loses weight and is dehydrated), which can be transitory, and is unaffected by other hormones in the pituitary gland. Perhaps the loss of blood explains the link between maternal anaemia (haemoglobin below 10mg/dl) and early termination of breastfeeding (attributed to lack of milk, or to the fact that the baby feeds too frequently and gains little weight).

However, there has been a published case study of a woman whose pituitary gland was removed because of a tumour, and who breastfed for three months. There is much we still don't know about the physiology of breastfeeding.

→ Sert, M., Tetiker, T., Kirim, S., Kocak, M. 'Clinical report of 28 patients with Sheehan's syndrome', *Endocr J* 2003;50:297-301

→ Willis, C.E., Livingstone, V. 'Infant insufficient milk syndrome associated with maternal postpartum hemorrhage', *J Hum Lact* 1995;11:123-6

Congenital prolactin deficiency

This is an extremely rare hereditary condition, and only half a dozen known cases have ever been recorded. Only half a dozen! I said before that a woman has more chance of winning the rollover lottery than suffering from hypogalactia. Well, she has more chance of marrying a prince than of suffering from congenital prolactin deficiency. There are more than half a dozen princes in the world.

The reason it is so rare is because, up until very recently, if a mother had no milk her children would die. The existing cases are a recent mutation; we know it is hereditary because we have seen it passed from a mother to her daughter. But the grandmother almost certainly didn't suffer from it.

Malnourishment

In our society, lack of food or water in the mother *doesn't* cause hypogalactia. Only severe malnutrition can affect the quantity or quality of a mother's milk. Even a restricted diet of 1,765 calories a day doesn't affect the production or composition of milk or the baby's weight gain (see page 177).

The baby of an American mother who purposefully restricted her diet to twenty calories per kilogram a day was seen to suffer from weight stagnation. But twenty calories per kilogram is extremely little, and the mother must have been skin and bone.

So get the idea out of your head that by eating more and better food and drinking a lot of liquid you will secrete more milk.

Galactogogues

Many traditional as well as modern drugs that claim to increase milk secretion have been promoted. No studies exist proving the effectiveness of specific herbs (alfalfa, cumin, etc.) or foods, but it wouldn't surprise me if some herbs actually worked.

There are studies showing the effectiveness of beer (not the alcohol, but some other ingredient), domperidone, metoclopramide and sulpiride; all these substances stimulate the production of prolactin, which is exactly what the baby does when he nurses. Why use drugs that may have side-effects when you can achieve the same result with frequent feeding and correct positioning? It is no coincidence that many of these studies were carried out on the mothers of premature babies, whose milk production usually decreases after weeks of using a breast pump, which stimulates prolactin less efficiently than a baby. Nowadays, the kangaroo method usually solves the problem, though some cases may still require drugs.

And yet, many drugs, herbal or popular remedies (specific foods that are said to 'stimulate your milk') are used completely unnecessarily. Some doctors automatically prescribe drugs if the mother makes the slightest complaint: 'I don't think I have any milk'. 'Here, take these pills', without bothering to discover whether their patient really has hypogalactia or not, and if so, which type. In cases of genuine hypogalactia, galactogogues are probably ineffective: hypothyroidism is treated with the thyroid hormone; in cases of placental retention the placenta has to be removed; they would be useless in treating mammary agenesis, and they have been tried without success in women with prolactin deficiency (the pituitary gland doesn't function, and therefore doesn't respond to stimulants).

Perhaps an illness will one day be discovered which responds to these drugs. An illness where the pituitary gland produces few hormones, and doesn't respond to the normal stimuli of frequent feeds, and these drugs will enable the breast to work perfectly and respond to prolactin. But such an illness, if it exists, hasn't yet been seen. How about trying these drugs as a last resort, just in case they work? Well, all right, but this would have to remain the exception.

If these drugs are frequently useless in treating cases of genuine hypogalactia, then what are they good for? For treating 'imaginary' hypogalactia; for reassuring mothers who think they don't have milk when they do. People place a lot of faith in pills and herbal remedies.

'I have much more milk after taking "x."' I find this difficult to believe. In order to believe it, I would need to see a chart showing that the baby's weight stagnated for several weeks, despite his nursing all the time, and that as soon as the mother took 'x' the baby happily started gaining weight. I have never seen such a thing (I assume it has happened at some point, but not to my knowledge). Generally speaking, there is no before and after with weight charts. Everything stays much the same.

Why then, does the mother think she has much more milk? I suggest that it is a question of perception.

Of the total amount of milk secreted in one day, the baby takes a part, another part is probably reabsorbed, and a tiny amount leaks out. In addition, a certain amount of the milk stays in the breast, as a reserve. And there is no more.

When the mother takes a drug or herbal medicine to increase her milk, what is it that increases? The amount the baby takes? No. If his weight gain hasn't suddenly increased it means he is drinking the same amount as before. Or perhaps the amount of milk produced and reabsorbed increases, which is completely pointless. Maybe the reserve of milk in the breast increases, so that instead of, say, 50ml, there is now 75ml, and the mother's breasts feel fuller? But it can't go on increasing, 75ml one day, 100ml the next, 125ml the next, and so on, otherwise her breasts would end up exploding. No. It increases to 75ml and remains there, and as the baby hasn't used it, the increase is superfluous. Or perhaps more milk leaks from the breast, and as a few millilitres is enough to soak a bra, the psychological effect is heightened. And this is all it is: mere façade. There appears to be more milk, but (fortunately) there isn't.

Herbs aren't always harmless. In Italy, there have been two reported cases of infant intoxication (low muscle tone, vomiting, and lethargy, requiring hospitalization) as a result of mothers drinking more than two litres a day of a herbal concoction supposed to increase milk supply (liquorice, fennel, aniseed and *Galega officinalis*). 'Goodness, two litres!' you might think. This sort of thing happens because, on the one hand women are told to 'take herbal medicine', and on the other they are urged to 'drink lots of water'. And they press on regardless, because herbs are 'natural' and therefore can't be harmful. Well, they can. However 'natural' they may be, some herbal medicines are extremely potent, and should only be used in the correct dosage to treat specific illnesses. People who are healthy don't need to take drugs, from a chemist or anywhere else.

→ Rosti, L., Nardini, A., Bettinelli, M.E, Rosti, D. 'Toxic effects of a herbal tea mixture in two newborns', *Acta Pædiatr* 1994;83:683

Chapter 9
THE MOTHER'S DIET

There are several things that worry mothers: what and how much they should eat, which foods they should avoid, and which are especially beneficial because they produce lots of good-quality milk, how much should they drink and so on.

Fortunately, the simple answer to all of those questions is: whatever they want. I will explain why in more detail.

How many calories

Obviously, breastmilk has to come from somewhere. Whatever the mother eats is converted into milk. Many years ago now, someone calculated how many extra calories a woman needs in order to produce all this breastmilk. It is easy to work out: 'x' millilitres of milk contain 'x' number of calories. By adding a percentage for the metabolism (in other words, how much energy is used to produce the milk), the figure they came up with, if I remember correctly, was 700 calories a day more than a woman normally eats. (Warning: in many books on nutrition what they call a calorie is, scientifically speaking, a kilocalorie i.e. one thousand calories.) This was the theoretical figure. But when real studies of real mothers were carried out (healthy, well-nourished mothers from Western countries, whose babies gained weight normally when exclusively breastfed) it was discovered that they didn't eat 700 kilocalories a day more, but scarcely 100 or 150 (and in some studies even less). This increase was sufficient for them to maintain their normal weight, their normal level of activity, and to produce all the milk their babies needed. Apparently, during breastfeeding (the same as during pregnancy), the body's metabolism changes, making better use of the food that is ingested, like a car that uses less petrol after it has been serviced.

Even so, a lot of books carry on giving the same advice as before. And some even convert these calories into specific food types: milk, bread, meat, pasta and so on. The mother who follows this advice won't manage to eat this much. And if she does, well, perhaps that explains where the idea that breastfeeding makes you fat came from.

In any case, the nursing mother doesn't need a book to tell her how much to eat. Animals all eat what they need without having to read a book, or ask a vet. Our nutritional needs change throughout our lives, but it doesn't occur to anyone to ask their doctor how much they need to eat when they become a teenager, or an adult, or when they get a job as a postman or an office clerk. How many extra calories does an office clerk who cycles to work in August need? Or how many fewer calories should a miner who spends his holiday sitting in a deckchair reading have? How much more or less we eat is automatic: when our caloric need increases (because we are growing, or because of increased activity) we are hungrier and eat more; when our caloric needs diminish, we are less hungry and we eat less.

So, there is no need for you to stick to a diet, or count calories, or anything out of the ordinary. Simply eat according to how hungry you feel, and ignore any preconceived ideas (a lot of women think that when they are pregnant they are 'eating for two', and that is what they try to do).

Is this method reliable? What if I get it wrong and eat too much, or too little? The only time it is unreliable in animals is when they are ill. However, we humans are so influenced by education, culture, social pressures and advertising, that occasionally we eat too little, and far more often we eat too much. But you can easily see this for yourself: if you get too fat, you need to eat less, and if you get too thin, you need to eat more. No one gains thirty kilos without having first gained one, two, three…, so you will have plenty of time to realise and take the necessary steps.

What to eat

Eat what you usually eat. There is no reason to change your diet because you are breastfeeding.

Ah, but shouldn't I eat a healthy balanced diet? That is what I said: eat what you always eat. Or is it that now you have a child you realise you don't eat healthily and feel you should do something about it?

A healthy diet consists of cereals (bread, pasta, rice) and pulses (lentils, peas, chickpeas, beans) complemented by a daily intake of fresh fruit and/or vegetables and from time to time some food of animal origin: fish, meat, eggs or dairy products.

Mixing grains and pulses is essential, because the proteins in them complement one another. Proteins are made up of amino acids, some of which our bodies are unable to produce, and we must consume them ready-made: these are the so-called essential amino acids. Animal proteins contain the right combination of all the essential amino acids, which is why they are known as high biological value proteins. Vegetable proteins, on the other hand, are considered low biological value proteins, because they are lacking in some essential amino acids. Unless the body has all these essential amino acids at once, it can't produce new proteins. It is like putting together a watch with a cog missing. If a single piece is missing, the rest won't work, our body can't utilise them, and eliminates them.

Fortunately, grains and pulses are lacking in different amino acids. Those lacking in one are present in the other, and together these proteins are as nutritious as any animal protein. Some of the staple meals our great-grandparents enjoyed (unless they were wealthy), such as bean stew, combined pulses and grains. The odd piece of cured meat, eggs or cheese was eaten just to be on the safe side, and these provided a greater variety of amino acids. Nowadays, the tendency is to eat meat every day and pulses only occasionally, so we have plenty of amino acids, but we don't eat enough fibre, and therefore suffer more from constipation and other problems.

'Will my milk be bad if I don't eat a healthy diet? Should I sacrifice myself for the good of my baby, and eat vegetables, (which I hate), and stop drinking soft drinks and eating sweets? Since my diet isn't very healthy, isn't it better if I bottle feed him, then at least I'll know what he's eating?' No, no, and no. You needn't sacrifice yourself by eating a healthy diet for the simple reason that the composition of your breastmilk has almost nothing to do with what you eat. And artificial milk can never be better than your own (see the section below entitled The cow's diet).

Milk proteins are produced in the breast and aren't affected by what you eat. The same goes for lactose. What you eat has a slight effect on the composition of the fat in milk, so that if you eat more vegetable oil and more fish, your breastmilk will contain more unsaturated fats, and if you eat more meat, it will contain more saturated fats. But even if you eat huge amounts of saturated fats, your breastmilk will still contain more unsaturated fats than cow's milk, and will still be acceptable for your baby. As for vitamins and minerals, a few, such as pantothenic acid and iodine, are affected by the mother's diet, while others, such as iron, sodium and vitamin C, won't vary however much of them she consumes. In any event, the vitamin and mineral levels in the mother's milk will only be abnormal if she has a deficiency. If you are healthy, your milk will be normal. So, eating more fresh fruit and fewer sweets won't improve your *baby's* health, but it will improve *yours*.

A nursing mother should eat healthily, as should a woman who is bottle feeding, a woman who has no children, and everyone else. This is why I say: eat what you usually eat. And don't worry if your diet isn't 'perfectly balanced'. Firstly, because there is no such thing as a "perfectly balanced' diet, and secondly, because health isn't, and can't be, the sole consideration when choosing your diet. Habits, personal preference, money and time also play a part. If I am prepared to risk injury because I like to do sport, why can't I risk an increase in cholesterol because I like fatty foods?

The cow's diet

What the mother eats, I repeat, has very little effect on the composition of her milk. But even if it did, it would be silly to think: 'Because I eat unhealthily, my milk must be so bad that I'd be better off bottle feeding my baby'. Do cows eat healthily? At best, cows only eat grass, which for them constitutes a healthy diet, although it is hardly 'balanced'. Cows don't eat meat, or eggs or fruit or milk. But the fact is, much as we hate to admit it, most cows don't eat grass. In recent years we Europeans discovered that our cows were being given compound feed made from diseased sheep, and other such delicacies. Do you suppose that artificial baby milk (infant formula) is made from special cows that feed in green pastures and are milked by rosy-cheeked Swiss milkmaids? Well, it isn't. Artificial baby milk is made from normal milk taken from normal cows, which no doubt live in huge sheds and eat compound feed.

Forbidden foods

Every country or region has its own forbidden foods, which women aren't supposed to eat during lactation. In Spain, these are usually garlic, onions, artichokes, brussel sprouts and asparagus, which apparently give milk a bad taste, and also pulses, especially beans, and broccoli, which supposedly give babies gas.

In other countries other foods are forbidden. In Norway, for example, nursing mothers are advised not to eat grapes or strawberries. A mother who had to abstain from eating every type of food forbidden by someone somewhere in the world at some point, would probably starve.

The only food that has been scientifically researched is garlic. A random double-blind study was made. This means using a treatment group that takes the 'drug' being tested (in this case garlic) and a control group that takes a placebo (a simulated drug that produces no effect). The two groups were divided by drawing lots, and neither the mothers nor the experimenters knew who had taken garlic and who had taken the placebo. The garlic was inside a capsule that had to be swallowed whole; the mothers in the control group took an empty capsule. The experimenters who had contact with the mothers only knew that they had to give mother A capsule no.1, mother B capsule no.2, and so on. And only those in charge of the research, who had no contact with the mothers, knew which capsules contained garlic and which didn't. These precautions are essential in clinical trials to prevent autosuggestion (on the part of patient or doctor) from distorting the results ('since I took the pill, it doesn't seem to hurt as much').

The study showed that the milk smelled of garlic, and when they analysed it in the laboratory they found essence of garlic. Also, the babies whose mothers had taken garlic nursed for longer during the subsequent feed. Apparently they liked it, which isn't so surprising since a lot of us adults like garlic, which is why we eat it.

Of course, some babies might not like it, just as others might not like artichoke. In theory, all mothers can eat everything, but if a particular mother notices her baby refuses to nurse for a few hours after she eats a particular food, he probably doesn't like it. This isn't a problem; he will nurse again once the taste has worn off, or when he has more of an appetite. This sort of thing is more likely to happen when the mother suddenly eats a large helping of a food she hasn't eaten for a long time. Because if the mother eats a food regularly, her baby will have become accustomed to the taste even before he is born, through the placenta and the amniotic fluid.

No doubt one or two clever readers will be thinking: 'Well, if babies nurse more when their mothers eat garlic, I'll eat garlic everyday and my baby will nurse more, and gain more weight'. If this reasoning were correct, it would be dangerous (infant obesity is already a serious problem in Europe, and particularly in Spain). However, fortunately it doesn't work like that. The babies nursed more during one feed, and then compensated by nursing less during the next. And besides, if the milk always tasted of garlic, they would get used to it, and would go back to feeding normally. This goes for all of us: if you are partial to haddock, you may want seconds one day. But if you eat haddock for breakfast, lunch, and dinner I can assure you, after a while your enthusiasm will wane.

→ Mennella, J.A., Beauchamp, G.K. 'Maternal diet alters the sensory qualities of human milk and the nursling's behavior', *Pediatrics* 1991;88:737-44

Mysterious gases
It is possible that in certain cases a baby might dislike the taste of something his mother has eaten, but the idea that it could give him gas is completely unfounded. It is completely impossible for a mother to give her baby gas by eating beans or broccoli.

These foods give adults gas because they contain certain carbohydrates, which humans can't digest, and therefore can't absorb. These carbohydrates pass whole into the large intestine, where bacteria ferment them, producing gas.

Obviously, since the body can't absorb these substances, they can't pass into breastmilk. Neither can the gas itself. Anything that passes from the digestive tract into breastmilk has to do so via the blood. And neither blood nor milk contains bubbles.

Consequently, you can eat as many beans as you want. But perhaps you prefer not to debunk the myth. This way, if during a gathering there is an embarrassing explosion, you can always say nonchalantly: 'That was my baby, I'm breastfeeding him...'

Foods that boost milk production

Many foods are also said to boost milk supply. Almonds, hazelnuts, sardines and cow's milk come to mind. I once heard someone mention alfalfa, which is apparently sold for human consumption (I suppose the reasoning being: 'Cows eat it, and they have plenty of milk…').

Some of these foods are indeed healthy and nutritious. Perhaps this was an old pretext our great-great-grandmothers, back when not everyone managed to eat every day, used to justify giving the best portion to nursing mothers. But today, in the West, where we eat more, more often, this myth sometimes turns against mothers, obliging them to eat things they don't like.

There is no food that you need to eat in order to have milk. Remember, different mammals have very different diets: cows eat grass, lions eat meat, seals eat fish, whales eat plankton and anteaters eat ants, and they all produce milk. Human beings are by nature omnivorous. This means you can eat what you like, and you will still have milk. So if you hate hazelnuts, don't worry: you can breastfeed for years without having to eat a single hazelnut.

Beer

The popular belief that beer increases milk supply has been shown to be true. Beer contains a component that increases prolactin levels. But, of course, in order to prove that the milk supply increased, it was necessary to express milk from two groups of women, one that had been given beer and one that hadn't. Because, remember, the only way to produce more milk is to extract more milk. Otherwise, women who don't have children (or whose children have been weaned) wouldn't be allowed to drink beer, because imagine the predicament if you started producing more milk. Although you have more milk, your baby's milk consumption won't increase (see page 28); the excess milk contains a substance that inhibits lactation, and production goes down again. Milk production is self-regulating.

Beer might have helped some mothers in the days when it was obligatory to breastfeed for ten minutes every four hours. But for women who breastfeed on demand, there is a much simpler way to increase prolactin secretion: frequent feeds. The mother doesn't need to make a conscious decision: 'I'll give her more feeds so I have more milk'. If the baby is hungry she will want to nurse more. And if she doesn't want to nurse more, it is because she isn't hungry. It is as simple as that.

The effect of beer on milk supply has nothing to do with alcohol. Wine, brandy and spirits don't have the same effect.

Don't do anything to boost your milk supply, including drinking beer. And if you do have the odd beer, make sure it is alcohol-free (see page 242).

→ Koletzko, B., Lehner, F. 'Beer and breastfeeding', *Adv Exp Med Biol* 2000;478:23-8

Cow's milk

One type of food that causes mothers a lot of problems is milk. Mothers are frequently told that in order to breastfeed they need, absolutely need, to drink a litre of milk a day. Some have even been advised to drink two, presumably because: 'too much is better than not enough'.

This is absurd. Other mammals don't need to drink milk in order to produce milk. Cows don't drink milk. If a woman needed to drink a litre of milk to produce an average of three-quarters of a litre of milk, then a cow would need to drink forty litres of milk to produce thirty litres of milk. How would farmers make any money? Who would bother breeding dairy cows if they had to give them more milk than they produce?

Humans are the only animals that drink the milk of other animals. Humans are the only animals that continue to drink milk after weaning age. In fact, there is a clever mechanism that prevents adults from drinking milk. Milk contains a special type of sugar called lactose, which doesn't appear in any other food of animal or vegetable origin. Lactose is produced in the breast; the mother's blood contains no lactose. Lactose can only be digested thanks to lactase, a special digestive enzyme found only in the intestines of baby mammals. Once lactation comes to an end, lactase stops being produced, and the individual is no longer able to digest milk. Milk produces wind, diarrhoea, stomach-ache: all the symptoms associated with lactose intolerance. It is thought that this is nature's wise way of ensuring that the milk goes to the right recipient: if adults were able to drink milk, many males (or dominant females) would see off the mother's offspring and start nursing themselves. But they can't, because it gives them a stomach-ache.

It seems that a few thousand years ago, some groups of people (mostly Indoeuropeans, and some African groups) domesticated herd mammals and drank milk from them. A genetic mutation allowed these people to produce lactase and digest milk all their life. Their descendants can also digest milk. However, the majority of humanity (Asians, Native Americans, and most Africans) *can't* digest milk. Lactose intolerance in adults isn't an illness. It is normal. The abnormal ones are those of us who *aren't* lactose intolerant.

Some claim this mutation has been advantageous because it has allowed us to exploit another source of food. Others observe with irony that it hasn't been all that advantageous, given how many more Chinese there are on the planet than Swedes.

Studies carried out in China to discover at what age lactase disappears from the intestine have found that in some children it disappears when they are three, whereas in others it is still present until they are twelve. After the age of twelve, almost no Chinese people are lactose tolerant. This is another clue as to how long it is 'normal' for human beings to go on nursing.

We Spaniards, with our mix of races, don't tolerate lactose as well as the Swedes, and it is estimated that fifteen per cent of Spaniards are lactose intolerant. Most people don't know they are lactose intolerant; they haven't been tested, or 'diagnosed' (how can you be diagnosed with something that isn't an illness?), they simply don't drink milk. It isn't always so clear-cut: some people tolerate small amounts of lactose, but too much of it gives them a stomach upset. They will usually drink a macchiato rather than a cappuccino. Some tolerate other dairy products, such as yoghurt or cheese. In Latin America, the number of lactose intolerant people can be much higher, depending on the country.

For those who are lactose intolerant, it can't be much fun being forced to drink a litre of milk a day. It must be sheer torture.

→ Yang, Y., He, M., Cui, H., Bian, L., Wang, Z. 'The prevalence of lactase deficiency and lactose intolerance in Chinese children of different ages', *Chin Med J* 2000; 113:1129-32

The vegetarian diet

A balanced ovo-lacto vegetarian diet is perfectly suitable for adults, children, nursing mothers and pregnant women. But it has to be properly balanced. Pulses must be eaten with grains so that their amino acids complement one another to form a high-value protein. Very little of the iron in pulses and grains will be absorbed unless they are accompanied by the vitamin C in fruit. An omnivorous diet (i.e. one that includes all food types, including meat and fish) usually contains plenty of nutrients, and so less care needs to be taken. Being a vegetarian doesn't mean eating a big salad and skipping the main course. You need to know about nutrition and to pay attention to the food you eat. You will find plenty of information on the Vegetarian Society's web page:

→ www.vegsoc.org

Most vegetarians are very sensible, and they often know more about nutrition than their own doctors. But there are some strange philosophical or religious groups who advocate bizarre and inadequate eating regimes, like the macrobiotic diet. The macrobiotic diet is progressive, and the so-called advanced stages are unsuitable for adults, and extremely dangerous for children, pregnant women or nursing mothers.

There are also those who do their own thing. Years ago I met a man who had reached the conclusion that apples were the only healthy food. Only apples. Apples all day every day. He imposed the diet on his wife, and on his two-year old son. Fortunately, the nursery school fed the child on the quiet.

Learn to differentiate between sensible and nonsensical information. Are proteins and nutrients mentioned, or calcium and iron, or is it about cosmic energy, the healing power of food, and 'toxins', none of which are ever named?

Veganism

A strict vegetarian or vegan diet that contains no eggs or milk is seriously problematic because it provides no vitamin B12.

No animal or plant is capable of making vitamin B12. Only bacteria can do this. Herbivores obtain this vitamin, which is essential to life, from the bacteria and insects they accidentally ingest while eating plants and leaves. It is the same in some traditional societies, which are exclusively vegetarian yet don't suffer from a vitamin B12 deficiency.

But we wash our vegetables thoroughly before eating them, and we should go on washing them, to avoid infection. And when we find insects in our rice or beans, we throw them away.

Plants contain no vitamin B12 at all. Meat, fish and milk and eggs do contain vitamin B12. Yoghurt and some cheeses have more vitamin B12 than milk, because they also contain bacteria.

In Spain, the only commonly eaten food enriched with vitamin B12 is breakfast cereal; you can see for yourself if you look at the label, and you can calculate how many grams of cereal you would need to cover the recommended daily intake. Royal jelly, tofu, miso and tempeh contain no vitamin B12. Neither does brewer's yeast, unless it has been enriched, meaning that vitamin B12 has been added during processing.

Despite the claims of those who market it, the algae Spirulina contains no vitamin B12. What it does contain is a molecule so similar to vitamin B12 that it gives a positive result when analysed, but this molecule has no effect on the body whatsoever. Worse still, it is suspected of blocking cell receptors, and impeding the uptake of the real vitamin.

Because vitamin B12 is so vital to the organism, our bodies have developed very elaborate ways of preserving it. A healthy person usually has enough reserves of vitamin B12 to last them three to four years. We don't need to eat meat every day, only occasionally. A strict vegetarian, who doesn't take vitamin B12 supplements, won't get ill for several years.

Vegans, as well as ovo-lacto vegetarians who eat few eggs or dairy products, will need to take vitamin B12 supplements all their lives – men and women alike, everyone. Most vegetarians are aware of this and take a supplement.

When you take a lot of vitamin B12 all at once, the body doesn't know what to do with it, and it doesn't get absorbed very well. The amount you need therefore depends on how often you take it:

- If you eat food that is enriched with vitamin B12, 3–5µg (micrograms) a day is enough.
- If you take a daily supplement in tablet form, you need

between 10 and 20µg every day. Chew the tablets well so that they are properly absorbed, or place them under your tongue (letting them dissolve in your mouth like a sweet).

- If you take a supplement once a week, 2000µg.
- If you haven't taken vitamin B12 for several months or years, you will first need to replenish your reserves by taking 2000µg daily for fifteen days, and then continue taking the normal dose, daily or weekly.

Vitamin B12 deficiency causes megaloblastic anaemia, so called because the red blood cell count is low and the cells are very big (unlike anaemia caused by iron deficiency, where the red blood cells are tiny). But it can also cause neurological problems and coma. This type of problem is more frequent in young children.

In Europe and the United States, children of mothers who are vegan or who follow a macrobiotic diet have been known to die from vitamin B12 deficiency. Children are normally born with reserves that last several months or years, but if the mother already has a vitamin B12 deficiency, her baby is born without reserves, and is already sick. Breastmilk is usually very rich in vitamin B12, but if the mother hasn't got any, it won't materialise out of nowhere.

If you are vegan and take regular vitamin B12 supplements, there is no problem; your baby will be born with reserves, and your milk will be as rich in vitamin B12 as that of any other mother. If your baby is breastfed, she won't need to take vitamin supplements.

If you are vegan, and you don't take vitamin B12 supplements, and you have only realised now you are pregnant, begin taking 2000µg a day immediately for fifteen days, and then carry on taking regular supplements. If you are due to give birth in a few weeks' time, don't worry: your baby still has time to 'soak it up' and will be born with sufficient reserves.

If, on the other hand, you begin taking vitamin B12 supplements shortly before or after the birth, your baby won't have reserves, and may already be ill. She will need a massive dose of vitamin B12. After that, if you continue taking the vitamin B12 supplements, your baby will be able to breastfeed normally and won't need any further supplements.

Remember that if you have been a vegan for many years, you will need a massive dose of vitamin B12 straight away. Even if you decide to start eating meat, it will take months for your vitamin B12 reserves to build up.

What if you are an ovo-lacto vegetarian? How many eggs and how much milk do you need? You need approximately three glasses of milk or four eggs a day. However, one glass of milk and one egg a day, plus a bit of yoghurt and some enriched breakfast cereal, is probably enough. If you eat less than this you should take a supplement, especially during pregnancy and lactation.

→ www.vegsoc.org/page.aspx?pid=807

→ 'Neurologic impairment in children associated with maternal dietary deficiency of cobalamin', Georgia, 2001. *MMWR Morb Mortal Wkly Rep* 2003;52:61-4 www.cdc.gov/mmwr/preview/ mmwrhtml/mm5204a1.htm

Vitamins and minerals

Nursing mothers only need to take two supplements: iodine, and, in the case of vegans, vitamin B12.

Iodine

Iodine is an essential trace element that enables the thyroid gland to produce thyroxine, the hormone that controls our metabolism.

A large part of the earth's soil is iodine-poor, because for millions of years rainwater has dissolved it and washed it into the sea. As a result, the earth's plants and animals (including freshwater fish) contain little iodine. Saltwater fish, on the other hand, is rich in iodine.

We used to think that iodine deficiency only affected people who, a hundred years ago, lived in isolated mountain areas, like Las Hurdes in Spain or the Alps in Switzerland, where they didn't have any fish. It was common in those places to see people with goitre (a lump on the throat, which is the thyroid gland hypertrophied, trying desperately to use whatever iodine is available) and cretinism (severe mental retardation due to a lack of thyroid hormone during infancy).

But this was merely the tip of the iceberg. In recent years, several studies have shown that all over Spain, even in coastal regions, a sizeable part of the population (approximately one third) suffers from iodine deficiency; this includes adults, children, and pregnant women. Similarly, in the UK, a survey published in 2011 found iodine deficiency (mostly mild) in 69% of schoolgirls aged 14–15 years old. The deficiency is slight, but it has been associated, in another British study, with an adverse effect on child cognitive development. It also produces a lot of mild cases of goitre, thyroid glands that have been forced to hypertrophy, and which as a result are on the verge of collapse. Many thyroid problems in adults (hyperthyroid as well as hypothyroid) stem from an iodine deficiency in early childhood.

In order to prevent this, everyone in the family, children and adults, should eat iodized salt. Don't buy salt that isn't iodized (in some countries, uniodized salt is available from the chemist on prescription, for rare conditions such as thyroiditis, where iodized salt is contraindicated). Sea salt contains no iodine unless it says 'iodized sea salt' on the packaging.

However, during pregnancy and lactation women need more iodine than usual: 300µg as opposed to the usual 100ug. Eating iodized salt is unlikely to increase your intake enough. And so in many countries pregnant women and nursing mothers are advised to take a daily supplement of between 100 and 200µg (ideally starting three months before getting pregnant).

As with a lot of other public health recommendations, the whole population is targeted, when in fact two-thirds of pregnant women probably have no need of iodine supplements. But finding out who does and who doesn't would require cumbersome and costly testing, whereas iodine supplements are cheap and completely safe. Even if you have plenty of iodine, taking 200µg more won't do you any harm. For this reason, it is best that all women take them.

The Spanish Department of Health has been recommending this supplement for women since 2004, but it is possible some doctors still don't know about it. They might even say iodine supplements aren't necessary, and tell you not to take them. Probably because the American books we doctors read used not to recommend iodine supplementation. For many years now in America all salt for human consumption, as well as many other food products, is enriched with iodine (while in most European countries iodized salt is optional, and so most processed foods and restaurant dishes contain no iodine, and deficiency is much more frequent). Americans don't usually suffer from iodine deficiency, because, unbeknownst to them, they all take supplements. Even so, the American Thyroid Association recommends now a supplement of 150μg for pregnant and lactating women in the US and Canada. Similar recommendations have been made in Australia and New Zealand, and also in the UK by the British Thyroid Foundation (http://www.btf-thyroid.org/index.php/campaigns/iodine). In Europe, iodine deficiency is much more of a problem than in America, and supplementation is more important. Speak to your doctor or midwife about it. Most (but not all) prenatal vitamins already contain iodine.

Kelp and seaweed contain a large excess of iodine that can be harmful, especially during pregnancy and lactation.

→ Morreale de Escobar, G. 'El yodo durante la gestación, lactancia y primera infancia – Cantidades mínimas y máximas: de microgramos a gramos', *An Es Pediatr* 2000;53:1-5

→ Domínguez, I., Reviriego, S., Rojo-Martínez, G., Valdés, M.J., Carrasco, R., Coronas, I. y cols. 'Déficit de yodo y función tiroidea en una población de mujeres embarazadas sanas', *Med Clin (Barc)* 2004;122:449-53

→ Dunn, J.T., Delange, F. 'Damaged Reproduction: The most important consequence of iodine defciency', *J Clin Endocrinol Metab* 2001;86:2360-3 jcem.endojournals.org/cgi/content/full/86/6/2360

→ Zimmermann, M., Delange, F. 'Iodine supplementation of pregnant women in Europe: a review and recommendations', *Eur J Clin Nutr* 2004;58:979-84

→ Vanderpump, M.P., Lazarus, J.H., Smyth, P.P., Laurberg, P., Holder, R.L., Boelaert, K., Franklyn, J.A.; British Thyroid Association UK Iodine Survey Group. Iodine status of UK schoolgirls: a cross-sectional survey. *Lancet* 2011;377:2007-12

→ Vanderpump, M.P.J. Iodine deficiency as a new challenge for industrialized countries: A UK perspective. *Int J Epidemiol* 2012;41:601-4 ije.oxfordjournals.org/content/41/3/601

→ Bath, S.C., Steer, C.D., Golding, J., Emmett, P., Rayman, M.P. Effect of inadequate iodine status in UK pregnant women on cognitive outcomes in their children: results from the Avon Longitudinal Study of Parents and Children (ALSPAC) *Lancet*. 2013;382:331-7

→ Public Health Committee of the American Thyroid Association, Becker, D.V., Braverman, L.E., Delange, F., Dunn, J.T., Franklyn, J.A., Hollowell, J.G., Lamm, S.H., Mitchell, M.L., Pearce, E., Robbins, J., Rovet, J.F. Iodine supplementation for pregnancy and lactation-United States and Canada: recommendations of the American Thyroid Association. *Thyroid*. 200;16:949-51.

→ Mackerras, D.E., Eastman, C.J. Estimating the iodine supplementation level to recommend for pregnant and breastfeeding women in Australia. *Med J Aust* 2012;197:238-42.

Vitamin B12

See the previous section under the heading 'Veganism'.

Iron

During lactation, a mother's iodine requirements triple, but her need for iron halves. The main cause of anaemia in women is repeated loss of blood during menstruation. During a large part of the lactation period, women don't have periods, and therefore they lose less iron.

So, if you didn't need to take iron supplements before you were pregnant, you will need them even less when you are breastfeeding.

If your hair starts falling out, it isn't because you have an iron deficiency, but for other reasons (see page 294).

If you suffer from anaemia, not only *can* you continue breastfeeding, you *should* continue breastfeeding. Breastfeeding helps cure anaemia more quickly. Obviously if you are suffering from anaemia, you will have to take an iron supplement. Your doctor will tell you the correct dosage.

Calcium

Calcium requirements don't increase during pregnancy. The recommended intake is the same for all women, whether they are breastfeeding or not. You either need lifelong supplements, or you don't need any at all.

For about the first six months of lactation, all women lose approximately 5 per cent of their bone calcium. This has been shown through bone-density testing, which measures the calcium in bones. It makes no difference how many calcium-rich foods you eat or how many calcium supplements you take, you will still lose bone calcium. Taking calcium tablets will only increase the amount of calcium you eliminate in your faeces or urine. This bone decalcification isn't caused by a lack of calcium in the diet, or by a loss of calcium through the milk. It is due to changes in the mother's hormonal balance and in her metabolism.

From the sixth month of lactation onwards, a woman's bone calcium increases again. This recalcification takes place without any need for calcium tablets or supplements. It is enough to eat a normal diet that isn't especially rich in calcium. Women who have breastfed for a year have more or less the same amount of calcium in their bones as women who haven't breastfed. We aren't sure what happens after this year, but we do know that in the long term breastfeeding helps prevent osteoporosis (although, out of ignorance, many people, and even some doctors, still say the opposite).

These long-term effects are ambiguous: some studies show that women who breastfeed for longer have more bone calcium; others that they have less, and still others find no difference at all. However, where all studies are almost unanimous is in comparing the risk of fracture. This is done using case-control studies: doctors find elderly women who have been hospitalised with fractures due to osteoporosis (humeral fractures, collapsed vertebrae, and above all the dreaded femoral fractures) and compare them with women of the same age who haven't suffered fractures. The women with no fractures had breastfed for longer.

It is curious that breastfeeding for longer doesn't appear to prevent osteoporosis so much as osteoporosis-related fractures (which is the real problem: osteoporosis wouldn't matter if it didn't increase the risk of fractures). Apparently, the risk of fractures doesn't depend solely on levels of bone calcium, but also on its placement in the bones, on the structure of the trabecules (microscopic mineral rods that shape the bone). It is like the construction of a bridge: you can't take a pile of steel and arrange it any old how. An engineer must decide where each girder goes. Perhaps the fact that during lactation a tiny part of the bone dissolves and then reconstitutes itself in some way renews the structure, replacing the old girders with new ones.

To sum up: breastfeeding doesn't weaken the bones, it strengthens them, and the longer a mother breastfeeds the better. Breastfeeding for two or three years doesn't 'wear out' the mother; on the contrary.

'What if lactation is closely followed by pregnancy, doesn't it end up damaging your bones?' It has been shown that even when the mother becomes pregnant within eighteen months of her last pregnancy, her bone calcium is still restored. The recommended daily intake (RDI) of calcium is exactly the same for women who are breastfeeding and for those who aren't. No experts say that women should take more calcium during lactation than at any other time in their lives. It is absurd to insist that nursing mothers should drink more milk, or eat more calcium-rich foods, or take calcium tablets.

Don't worry if you don't drink milk. Neither do the majority of other women (see page 165). There are many other calcium-rich foods: green leafy vegetables, broccoli, and small fish with edible bones. Lionesses only eat meat, and they also have bones, and get pregnant and breastfeed. And so do deer, which only feed on grass, and female bats, which only eat insects. Your diet would need to be very strange indeed for you to have a calcium deficiency, and if this were the case, you would have to change your eating habits (or take supplements) not just while you were breastfeeding, but for the rest of your life.

If you have backache, or your legs are sore, or you feel tired, this isn't due to calcium deficiency, or because you are breastfeeding, and weaning your baby won't help. Osteoporosis doesn't hurt unless you have a fracture; the back pain some elderly women suffer from is due to collapsed vertebrae. And this only happens with advanced osteoporosis. It is impossible for a fracture to be caused by the 5 per cent loss of bone calcium during the first six months of lactation. Your aches and pains may have other causes, some related to motherhood (chores, carrying around extra weight, lack of sleep) and others not.

→ Sowers, M., Randolph, J., Shapiro, B., Jannausch, M., 'A prospective study of bone density and pregnancy after an extended period of lactation with bone loss', *Obstet Gynecol* 1995;85:285-9

→ Melton, L.J. 3rd, Bryant, S.C., Wahner, H.W., O'Fallon, W.M., Malkasian, G.D., Judd, H.L., Riggs, B.L., 'Influence of breastfeeding and other reproductive factors on bone mass later in life', *Osteoporos Int.* 1993;3:76-83

→ Cumming, R.G., Klineberg, R.J., 'Breastfeeding and other reproductive factors and the risk of hip fractures in elderly women', *Int J Epidemiol* 1993;22:684-91

→ Prentice, A., 'Maternal calcium metabolism and bone mineral status', *Am J Clin Nutr* 2000;71:1312S-6S www.ajcn.org/cgi/content/full/71/5/1312S

How much liquid?

It is logical that nursing mothers need more water. But you needn't force yourself to drink a specific amount. You will automatically drink what you need, like any other healthy person. If, in addition to breastfeeding, you do exercise, and the weather is warm, you will get thirstier still.

Sometimes mothers are advised to drink a lot of water in order to have more milk. Of course, this doesn't work. Farmers have been experimenting with this for hundreds of years, giving cows more to drink, but they don't produce more milk. It only works the other way round: first you milk the cow, then you add water to the milk, and then of course you have more milk. Before you protest: 'But women aren't cows', you should know that scientific experiments have been done with women, where they were asked to drink several litres of water a day for weeks and their breastmilk didn't increase.

In some parts of the world, there is a popular belief that when a mother drinks water while her baby is nursing, the water travels straight to her breast, through some duct which scientists haven't discovered yet, and that instead of getting milk, the baby gets water. This is obviously not true. But it is a mistake that can cause discomfort, because the hormone oxytocin makes you thirsty, and mothers often feel thirsty while their babies are nursing (and during labour). You can drink as much water as you like while your baby is nursing.

Allergy prevention

Lactation reduces the risk of various atopic diseases. The American Academy of Paediatrics used to suggest that if a mother had a strong family history of allergies, she should stop drinking milk, and eating eggs, fish and nuts during pregnancy. However, there is no clear evidence that this actually reduces the risk of allergies.

In one study, mothers stopped drinking milk and eating eggs, without any visible benefits.

In another study, mothers stopped drinking milk and eating eggs and fish for the first three months. Their babies had fewer skin allergies up until six months (11 per cent compared to 28 per cent), but at age four the difference was less, and at age ten there was no difference. Other types of allergy didn't diminish either. Is it worth following such a restrictive diet because it might reduce the incidence of skin allergies for a few months? Only you can decide. But before you do, bear in mind how difficult it would be to follow a diet without milk or eggs, how many recipes, or prepared foods contain milk and eggs: biscuits, cakes, pasta, breaded fish and meat, pizza and so on. If you were to half follow the diet, it would probably have no effect.

→ Zeiger, R.S. 'Food Allergen Avoidance in the Prevention of Food Allergy in Infants and Children', *Pediatrics* 2003;111:1662-71
   pediatrics.aappublications.org/cgi/reprint/111/6/S2/1662

Losing weight

One of the supposed benefits of breastfeeding is that it helps mothers to lose weight. This is true, but sometimes expectations run too high, and can lead to frustration.

Weight increase during pregnancy depends on several factors: the weight of the baby, the placenta and the amniotic fluid, how much the womb grows, increase in blood volume… and a little bit of fat stored for use during lactation. Nature predicted that mothers would have difficulty hunting and gathering (or whatever our ancestors did to find food) whilst carrying a baby. Logically, the mother who doesn't breastfeed will have more trouble getting rid of this surplus fat. She will have to burn it up by doing exercise. Breastfeeding, on the other hand, can be done sitting comfortably in a chair. It is like a natural form of liposuction.

Indeed, nursing mothers have been known to lose approximately half a kilo a month for the first six months. However, don't imagine it is all plain sailing: a lot of mothers don't begin to lose weight until they have been breastfeeding for three months.

If you have gained a lot of weight during pregnancy, it won't be enough simply to breastfeed and everything will go back to normal. You will need to do exercise and watch what you eat.

Obviously it isn't a good idea during lactation (or at any other time) to follow silly, unbalanced miracle diets, to skip meals, only to eat grapefruit for a week, or to try to lose five kilos in a week. On the other hand, it has been shown that if you follow a controlled, balanced diet, with the aim of losing five kilos in ten weeks, it has no effect on the amount or composition of the mother's milk. The baby carries on gaining weight while the mother gets slimmer.

Some have warned of the hypothetical danger that losing weight during lactation releases some of the pesticides stored in the mother's fat (sadly, we all have pesticides inside us), which transfer to the milk and contaminate the baby. But this doesn't happen. A study has shown no increase in pesticide levels in breastmilk when a mother loses weight.

As at any other time in life, if you want to stay slim you must exercise as well as diet. Dieting on its own will only make you lose muscle mass. Dieting and exercising maintains (or even increases) muscle mass and burns up fat. Losing muscle mass is bad, and the body usually tries to regain it as soon as possible. In addition, muscle tissue is highly active, and burns up calories even when you are resting, whereas fatty tissue is inactive and burns no calories. This is why people who lose weight through dieting, but without exercising, usually put weight back on quite quickly.

After giving birth, it is a good idea to start following a postpartum exercise routine. Your midwife will show you how to do pelvic floor exercises. Doing abdominal exercises before strengthening the pelvic floor can exacerbate certain problems, such as incontinence.

→ Lovelady, C.A., Whitehead, R.A., McCrory, M.A., Nommsen-Rivers, L.A., Mabury, S., Dewey, K.G. 'Weight change during lactation does not alter the concentrations of chlorinated organic contaminants in breast milk of women with low exposure', *J Hum Lact* 1999;15:307-15

→ McCrory, M.A., Nommsen-Rivers, L.A., Mole, P.A., Lonnerdal, B., Dewey, K.G. 'Randomized trial of the short-term effects of dieting compared with dieting plus aerobic exercise on lactation performance', *Am J Clin Nutr* 1999;69:959-67 www.ajcn. org/cgi/content/full/69/5/959

Chapter 10
GOING BACK TO WORK

There are many things you can do when it is time to go back to work. And it is impossible to say in absolute terms that one course of action is better than the others, because there are a lot of factors to take into consideration. Needless to say, we all want what is best for the baby, but also what is best for the mother, for the whole family, for the family finances. No one can decide for you, because no one knows your situation.

A note: my remarks in this chapter relate to maternity leave and benefits as they are in my home country of Spain. Arrangements for maternity leave vary significantly from country to country. It may be interesting for English-speaking readers to compare the Spanish provision with that of their own country. Up to date information about the UK can be found at www.gov.uk, and for the US at www.dol.gov. The majority of my comments, however, will apply to all countries.

Practical considerations

Maternity leave

At the moment, maternity leave in Spain is only sixteen weeks. In the case of twins and triplets, this is extended to eighteen and twenty weeks respectively (they could have made it sixteen weeks per child; twins aren't exactly common, and women don't have them on purpose in order not to work).

If you have been off work during pregnancy for medical reasons, you still have the right to sixteen weeks maternity leave after you give birth.

The law allows the father to take up to ten of the sixteen weeks' leave in place of the mother. Special circumstances aside, I don't

think this is ideal if you are breastfeeding, or the best thing for
the baby.

Breastfeeding breaks

For nine months, you have the right to an hour's break a day for
breastfeeding, with full pay. This can be a break of one hour, or
two breaks of half an hour. Although it is called the 'breastfeeding
hour', obviously you don't have to be breastfeeding; mothers who
are bottle feeding have the same right. You can also choose to begin
work late or leave work early, but then, for some reason no one has
ever been able to explain to me, one hour becomes half an hour.
Given that taking an hour off in the middle of the day is usually more
inconvenient for an employer than arriving late or leaving early, you
can probably negotiate: 'If you don't let me leave work an hour early,
I'll take my breastfeeding break between eleven and twelve, when
things are at their busiest, just to be difficult' (this is what you will be
thinking, and what your employer will think you are thinking. Of
course, you will express it in more diplomatic terms).

You have the right to choose when you take your breastfeeding
break: a primary school teacher who was forced to breastfeed during
break time went to court and won her case. A woman doctor also
won a case in which she argued that a one-hour breastfeeding break
corresponded to an eight-hour working day, and that when she was
on twenty-four hour duty, she had the right to three hour-long breaks.

There are several ways in which the breastfeeding break can
be used to the best advantage. If your work is close to where you
live, you can pop home and breastfeed your baby. If it is far away,
try to find a nursery or childminder near where you work, so you
can breastfeed her on your way to and from work. This way you
will spend less time away from your baby. You could also arrange
with the child's grandparents, or a childminder, whoever is caring
for the baby, to meet you in a park or a café near your work. Other
mothers use the hour to express their milk.

It is also possible to save up the hours from the breastfeeding
breaks and exchange them for an extra month of maternity leave.

Working part-time

Up to the age of six years, both the father and mother (either
separately or at the same time) can ask to work part-time (from

between a third and a half fewer hours with the corresponding reduction in salary). You have the right to decide how you organise your day. Some mothers prefer to work two or three hours less per day, others prefer to take one day off a week (for example, the day when no one can mind the baby). Remember, they aren't doing you a favour; this is your legal right, and a costly one at that, because you are losing part of your salary. Theoretically, with the money saved, your employer can afford to pay someone to make up the hours. You aren't 'letting anyone down', and you mustn't try to do in six hours what usually takes you eight. This reduction must also involve effective working hours, and not simply be taken off time spent in training, meetings or lunch and coffee breaks.

Unpaid leave

Up until their child is three, a father or mother or both can ask for unpaid leave for periods of varying duration. Employers are obliged to keep your job and your shift open for you for the first year. After that, it depends on the goodwill of your employer; if they want to make life difficult for you they will doubtless find a way.

You don't have to fix in advance the date you return to work. When you decide you want to start work again, you simply give your employer two weeks' notice.

Obviously, not being paid is a huge, though at times unavoidable, inconvenience. However, try not to regard it as money wasted, but as money well spent. A lot of people spend a month's wages on a holiday, or fifteen months' wages on a car, or 200 months' wages on a house. Why not spend two, or ten, or twenty months' wages on caring for your child? After all, it will only happen once or twice in your life. Very few Spaniards these days have a third child.

When making a thorough financial appraisal, other factors should be included in the equation. Besides buying time with your child, you are also buying time with your family and friends, time to read, to go for walks, to think, to live. ('I won't have much time for reading when I have a baby', you will be thinking. This is true. You won't have much time. But you will have even less time if you work an eight-hour day, and take care of your baby the rest of the time.) You are buying the freedom to be with your child, instead of worrying about her from afar ('I wonder what she's doing now? Is she crying? Has she been sick again? I should have taken her temperature this morning…'). You are buying, in many cases, the peace of mind that comes with forgetting about work, employers, fellow employees, rivalries, measurable goals, overtime, the sour looks you get whenever your baby is ill. Your income will go down, but so will your expenditure: daycare, childminders, transport, and meals (it is cheaper to eat at home every day than to eat out).

It would be wonderful if all children – whether breastfed or bottle fed – could stay with their parents until about the age of three. This is the age (which varies, of course) at which children usually stop crying when their parents leave them, and are happy to go to nursery. Note that I said *with their parents* not *with their mother*. I am not suggesting mothers stop working for three years. Fathers also have the right to escape the tyranny of work in order to spend time with their children. By the age of one, or one and a half (or, with any luck, earlier) children usually feel quite happy to be left with their father. Breastfeeding stops being an issue when the baby starts eating solids. In many families, mothers and fathers take turns: the mother takes a year's unpaid leave, and then the father takes another (more or less, depending on the finances). Taking a year off work each isn't the same as taking two months off work each. Babies have great need of their mothers during the first twelve months. After that, up until the age of three, they have great need of both parents. Then, between the ages of three and thirty, they still have need of both parents, but the need isn't so great.

If your finances won't permit you to take three years, or one year, or even six months' unpaid leave, consider at least taking one or two months. Four months' maternity leave is not long enough, because most babies don't move on to solids before six months old. Once a baby is already on solids, everything becomes easier: there is no longer any need to express milk, leave it in the fridge, heat it up. When the mother isn't there, the baby can eat rice, banana, chicken and other foods.

Taking your baby to work

In Spain we have a law with the pompous title: 'Law for the reconciliation of work and family life'. Despite having read it inside out, I don't see where reconciliation comes into it. Basically you must choose between work and family life. If you choose family life, you take unpaid leave; if you choose work you put your child in nursery or with a childminder.

I understand the word 'reconcile' as meaning to be able to do both things at once. The way people have throughout the history of humanity. Because we would be fooling ourselves if we thought that working women were a recent phenomenon; women have always worked.

'Yes', someone might object, 'but they worked in the home, not outside the home for a wage.' Well, yes, women working outside the home for a wage is a relatively recent phenomenon. With the advent of the industrial revolution, husbands went to work at the factory or at the office while their wives stayed at home cleaning and cooking. But before that, for hundreds of years, peasants and craftsmen worked in the house or next door to the house, and the differences between men and women's work were quite blurred. Neither fathers nor mothers left their children to go off to work. It was only about 200 years ago that fathers were snatched from the home, and about fifty years ago that production methods abducted mothers, too, leaving babies to be looked after by strangers.

In many parts of the world, mothers still work in the fields, walk for miles to transport water or firewood, buy or sell in the market, weave or cook, all the while carrying their baby on their back. Of course, a woman carrying a baby works more slowly, and has to take frequent rests to look after him. She isn't as productive. But in many societies this isn't an issue, because their priorities are very clear: first and foremost you attend to your child's needs, and then to your work as best you can. The motto in our society appears to be the opposite: first and foremost you attend to your work, and then to your child's needs as best you can.

This may change. In fact, I am quite sure it will. Our current economic system is too stressful; it clashes too strongly with our biological needs. Of course, many workplaces are too dangerous, or too impractical, to accommodate a baby. But many others don't 'allow' babies, not for any logical reason, but out of habit. There will come a day when the hotel receptionist, the tax inspector, the cinema usher or the travel agent will attend to us holding a baby in her arms. Telling a mother: 'You aren't allowed in here with a baby', will seem as incongruous as telling a pregnant mother 'You aren't allowed in here with a womb'. One day, our grandchildren will be surprised when they see people in films going everywhere without their children. And this will only be a first step, because one day, parents will be given the choice of reconciling work and family life. One day, we will see children running around offices and shops, the way they once ran around the fields and artisans' workshops.

Who will look after my baby?

Regardless of whether you work full-time or part-time, or whether you return to work after four or twenty months, someone will have to look after your baby when you aren't with him. This is a very important decision, far more important, for example, than choosing a school for you child when she is older.

First of all, babies and young infants have a far greater need for affection. It isn't enough for someone to 'look after' or 'watch over' your baby; your baby needs to form a strong emotional bond with the person caring for her. Secondly, the trust you place in your baby's caregiver is far greater, because your ability to supervise or control that person is very small. A six-year-old can tell you if she has been hit; a two-year-old can't.

I think all parents would agree that our children are our most cherished treasure. Act accordingly. Would you entrust the person caring for your child with the keys to your car or your house? Would you give them your credit card and your pin number? If not, how can you trust them with your child?

Ideally, of course, it is the father who looks after the baby while the mother is out. If the father devotes himself 100 per cent to looking after the baby from the very beginning (if he gives her all his time and attention), the bond between father and baby can be so strong that the baby will accept him completely as a mother substitute. This means she won't (often) cry or get upset when her mother is absent for a while. Some couples manage to share the task of looking after their children, by working different shifts, or if possible working part-time.

Other relatives (such as the baby's grandmothers) are the next best option. They are people you can trust implicitly, and with whom the baby is probably already familiar. They also have experience of caring for children (you are living proof that your mothers didn't do a bad job). Besides, relatives are for life; the bond your baby makes with them will last forever, and they aren't going to vanish from her life the way a professional childminder will.

Some women hesitate to ask their mothers, for fear they may be taking advantage of them. Of course there are those who do take advantage; some grandmothers are shamefully exploited. Does your mother want to look after your baby? Would it entail her giving up other activities or neglecting other duties? Is she still young and fit enough to look after a baby? On the one hand there are exploited grandmothers, and on the other, grandmothers who would like nothing more than to look after their grandchild, who would feel more rewarded, more useful, and more alive. And then there are the children, who because of the qualms of parents who don't want to be seen to be taking advantage, or to be frowned on by siblings, end up in nursery. Perhaps you would feel better paying the money you would otherwise spend on childcare to your mother; this way you wouldn't feel as if you were taking advantage of her, and at the same time you would be helping her financially without offending her (some pensions don't stretch very far). Of course, in some families offering or accepting money would be considered bad taste; questions of pride differ from family to family.

Another supposed drawback to grandmothers is the idea that they 'spoil' their grandchildren, and let them get away with everything. This is nonsense. No grandmother (or mother, or father) can let a child get away with everything. Of course they won't let their grandchild set fire to the house, or jump out of a window, or play with a knife. Nor will they allow him to break vases, smear paint on the walls or tear the pages out of books. What, then, do people mean when they talk about 'spoiling' a child, being too lenient? Do they mean the grandmother will pay 'too much' attention to her grandchild, tell him 'too many' stories, sing 'too many' songs to him, play with him, smile at him, tickle him…? Because this is exactly what babies need. It is impossible to pay too much attention to a baby, because a baby needs constant attention.

'But what if she gives him all her attention, and then we aren't able to, won't he suffer?', some parents will ask. This argument is doubly wrongheaded. Firstly because if both parents work (and this is why they leave the baby with the grandmother), surely they will be eager to play with their baby when they get home. Secondly, if they really have no time for him in the evening, then it is just as well the grandmother is with him in the morning otherwise the poor baby would get no attention all day.

Although it is customary for grandmothers to babysit, more and more grandfathers feel perfectly at ease changing a nappy. And there may be other relatives: a sister or a cousin who is unemployed, a sister-in-law who is looking after her own baby, or an aunt.

Sometimes two or three women friends come to an informal arrangement: one takes unpaid leave and looks after all their babies while the others work, and they divide up their wages.

Sometimes it is necessary to find someone outside the family. This could be a nursery, or a childminder who looks after the baby either at your house or at her own house.

The American Academy of Paediatrics suggests the following standards, among others, for nurseries (known as 'daycare' in the US):

Under twelve months: three children per carer.
Thirteen to thirty months: four children per carer.
Thirty-one to thirty-five months: five children per carer.
Four to five years: eight children per carer.

In Spain, the law allows eight babies of under one year old per carer! How do you think one person can look after eight babies? As you know, it is enough trouble looking after one! By the time you have changed all their nappies and fed them, it is time to start all over again. The amusing thing is that a lot of people insist you leave your baby in nursery because 'she will get more stimulation there'. You will be lucky if the carer has time to take her out of the cot from time to time!

One of the other standards suggested by the AAP is that parents be allowed to observe the care given to their children. And this is something that has always surprised me about nurseries: their secretiveness. Few Spanish nurseries allow parents inside, not even when they come to pick up their children. A nice young woman ushers the children in, or out, while their parents wait outside. I mean to say, you are their parents, and they aren't even three years old. This isn't a boot camp! Parents should be allowed to enter the nursery at any time during the day, without asking permission, and to remain in the classroom with their child as long as they want. Absurd arguments are used to justify denying parents this basic right: the child gets upset, and it interferes with the teacher's work. Parents are allowed to come and go as they please in hospitals, where the work people do is a lot more difficult, and where the child has many more reasons to get upset. Mothers are even allowed into intensive care, with certain restrictions; and yet their child's day nursery is off limits. Pay no attention to the catastrophic scenes they will evoke of hordes of fathers, mothers and grandmothers all crammed in to a tiny room with eight children all day; the reason you leave your child at a nursery is precisely because you can't be with her the whole time – what is wrong with you having a spare moment once a week to pop in and see her? When I come across a nursery that won't allow parents inside, I ask myself what it is that they don't want us to see.

How do you choose a nursery for your child? It is important to find out how many children there are per caregiver, and it is even more important to know what sort of care your child will receive. This will depend on the character of the individual caregiver. Visit the nursery. Do the children of between one and three have enough space to run around, do they have fun toys to play with, or are they made to sit down and do 'educational' activities? Children this age don't need to learn about shapes and colours; what they need is attention and affection. Do the caregivers seem kind and affectionate? Can you drop in and see the children, and watch their carer in action, even if you are only watching through a window? Many nurseries take the children out to the park every day; this is a good opportunity for you to see the sort of care they receive.

A childminder will care exclusively for your child (and possibly two or three others, if she looks after him at her house), but this costs more. In Spain some local councils provide training and supervision for women who look after children in their own homes. In many cases, it is up to parents to choose and supervise a childminder, and this can be a very delicate task. Don't hesitate to ask a lot of questions, and to demand references. Also, talk to the parents of other children the childminder has looked after. Some nurseries may be able to recommend a student of childcare who is training with them.

It is important for the childminder to commit for a medium term of at least one year, ideally until your child is able to start school. Of course, unforeseen events can happen, and of course you won't be able stop the person from leaving. But you can at least make sure she has the intention of caring for your baby for a while. It isn't good for babies to change childminders every few months. Someone who only wants to work for a few months while they try to find a better job should be looking after older children, not babies.

→ American Academy of Pediatrics Committee on Early Childhood, Adoption, and Dependent Care, 'Quality early education and child care from birth to kindergarten', *Pediatrics* 2005;115:187-191 aappolicy.aappublications.org/cgi/reprint/ pediatrics;115/1/187.pdf

Meeting the childminder

It is important for your child to meet the person who is going to look after him in advance. If it is his grandmother or another family member, he will probably already be familiar with them. But not necessarily: if he only sees his grandmother from time to time, she will be as much of a stranger to him as anyone else.

Try to arrange a transition period before you go back to work. If you plan to use a childminder, employ her a few weeks in advance. If you are going to use a nursery, start going there a few weeks before you begin work. But take note: the idea isn't to leave your baby for half an hour with the childminder, or at the nursery, and the next day leave him for an hour, and so on. This would be a gradual change, and although it might be slightly less bad than a sudden change, it is still far from ideal. In addition, by making this gradual change you have brought forward the separation by two weeks, so you haven't achieved anything.

The idea is for mother, baby and childminder to be together for a while, or for you to be able to spend a few hours with your child at the nursery, or for the childminder to come to your house or accompany you and your baby to the park for a few hours every day. Some nurseries already allow mothers in during this period, and hopefully all nurseries will soon realise that not only can they 'allow' it, but that it is also in their interests.

When the baby sees the childminder with his mother, in some sense he classifies her as 'mummy's friend', and transfers some of his trust to her. In addition, since he is happy and contented (because he is with his mother), he is more likely to be open to new people and places, and he will enjoy the experience. In contrast, the child who is left alone at a nursery for the first time immediately starts crying. If he associates new people and places with his distress, he may develop an aversion to them. He will end up getting used to it, but the process will take much longer. In his memory, the beginning of term will always be associated with tears and upset.

When (in Spain) children start school aged three, it is precisely the ones who haven't been to nurseries who usually cry the least. At that age, children are normally ready to be separated from their mothers for a few hours, and they don't get upset. But many children who went to a nursery retain the memory of their suffering on that first day a year or more before.

The transition period also helps you to be sure you have found the right childminder. If you discover something about her that you don't like, there is still time for you to find someone else.

What will she eat when I'm not there?

There are several possibilities. For example, a carer can feed her formula from a bottle. In mentioning this first, I am not suggesting it is the best option, only that it is an option. I have seen many mothers wean their babies before going back to work (sometimes a month before), because, they argue: 'I won't be able to breastfeed her when I'm working'. One mother I knew decided not to breastfeed her baby at all, not even for a day, because she decided it wasn't worth it for four months. It is true that you won't be able to breastfeed your baby at work (not until women are allowed to take their children with them to work), but you can breastfeed her in the morning and evening, during the night, and on weekends. If you are planning to give her formula anyway, why not also breastfeed her in the evenings? That way you will spare your child one more upset (babies don't like their mothers leaving them, and they don't like being weaned either). Weaning them and going back to work is a double blow. Your milk will make her more resistant (not completely, of course, that would be impossible) to the many viruses she will be exposed to at nursery. And you will feel better, after being away from your baby the whole day, if you can breastfeed her when you get home.

You can also express your milk. As this takes a bit of explaining, I have given it a subchapter of its own (see page 192).

You can give your baby other things than milk. Remember, food is just as nourishing no matter what time of the day it is eaten. I say this because the custom in Spain of giving babies fruit in the afternoon and vegetables in the evening is so deeply ingrained in some people, that many mothers express their milk and leave it in the fridge for the grandmother to give to the baby during the morning, and when they get home they feed him fruit. There is no reason for the grandmother not to feed the baby fruit, chicken, meatballs, lentils or any other kind of food, and then when the mother gets home she breastfeeds him as much as possible. This is why I think it is such a good idea to take a few months' unpaid leave, because after six months the baby can eat solids and everything becomes a lot easier.

If you go back to work when your baby is four to six months old, and you don't want to or can't express your milk, it is better to start your baby on solids a little early than to give her formula. The reason for this is that milk and other dairy products, or products made with milk (including cereals made with milk and yoghurt) are the main cause of food allergies in young children. It is safer to feed your baby boiled rice or mashed banana. (I mention these because they are relatively high in calories, and if the idea is for the baby to go for a few hours without nursing, boiled vegetables and apple, which are largely made up of water, won't do the trick). Until she is six months old, breastfeed her as often as you can, and only give her solids when it is absolutely necessary.

And now comes the most entertaining part. After racking your brains to think of something your baby might eat, I have to inform you that she probably won't eat anything.

Older babies, who are already eating substantial amounts of solids, will probably carry on eating when their mother goes back to work. But babies of between four and six months (and many until eight or ten months) who are almost exclusively breastfed, will probably refuse to eat at all. They won't accept the bottle, not even when it contains breastmilk – less so than when it contains formula. They won't take milk from a cup, or from a dropper. They won't eat banana or boiled rice. They won't eat anything. If you have a reduced working day and are only away for five or six hours, your child probably won't eat during that time. But even when the mother works an eight-hour day (nine or ten including journey time), many children will still refuse to eat. They simply don't eat during the day, and spend most of the time asleep, and then they make up for it by feeding like crazy in the evening and at night. This is why a lot of working mothers decide to have their baby in the bed with them, as it is the only way to get some sleep and let the baby feed as much as she likes.

It is a good idea to top her up before you leave the house. Set your alarm so that you have time to nurse her in bed, and then after you have had your shower, got dressed and had breakfast, let her nurse again just before you leave the house. Or, if you are going to leave her at nursery, try to find one near to where you work and breastfeed her on the train or bus.

Of course, some babies will eat while their mother is at work. They will accept solids, milk, the bottle, everything. The problem is, we can't know in advance whether a baby will eat or not. And so it is always a good idea to be prepared. Leave the childminder with clear instructions about heating milk, mashing banana and so on, and also warn her that the baby might refuse to eat, or only eat a few spoonfuls, and not to worry or panic or try to force her.

Becoming used to feeding

While it is an excellent idea to acquaint your baby with the childminder before you go back to work, trying to accustom her to the bottle or the spoon in advance is a waste of time.

If the bottle contains formula, or you put her on solids when she could still be exclusively breastfeeding, her nutrition will suffer. And if the bottle contains expressed breastmilk, or you try to feed her breastmilk from a cup, it is a waste of energy and can be counterproductive because of the anxiety it causes.

When you bottle feed a baby for the first time, one of two things can happen: the baby either takes the bottle or she refuses it. (Incidentally, she is more likely to take the bottle when you aren't in the house.) If you give your baby the bottle a month, or a fortnight before you go to work, and she takes it willingly, what have you gained? She would most likely have done the same a fortnight later. All you have achieved is to substitute something relaxing and wonderful (breastfeeding) for something far more cumbersome (expressing your milk and putting it in a bottle).

On the other hand, if you give her the first bottle and she refuses it, spits it out and gets upset, what can you do? Block her nose so she opens her mouth, and try to force-feed her? You will only succeed in making your last two weeks at home a nightmare for you both, instead of a joy, and your baby will develop a genuine aversion to the bottle. Leave the house for eight hours so that the baby understands she isn't going to be breastfed, and accepts a bottle from her grandmother? In this case, what is the point of having sixteen weeks' maternity leave, if after twelve or fourteen weeks you leave her alone with her grandmother? You may as well go to work, instead of wasting eight hours out of the house; at least you would be doing something useful.

Don't try to habituate your baby in advance. Simply wait until the day you start work, and see how it goes. If your baby goes to sleep, she should be left in peace. If she wakes up and seems happy, the childminder can play with her. If she wakes up and seems hungry, the childminder can try feeding her whatever you have agreed on, from a cup, a bottle or with a spoon. If she eats, good, if not then it doesn't matter; it simply means she isn't hungry and prefers to wait until her mother comes home.

Expressing your milk

Expressing milk is an art. How easy do you think it would be to milk a cow? Well, expressing milk from a breast (even if it is your own) is no less of an acquired skill. It can be done quickly and easily once you know how, but it takes a bit of learning. It is a good idea to practice for a few weeks, at least, before D-day.

You can express your milk by hand or with a breast pump. Expressing by hand has many advantages: you don't have to buy a pump and you don't have to wash it, and you can do it anywhere. Mothers who are familiar with both methods usually agree that doing it by hand is easier and less painful than using a pump. The only inconvenience is that you have to learn how to do it, and that in our mechanised society using a pump is considered more 'sophisticated', and many women regard with trepidation the idea of expressing their milk by hand.

When you read about how to express your milk by hand, it will no doubt seem unnecessarily complicated. Remember that things will be a lot easier if you take some unpaid leave and go back to work when your baby is a little older and able to eat solids.

I am referring here to working mothers, and therefore to healthy babies of several months, who will continue feeding mostly from the breast. The situation is slightly different for a baby who is premature, or sick and in hospital. If your baby falls into either of these two categories, follow the advice they give you at the hospital.

Getting the milk out

First wash your hands. You needn't wash your breasts, unless for some reason they are particularly dirty.

It is a good idea to massage your breasts gently from the base towards the nipple. Women with large breasts sometimes lean forward and shake them with their hands. Touch your nipple (over your clothes is best, as fingers, even if you wash them, have many more microbes on them than nipples) in order to stimulate the milk ejection reflex. If your baby isn't with you, look at a photograph of her or a piece of clothing that reminds you of her, as this helps stimulate the reflex.

If you are expressing your milk by hand, make a 'C' with your thumb and fingers and place them a few centimetres from the base of the breast (for many women this means outside the areola, but inside for those whose areola is very large). Begin by pressing with your fingers away from your nipple (towards your ribs) and then squeeze your fingers together, compressing the breast firmly between thumb and forefinger. It isn't a good idea to let your fingers slide over the skin as it can end up chafing. Change the position of your fingers, moving round the nipple, and keep doing this while the milk is coming out. When the milk has almost stopped coming out, change breasts. You can probably find another mother, either through a mother's group or through your midwife, who knows how to express milk and can give you a demonstration.

If you prefer to use a breast pump, there are several different models. There are manual ones, in the shape of a giant syringe with a stopper that moves in and out, battery-operated ones, and small electric ones, which you may be able to have on loan or hire from a hospital, mother's group or a mail-order company. Hospitals sometimes have enormous electric pumps, which you can't use at home as they are too expensive. Each model has several different manufacturers. Find out from other mothers which one they used, and whether it worked well for them. Read the instructions that come with the pump; it would also be helpful to find a mother who has used the same model.

There is one model of breast pump I don't recommend: it is shaped like a trumpet, or bicycle horn, with a rubber bulb, which you squeeze and release. Most mothers agree that it is very painful and doesn't express much milk.

Whether you are expressing by hand or with a pump, it is normal on the first day for nothing to come out. Above all, don't be disheartened. I have heard one mother say: 'I tried using a breast pump and nothing came out, so obviously I have no milk', despite having a big bouncing baby who was clearly getting food from somewhere. If no milk comes out, it just means you aren't doing it properly. This is why you have to start practising a few weeks in advance.

Don't pulverise your breasts. It is better to try expressing milk several times a day (as often as you can) for five or ten minutes, than keep insisting for a whole hour, because you have decided on the first day not to give up until you have expressed 100ml. You may try for an hour and find you still haven't managed to express that amount. No, the aim on the first day is to express a few drops, and with any luck a few millilitres. If by any chance your milk comes out easily, this is wonderful and you are extremely lucky. The ease with which a woman expresses her milk has nothing to do with the amount of milk she produces, or with how easily her baby draws her milk out when nursing (although you can be sure that your baby does it a thousand times better than you).

For the first couple of days, you can discard the few drops of milk that come out (or add them to your coffee). When you begin to express larger amounts, 40–50ml at a time, you can begin freezing it.

You will usually keep the milk you express for the following day. There is no need to freeze this milk. It can be kept in the fridge. Any milk you aren't going to use the following day can be frozen for emergencies, for example if one day you are unable to express enough milk, or your baby wakes up very hungry and uses up all the milk in the fridge. If you have to use that reserve of frozen milk, you can replace it with the milk you express on Friday or Saturday (see below).

When should you express your milk? Whenever is most convenient for you. Some mothers express their milk at work and take it home with them every day. In order to do this, you will need a nice, clean place, time to do it (you can split your breastfeeding break into two thirty-minute periods), a fridge (or a portable fridge) where you can store the expressed milk (this has to be hygienic, i.e. not a fridge which dozens of people have access to, or where things you wouldn't want to keep around food are stored), and a cool bag for taking it home in (you can use one of those bags for frozen food, and store the milk in it with an ice pack).

Other mothers can't or don't want to express their milk at work, or they only need to express a little because their breasts are too swollen, and they have to discard it anyway because they can only express it in the bathroom, and quite frankly... Don't worry, you can also express your milk at home every day. In theory, it doesn't matter whether you do it before or after you breastfeed, or between feeds. Whatever works best and is most convenient for you. If you have mastered the hand technique, it might be a good idea to express the milk from one breast while your baby is nursing from the other; this way you make use of the oxytocin, and the milk comes out more quickly. When you have finished, change sides, placing your baby on the breast you have just expressed (there will always be some milk left, and remember, it has more calories), and you can try to express milk from the breast she has just been feeding from (again, some milk will usually come out).

If you express milk from the breast your baby has just been nursing from, make sure you wipe her saliva off first.

Some women express all the milk they need in one go. Others have to repeat the procedure two or three times, or more, in the space of an afternoon. Remember that expressing milk works exactly the same way as breastfeeding: the more you do it, the more milk will come out. If you find it easy to express 50ml, say, but in order to get 100ml you have to squeeze a lot, and it ends up taking ages, don't persist; it is better to express 50ml and then an hour or two later express another 50ml.

There is no need to boil or sterilise the breast pump or the bowl you keep the milk in. Simply wash them as you do the crockery and cutlery you, your child and the rest of the family eats from. If the breast pump has tubes or places that are difficult to get to with a brush or sponge, it is important to rinse them immediately after use so that the milk doesn't dry on them.

Conserving your milk

There has been much discussion about whether it is better to keep breastmilk in plastic or glass containers. You may read about cells sticking more to one, or immunoglobulin sticking to the other. In fact, it makes no difference. Even if breastmilk loses some of its immunoglobulin, it is still much better than artificial milk, which has none. Use whatever containers you have at hand, whether glass or plastic. What matters is that they are easy to clean, and sealable. If they are made of plastic, make sure they are suitable for storing food (look for a cup and fork logo). They should be big enough to contain one feed of 150–200ml. If they are too small, it doesn't matter, you can use several, but if they are too big it will take up unnecessary space in your fridge. Label them with the date when the milk was expressed.

Breastmilk can be kept in the fridge for up to five days. In fact, it is a good idea during that time not to freeze it, because the immunoglobulin and other factors will attack any microbes, which instead of multiplying will decrease. Normally, though, you will only keep it in the fridge for a day or two. Most mothers express their milk every day for the following day, from Sunday through to Thursday, and keep a small frozen reserve in case one day they don't express enough milk, or their baby is still hungry. This reserve will build up over the practice period, before they go back to work. If the reserve gets used up, it can be replaced with what you express on Friday and Saturday.

If you express your milk several times a day, you can keep it in the same container, adding it to the milk already cold or frozen.

Don't mix milk that has been expressed on different days; use a fresh container for each day. If you are planning to freeze the milk, put it in smaller containers of less than 100ml, even if you have to fill two or more of these in the same day. As it is meant for emergencies, you probably won't need a large amount all at once. If your baby has her usual 150ml and is still hungry, she won't need another 150ml. And if you thaw a large container, you will have to discard the leftover milk (or drink it yourself).

The length of time you can keep the milk frozen depends on how good your freezer is. Roughly speaking it will keep for longer than a steak in the same freezer. Meat is dead flesh. It has been dead for days, and a lot of different people have handled it in the slaughterhouse, in the truck, in the freezer, in the shop, so that when you froze it, it was already covered in microbes. Breastmilk on the other hand is expressed and then frozen, and it is still full of immunoglobulin.

Some women's milk changes after it has been frozen for a few days, and gives off a strange smell, like rancid fat. This is due to the lipase (a digestive enzyme in breastmilk that aids the baby's digestion) acting on the fats in the milk, and starting to digest them. This problem can be avoided by scalding the milk just after you express it: heat it up until tiny bubbles appear at the sides of the pan, without letting it boil, and then immediately cool it. Doing this supposedly heats the milk to 80 degrees Centigrade.

→ Pardou, A., Serruys, E., Mascart-Lemone, F., Dramaix, M., Vis, H.L. 'Human milk banking: influence of storage processes and of bacterial contamination on some milk constituents', *Biol Neonate* 1994;65:302-9

How to heat up breastmilk

Some books recommend thawing the milk slowly, taking it out of the freezer the day before, and leaving it in the fridge. This has always seemed silly to me. First of all, it means the milk sits for a whole day half-frozen, and is therefore less well preserved. And secondly, if frozen milk is for emergencies, how is it possible to foresee the need for it one day in advance?

In order to thaw the milk quickly, some books recommend placing the container under a running tap, cold at first and then gradually hotter. Thawing it in this way involves leaving the tap running for a long time, which uses a lot of energy, and above all is a waste of water, which is real crime against nature.

I used to advise people to thaw milk in a bain marie, but with the gas turned off. In other words, heat water in a pan, and when it is hot, but not too hot to put your hand in without burning yourself, turn the gas off and place the container of frozen milk in the pan. If the water is too hot, a glass container could crack because of the sudden change in temperature. This method is quick, efficient and environmentally friendly, but I no longer recommend it for fear of accidents. Given that by definition the mother isn't around, it is usually the grandmother who carries out the operation (and her reflexes aren't as quick as they once were) or the father (who is 'klutz' in the kitchen), and if the baby is crying because he is hungry it might make them anxious. They may try to console the baby with one hand while thawing the milk with the other. The hot water could scald the baby, or he might touch the gas ring, which is off, but still hot, and so on.

This is why I now recommend the following method, which is quick, environmentally friendly and accident-proof. Fill a large pan with hot water from the tap, place the container in it and wait. If the water goes cold change it as often as necessary.

You can also thaw or warm up milk in a microwave. Some books advise against it because it destroys the immunoglobulin; but not all of it is destroyed, and in any event formula has no immunoglobulin either. It doesn't matter if an older baby gets a little less immunoglobulin in one of his daily feeds (it would be different in the case of a premature baby, who needs this immunological defence). If the milk is heated to the right temperature, without being allowed to boil, it alters very little. In fact, the problem with microwaves isn't that they alter the milk, but rather that they can scald the baby.

Microwaving is the only method of heating things up that allows the centre of something to get hotter than the surface, and in an uneven way, so that one part can be much hotter than the rest. More precisely, a bottle may feel warm to the touch, but some of the milk inside can be almost boiling. When microwave ovens first appeared, and nobody really knew how they worked, there were several cases of scalded mouths and throats, and experts advised against heating babies' bottles in the microwave, whether they contained formula or breastmilk.

However, if you use the microwave sensibly it is perfectly safe. Remember that if you keep the timer and temperature settings the same to heat up a large or a small amount of milk, the larger amount will heat up more slowly. It is better to use a medium to low setting, because the milk will heat up more slowly, and you can control the temperature more easily. Heat it for a few moments, check the temperature, and then if necessary heat it some more. Most importantly, make sure that you give it a good shake before giving it to the baby to mix the heated milk through, and test it by putting a few drops on to the back of your hand or your inner wrist, the way the temperature of baby milk has always been tested.

Once it has been thawed, use the milk within twenty-four hours.

How to feed a baby expressed milk
It is normal for breastmilk to separate and for the cream to float to the top. Just give it a good shake.

Some babies will take their mother's expressed milk from a bottle, and then switch to breastfeeding without any difficulty. Others, even if they have been breastfed for months, pick up bad habits and start nursing in an incorrect position, which can lead to rejection of the breast, painful nipples and cracks. There are also many, many babies who are used to breastfeeding, and refuse the bottle completely.

With one thing and another, the bottle isn't usually the best option. Try it if you want, but you will probably find it easier to feed her from a cup. You can also use a spoon, a syringe or a dropper; these methods can be good for giving small amounts of supplement to a newborn; but feeding 150ml or more to a bigger baby with a teaspoon can be excruciating.

Feeding a baby from a cup sounds strange in our culture, and your female friends and relatives will probably be shocked. But it can be done. It is the custom in some countries to feed babies who are hospitalised from a cup, even premature babies. In some studies, where the nurse is familiar with the technique, premature babies feed more quickly and spill milk less from a cup than from

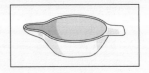

Figure 15: A paladai.

a bottle (other studies show the opposite, but I suspect this is because the nurses hadn't mastered the technique).

The ideal vessel should be small and have a pouring spout, like some saucepans or lemon squeezers. In India they use a traditional cup called a *paladai* (see *Figure 15*). You may find a similar vessel, or perhaps a toy saucepan. Otherwise, a small wine or liqueur glass will do.

First hold the baby upright. If you are right-handed, it is probably more practical to sit the baby on your left thigh and hold on to her with your left arm while you give her the milk with your right hand. Half-fill the cup, and place it in the baby's mouth so that it is touching the corners of her mouth; if you don't touch the corners of the mouth the milk will easily spill. Then tip the glass until the milk reaches the rim. Some babies drink like grown-ups, others like cats, with their tongue.

I have described the technique as though you were going to do it yourself, but in fact someone else is going to do it while you are at work. As I said above about bottles: it isn't necessary or a good idea to accustom your baby to feeding from a cup before you go back to work, but it is necessary to explain the technique properly to the baby's grandmother, or whoever will be giving her the milk.

The amount should be however much the baby wants. Any milk left over in the bottle or glass will be mixed with the baby's saliva, and is a haven for bacteria, so it is best to throw it away. This is why it is best to give her 50ml, and if she finishes that, another 50ml, rather than to start with 200ml, because if she only takes 50ml and then falls asleep, you will have to throw the rest away, and two hours later she might wake up wanting more.

If the baby seems hungry, but is having difficulty feeding from the cup or bottle, try thickening the milk with some cereal and feeding it to her with a spoon. This is a good way of 'eking out' the milk if one day there isn't enough in the fridge. If the baby refuses the cup or the bottle, and doesn't seem hungry, remember that this is normal, and you shouldn't worry, or try to force her to eat.

Political considerations

In Spain, maternity leave is only sixteen weeks. Well, in fact, the law only guarantees six. Convention C103 of The General Conference of the International Labour Organization of 1952 recommends twelve weeks of maternity leave, so sixteen wasn't that bad. However, the new convention C183 from the year 2000 (which the Spanish government, and those of the UK and US, had still not ratified by 2012 – I am not sure what they are waiting for) recommends fourteen, and in the Maternity Recommendation R191 it says: 'Members should endeavour to extend the period of maternity leave referred to in Article 4 of the Convention to at least 18 weeks'. However, in Spain, the 'Law for the reconciliation of work and family life' of 1999 established that only six out of the sixteen weeks are 'compulsory', and that the father may take the remaining ten weeks in place of the mother. So in Spain, mothers in fact have only six weeks' maternity leave guaranteed, far fewer than the eighteen or more weeks most European countries allow.

Needless to say, this development was presented (and apparently accepted) as an important advancement for women's liberation. At last we would all be equal, and fathers would take part in looking after the children.

But how can an encroachment on women's rights be seen as an advancement? They weren't awarding fathers sixteen weeks' leave to equal the mothers' sixteen weeks, but clawing back leave from the mother and awarding it to her partner. This was an attempt to imitate a law passed a year earlier in Sweden, where the circumstances are very different: maternity leave in Sweden is twenty-two months, so there is more to share!

The fact that these sixteen weeks aren't 'compulsory' means they are neither an advancement nor a liberation. Negotiations between employee and employer can't take place on equal terms because the employer has far more bargaining power. This is why employees' rights must be 'compulsory', established in law or in conventions: the forty-hour week is compulsory, wages are compulsory, holidays and bonuses are compulsory. If they weren't, if an employee could 'volunteer' to work a fifty-hour week (for the same pay) or only take two weeks' paid holiday, imagine the sort of pressure employees would be under? Well, some women still get that pressure: 'You're not taking the whole sixteen weeks, are you! You know how busy we are, and besides, I can't find anyone to replace you. Take two months' leave, and let your husband take the rest. Remember you're up for promotion…' And for his part, the father may suffer the same pressure: 'What? A month's paternity leave! You're kidding, right? That's women's stuff! Yes, I know, you have a legal right, but don't expect any favours afterwards…'

A few years ago in Spain, a petition was signed demanding six months' maternity leave (six months was a first step towards catching up with the rest of Europe). Nothing came of it.

I have explained, according to the usual methods, how to express your milk, and leave it in the fridge, how to freeze and thaw it etc. And yet I am still not satisfied.

Expressing breastmilk is sometimes seen as 'the solution' that allows mothers to combine work with breastfeeding, that allows working mothers to continue to breastfeed their baby. I have read it so many times, and repeated it so many times: the importance of having a special room at work for expressing milk, with a fridge, of having a crèche in the workplace.

Until one day I became indignant. What kind of a solution is this? It seems more like a mockery. Like saying to a mother: 'Leave your milk, which is the most important thing, in the fridge, and go off to work. Your baby will be fine as long as she gets your milk'. As though a mother's milk were the only (or the most important) thing a mother gives her baby.

Well, it isn't. I am supposed to be pro-breastfeeding, but if I were a baby I would far prefer my mother to stay at home and bottle feed me than to go off and leave somebody else to feed me her milk. Expressing milk isn't a solution, it is merely a stop-gap measure for what is a serious socio-economical problem; a completely wrong-headed way of organising work that puts the needs of children and mothers at the bottom of a list of priorities.

Of course it is often impossible for a mother not to be separated from her child, and clearly in such cases expressing your milk can be useful. But we mustn't see it '*the* solution', otherwise we (and those who govern us) will stop searching for a proper solution. Why give mothers longer maternity leave when it is much cheaper to hand out pamphlets telling them how to express their milk?

Chapter 11
COMPLEMENTARY FEEDING

A useful summary

You may have noticed that I don't like to say things 'just because', but rather to provide an explanation. The less what I say chimes with what 'everyone else' says, the longer that explanation has to be.

I realised that this chapter about solids was becoming very long, and might not prove all that useful, so I decided to begin by explaining a few useful things. Those who want to know why will find explanations in the following sections.

A few important details (That needn't be articles of faith)

- Never force a baby to eat.
- Until your baby is six months only feed her breastmilk: no baby food, no juice, no water, no herbal teas, not even juice freshly squeezed at home. There are some exceptions: if, when she is four to six months old she sees her parents eating and asks for solids, you can give her a little. If the mother works and can't or doesn't want to express her milk, it is better to start her on solids than to give her formula.
- At six months, begin to offer her solids after she nurses (without insisting). When she is ready she will start eating solids before nursing.
- Don't skip a feed in order to give her solids; until she is one year old she should nurse five to seven times a day (or more). Your baby will gradually reduce the number of feeds herself, until she is only nursing once or twice a day, but this shouldn't happen in the first year. Obviously, if you are a working mum, she will inevitably miss a few feeds, but she can make up for this by nursing more often

in the evening, and during the night.

- In the first few weeks, offer her one new food at a time, in small amounts, and with a few days in between.

- While she is still nursing, before she turns seven months, start giving her gluten (wheat, barley, rye or oats); for a month or more only in tiny amounts (that means most of the cereals she eats will be gluten-free).

- If she is breastfeeding on demand, she will be getting enough milk, of the best quality. She won't need any other milk or dairy products, so don't feed her yoghurt (even if it says on the label that it is suitable for babies) or milk-based baby foods. If you are using powdered cereals, make sure they contain no milk and don't add milk to them (dissolve them in hot water or broth). I am not saying this because I am anti-milk, but because the milk used in baby foods frequently causes allergies.

- Drain her foods; don't fill her tummy with soup, or broth, or the water from boiling.

- Allergenic foods (in particular milk and other dairy products, eggs, fish, peanuts and other nuts): for years parents have been advised to delay feeding them to babies, especially if the child has a history of allergy. Experts have recently concluded that there is no concrete evidence to suggest that delaying the introduction of these foods prevents allergy, not even in children with a history of allergies. Still, given we have to start somewhere and we can't introduce them all at once, it might be a good idea to begin with the least allergenic.

- Don't add sugar to the baby's food. Or salt (or if you do, only a little and make sure it is iodized).

- Keep breastfeeding your baby until she is two or older.

- The order in which you introduce solids is unimportant. There is not an age for meat, an age for fruit, etc. But don't delay meat: it's rich in iron, the only thing that your baby really needs on top of breastmilk.

- Once your baby is a year old, she can eat anything, unless for specific medical reasons (obviously within reason; there is no need to feed her fifty new types of food on her first birthday).

A few useful tips

(The following are personal preferences. If you don't like them, feel free to do things differently.)

Nursing babies prefer to eat what their mother eats, rather than specially prepared baby foods.

There is no need to blend her food (with a stick blender or food processor). Blenders were only invented a few decades ago, and prior to that I don't think any child suffered from malnutrition due to a lack of blended food. You can try placing some of the food on your plate within easy reach of your baby:

- Apple or pear, grated (but not too finely), or very thinly sliced (so they droop in your fingers).
- Banana, very thinly sliced or mashed with a fork. She can also can hold the banana and nibble the end.
- Orange or mandarin; she can suck on a segment while you hold it (so it doesn't choke her).
- Boiled vegetables mashed with a fork or diced into finger-sized chunks. Mixed vegetables are ideal, though you might want to peel the peas the first few times.
- Chicken or meat (poached, roasted, grilled or fried – but not in batter if she hasn't started eating eggs yet): you can cut the meat into narrow strips against the grain (she will probably only eat one or two strips). You can also fry some plain minced meat in a little oil in a pan, which will form into finger-sized lumps.
- Plain boiled rice. If you add a dash of olive oil she will probably like it more, and it will provide a few more calories. A few days later try adding some fried tomato.
- Bread: she can gnaw on a crust.
- Pasta: babies can take spaghetti or macaroni with their hands; if you prefer to spoonfeed, you can use alphabet soup, but drain off the liquid first.
- Pulses: boiled and mashed. To begin with you should remove the skin on chickpeas and beans.

Most days you won't need to cook special food for your baby. It will be enough to plan your meals with her in mind, and leave aside a portion without any salt or spices or any ingredients your baby shouldn't eat. For example, you can cook lentils with chorizo, or rice with rabbit; just take out the chorizo (which she probably won't like because it is spicy – though you never know) and the rabbit (because it has too many small bones). On the other hand, if she hasn't started eating fish, don't give her rice that has been cooked with fish (like paella) because, even if you don't give her any of the fish itself, the rice could trigger an allergic reaction. Remember, it only takes a tiny amount: I have seen babies come out in hives just from licking a dairy ice cream. Cheap pasta is made from durum wheat, but the more expensive kind contains egg. Most cakes and biscuits contain some milk, so make sure to always read the list of ingredients.

In Spain it used to be customary to introduce foods by month: 'Fruit after so many months, cereal after so many months, vegetables after so many months …' These were often mixed: four types of fruit, four types of vegetable, endless types of cereal. It is probably a good idea to introduce foods one at a time, at least to begin with (some people insist on introducing one a week, but it needn't be exactly one week). A lot of mothers try to combine traditional and modern approaches: so, for example, they start with apples, and a few days later they introduce bananas, then pears, then oranges, and so on. However, there is no need to set aside a special month for each food group. It is probably best to give your baby as varied a diet as possible in as short a time. For example, start with rice, then chicken, then peas, then banana. But you could just as well make that chicken, apples, carrots, rice, or pears, rice, lentils, chicken. Regardless of the order, the fact is that by the time your baby is seven months old, she will have a variety of foods to choose from.

The vitamin C from fruit or tomatoes helps the body absorb the iron in cereals, vegetables, and pulses more efficiently (without vitamin C, the iron content in vegetables is difficult to absorb). In order for this to happen, the different foods need to be in the stomach at the same time. This is why it makes no sense to separate the baby's food into types (cereals in the morning, vegetables at lunch, fruit in the evening), and what we adults do is far more sensible: the vitamin C in salad or fruit helps us to absorb the iron in the main meal.

In some countries, in order to give babies only small amounts of gluten, baby foods are wheat-free (barley, rye and oats contain far less gluten than wheat). The most recent recommendations suggest starting babies on gluten before seven months, but this could change. To my knowledge, all baby foods in Spain that contain gluten also contain wheat. You can mix the two together: a teaspoon of baby food containing gluten and the rest gluten-free. Or, if you are feeding your baby cereals prepared at home, you can give her a 'dish' of boiled rice and let her gnaw on a crust of bread every day. For the first month at least, she should eat very little gluten; after that she can eat as much as she likes.

One mother wrote out what her ten-month-old daughter Nuria ate (in addition to breastfeeding, which her mother claimed accounted for 95 per cent of her diet). I have copied it out in its entirety, as it is the perfect example of a balanced diet:

With her fingers:
- Orange and mandarin segments (she used to spit them out after sucking out the juice, now she eats nearly everything; she eats roughly half an orange or mandarin a day, in two stages, and nearly always with other food).
- She is gradually beginning to eat a few slices of other kinds fruit.
- Bread or toast: she tears bits off herself, and chews and swallows them.
- Boiled rice with a tiny bit of olive oil on it; she eats it a grain at a time, but she might eat about twenty altogether; occasionally I put peas or green beans in the rice and she eats some of them.
- Chicken; she tears the meat of the chicken thigh and also eats some of it.
- Four or five pasta quills.
- About 1/6 of a slice of ham.
- Lately some of the soft parts of cured ham.
- Occasionally she nibbles at a homemade French fry or eats chickpeas one at a time.

From a spoon (me guiding it at one end while she clutches it in the middle: she has never let me put the spoon in her mouth on my own, not even when I fed her puréed baby food):
- Occasionally, four teaspoons of (unpuréed) ratatouille made from onion, tomato, pepper and courgette.
- Occasionally lentil stew (unpuréed).

Thousands of desperate mothers of two or three year-olds, who will only eat puréed food if their mother feeds it to them, and who 'if there's a bit that hasn't been puréed' choke on it, will look with envy at the mother of Nuria, who at ten months eats all kinds of 'proper' food, and even feeds herself. And yet Nuria's mother writes to me, concerned because her daughter refuses to let her mother feed her 'baby food'.

How clever children are! Nuria prefers the healthy, varied, simple diet of adults to baby food. She prefers to eat with her fingers than to be fed by her mother. And she is eating what she needs: four teaspoons of vegetables or five pasta quills, or twenty rice grains, and the rest she gets from nursing. The main aim of complementary feeding is to gradually accustom children to eating normal, adult food. A baby who happily eats half a pasta quill with her fingers has made an important step in the right direction; months later she will eat five pasta quills, and years later a whole plateful. In contrast, a child who eats a whole jar of puréed baby food made of 'nine cereals', which his mother has to struggle to feed him using subterfuge, hasn't made any progress at all. He isn't learning to eat on his own, or to chew, or to enjoy eating, or to eat the kind of food eaten by adults (who clearly don't eat 'nine cereals'). And besides, eating a lot of cereals (or fruit or vegetables) means he is nursing less. And this isn't good for him, because breastmilk is far healthier and more nutritious than any other type of food with which they try to substitute it.

Almost any child will eat the way Nuria does if, from the beginning, they are given half a chance. Children at her age like to do things for themselves, and they want to try the food they see their parents eating. But if we don't let them experiment, because it takes too long, or because we want them to eat more, and not to make a mess, and we hold down their hands (so they don't get in the way) and put the spoon in their mouths, it will probably take them years to start eating independently.

Google 'baby-led weaning' and you will see what a wealth of information there is on the subject. And if you look on Google images, you will see dozens of babies happily eating normal, unpuréed food, with their fingers, from the very start.

Free yourselves from puréed food.

The naming of things

Any food you give a baby besides breastmilk or artificial milk is a complementary food. This includes purées, juices, sugar water, sweetened herbal teas, biscuits, or a bottle with a tablespoon of added cereal. You may think that sugar water doesn't count as a food, but in fact it contains a lot of calories. It isn't a very good complementary food (in fact, it is dreadful), but it isn't plain water.

I like the word 'complementary', because it clearly implies the existence of a 'primary' source of nourishment (guess which one), to which everything else is secondary. However, 'complementary food' is a bit of a mouthful, so from now on I will refer to 'solids' in the generic sense. By this I don't just mean puréed food eaten with a spoon, but also bite-size chunks that babies can clutch with their fingers, or anything the baby drinks besides milk. In fact, because I think it is better for babies to avoid puréed food from the outset, I will try to avoid referring to it at all.

Some know-it-alls may read: 'start introducing solids from six months' and argue that juices and cereals from a bottle are liquids not solids, and are suitable for a baby of two to three months. This isn't true. Before six months, the recommendation is to give babies nothing but milk: no solids, no liquids, no gases, nothing. Other mothers take this to the opposite extreme and define 'solids' in the strictest sense, excluding puréed foods; a mother once told me that her two-year-old still wasn't eating 'solids'!

Speaking of cereal from a bottle: it isn't a good idea. A baby who is breastfeeding should never be bottle fed; and a baby who is bottle feeding shouldn't be given cereal or anything else from his bottle. His bottle should only contain milk, and should only be used for a year. At six months it is a good idea to give him some of his feeds from a cup, so that at twelve months he will be able to drink from a cup by himself and can stop using bottles.

Of course, babies take more cereal more quickly from a bottle, but as I already mentioned, we don't want them eating too many solids. A baby's primary food is milk, and the more flour, fruit or vegetables he eats the less milk he will take. The aim is for the baby to learn to eat normally, and a baby who eats solids from a bottle isn't learning. I see more and more children of two and three who only eat solids from a bottle. I have even seen bottles containing vegetables and fish!

A bit of history

Throughout the twentieth century, the recommended age for starting babies on solids underwent significant changes. In *Figure 16* you can see the recommendations in various books by Spanish doctors (who weren't crazy scientists, but were making the same recommendations as their English, French and German colleagues at the time).

At the beginning of the twentieth century, babies started eating solids at twelve months. Up until then they were exclusively breastfed. In those days almost all babies were breastfed: the poor babies by their mothers and the rich babies by a wet nurse. In the worst-run orphanages (the best ones hired wet nurses) babies were fed on artificial milk, with dire results. Mortality rates were extremely high.

Cow's milk contains a lot of proteins and minerals, which a baby's kidneys are unable to eliminate, and it has to be diluted with water. But cow's milk also contains less lactose and fewer fats than human milk, and diluting it makes this worse. As there was no way of mixing fat into milk (the fat floated on the surface), they tried to compensate by adding plenty of sugar. And this was the way babies' bottles were prepared: so much milk, so much water, so much sugar. As time went on, other ingredients were added, until it became too complicated to prepare at home, and it had to be made up by a chemist. And that is why, to this day, artificial baby milk is referred to as 'formula'.

Some children survived thanks to these concoctions, but they had problems. There was no such thing then as industrial pasteurisation, where milk is boiled at the lowest temperature

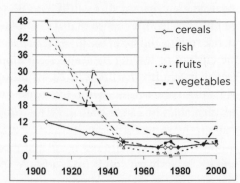

Figure 16: Recommended age for the introduction of the different food types, according to various Spanish books about childcare.

possible in order to destroy the bacteria while preserving vitamins. Milk was boiled at home, (fresh milk was responsible for the transmission of various diseases, including tuberculosis), and the vitamin C in it was destroyed. Babies who only received these primitive homemade formulas suffered from scurvy as a result of vitamin C deficiency. The iron in cow's milk is difficult to absorb, and diluting it with water lowered the iron content, so that these same babies also suffered from anaemia. Our main source of vitamin D comes not from our diet, but from the sun; when it is exposed to sunlight, our skin produces vitamin D. However, children kept in orphanages weren't taken out much, and they also suffered from rickets. What was the solution to these problems? Giving them fruit, especially orange juice, which prevents scurvy, iron-rich foods like red meat, and especially liver, which prevents anaemia, and foods rich in vitamin D like liver and fish, which prevent rickets. In 1920 a scientific study was made of the children in an orphanage, who were fed on a variety of solids from the tender age of six months, with, it would seem, remarkable success.

As a result of the First World War (and later on the Second World War), factories and offices opened their doors to women; the men were busy killing each other. This was the end of the age-old, noble profession of the wet nurse, which up until then had been one of the few ways a woman had of earning money. A wet nurse can't take the weekend off, leaving her charge to suck his thumb. A wet nurse worked twenty-four hours a day, seven days a week, 365 days a year, including on Christmas Day. Needless to say, the wet nurse slept with her 'customer' and nursed him at night. The babies of wealthy people didn't sleep with their parents (unlike the babies of poor people, who all slept together in one room). But don't imagine for one moment they slept alone; the custom of leaving babies to sleep alone in a room is a very recent invention. In English, the children's bedroom is called the 'nursery' from the word 'nurse', in French *nourrice*, and in Spanish *nodriza*. Every time the child woke up during the night, the wet nurse would suckle him: naturally, she wasn't being paid to leave him to cry. (Incidentally, before the advent of nursing schools, if anyone at home became ill, it was the wet nurse's job to look after them.)

So, the profession of wet nurse was one of the most arduous professions a woman could have. Who would want to look after another woman's child out of choice? Who would want to be a wet nurse when they could be a factory worker, a secretary or a telephone operator? There came a time when only women who were otherwise unemployable resorted to being wet nurses; women who were uneducated, in poor health, or of questionable morals. In the 1920s and 1930s, paediatricians began to warn of the dangers of leaving your child with a wet nurse, and even began to employ the derogatory term 'mercenary breastfeeding'. People with a lot of money would pay a fortune for the services of a trustworthy wet nurse. Women from the upper middle classes, who weren't millionaires, could no longer find reliable wet nurses, yet they weren't able to breastfeed themselves. There was a strong social prejudice that prevented a 'lady' from breastfeeding. Even today, many readers will have heard their own relatives reproach them for going round with their breasts hanging out all day! If people in the twenty-first century still dare to talk like this, imagine what they might have said in the 1930s. And so, women who enjoyed a certain social status (the architect's wife, the solicitor's wife... the doctor's wife!) began to bottle feed their babies. And their babies (the only ones who ever saw a doctor, because there was no national health service) began to suffer from scurvy, rickets and anaemia.

Paediatricians, who were understandably alarmed, came up with the most appropriate solution: to bring forward the introduction of solids progressively, to four months, two months, one month... One American expert in the 1940s even recommended sardines, tuna fish and prawns for babies of a few weeks old, while in Spain it was suggested that orange juice should be fed to babies over fifteen days old.

In the meantime, the old 'formula' prepared at home or by the chemist had become a thing of the past, and bottles were now filled with industrially produced artificial milk. Industry invested in perfecting its own product; the milk was enriched with vitamin C and D, as well as iron and dozens of other ingredients; if you have a tin of baby milk handy, look at the contents and you will see. Even today, advertisements for baby milk focus on the latest added ingredients; 'extra', 'enriched', 'fortified', with nucleotides, long-chain fatty acids and so on. As more and more nutrients were added to infant formula, so the need for solids diminished. Besides, the dangers of introducing solids too early became evident, in particular the risk of allergy (this had always existed, but had previously been considered a lesser evil; what did a few cases of allergy to fish matter compared to preventing hundreds of cases of rickets?) And so the introduction of solids was once again pushed back: to three months, to four months to 'between four and six months', to six months.

For years now, WHO, UNICEF, the AAP (American Academy of Paediatrics), the AEP (Asociacion Espanola de Pediatria) and the NHS in the UK have recommended exclusive breastfeeding until six months old, and after that introducing solids in addition to breastmilk.

We are creatures of habit, and we resist change. The age for introducing solids wasn't brought forward at the exact moment when wet nurses began to disappear, nor was it pushed back the moment baby milk was enriched with vitamins. In both cases, there was a delay of about twenty years, between when the need arose and when the solution was presented in books on motherhood. Despite this all-too-human delay, the astonishing changes we saw in *Figure 16* weren't the fads or whims of ignorant doctors, but rather the rational response of respectable, competent scientists to the needs of children at every moment.

The problem is that these changes, which reflected the changes in artificial milk, were also applied to babies who were being breastfed, even though breastmilk hadn't changed at all. Today's breastmilk is the same breastmilk our great-grandparents were fed on, exclusively, for a year. And they fared quite well on it.

A hundred years ago, scientific studies weren't as rigorous as they are now. Perhaps our great-grandparents, who were breastfed exclusively until they were a year old, weren't in perfect health. But they were certainly healthier than the children who ate other things – a fact paediatricians at the time were able to verify. Then again, of course, drinking water wasn't always safe, milk wasn't pasteurised, meat and fish weren't refrigerated and so on. Complementary feeding certainly isn't as dangerous now as it was a hundred years ago.

So we can't claim that exclusive breastfeeding for twelve months is best. Maybe scientists back then were mistaken. Or perhaps they were right, and at the time twelve months was the best advice, but today it is no longer true. In any event, after looking at *Figure 16*, I find it hard to believe that we have finally arrived at the absolute truth about feeding babies. If today's experts no longer agree with what other experts said twenty years ago, what will experts in twenty or fifty years be saying? I doubt this is the end of the debate, and personally I suspect the age for introducing solids will be pushed back even further. This is only my personal opinion; in the meantime, let us all agree on six months.

Why six months?

When deciding what the ideal age is for starting a baby on solids, there are two criteria to consider: one is theoretical, the other empirical.

The theoretical one goes something like this: 'Babies of "x" months old need so many milligrams of vitamin "x"; since breastmilk only contains so many milligrams, from "x" months' old onwards, babies need to eat other things.'

The empirical one is this: 'We compared 100 babies who were fed exclusively on breastmilk for "x" months with another 100 babies who were fed exclusively on breastmilk for "y" months. We compared their weight, their size, their psychomotor development, number of infections, incidence of anaemia etc., and concluded that the babies who were fed exclusively on breastmilk for "x" months had a better result than those who were fed exclusively on breastmilk for "y" months'.

Theoretical nutrient requirements in infants

The problem with theoretical arguments is that there isn't enough data to back up them up. We could almost say that we have no idea. To the basic question 'How many calories does a baby need?', *Table 2* provides several different answers.

AGE (months)	FAO/WHO/ UNU (1985)	WHO/ UNICEF (1988)	BUTTE (2000)
6–8	784	682	615
9–11	949	830	684
12–23	1170	1092	894

Table 2: Recommended daily intake (kcal), data from various authors compared by Dewey and Brown (2003)

I am only comparing figures taken from reliable, up-to-date sources. I dread to think what would happen if we started looking at all the books published in the last fifty years. Because of the methodology employed, Butte's figures seem to me the most consistent. Will these be the definitive ones, or will they change again in a few years time? Will they go down further or will they go up again? If Butte's figures are correct, what are the consequences of experts having recommended for years that babies be given 25 per cent more food than they needed? (Here is one for starters: babies refuse to eat that amount, and doctors' surgeries are full of babies who refuse to eat).

Of course, not all children eat the same amount. These figures are only an average, both in time and in space. In time, because a baby's caloric needs obviously don't jump from 684 to 894 calories overnight. They change gradually, and probably in a non-linear fashion – meaning that there may be periods when his caloric needs increase sharply, and other periods when they barely increase at all, or even go down. In space, because caloric needs are or should, by definition, be the average needs of the whole population. Anything between two standard deviations above or below the mean is considered statistically 'normal' (which is not the same thing as medically normal); 95 per cent of the medically healthy population will fall into this interval. Five per cent of healthy people (and a lot of sick people) are still outside these +/- 2 standard deviations.

AGE	BOYS	GIRLS
3 months	328–728	341–685
6 months	491–779	351–819
9 months	504–924	459–589
12 months	479–1159	505–1013
18 months	804–1112	508–1168
24 months	729–1301	661–1273

Table 3: Variability of energy needs (two standard deviations below and above the mean) according to age, sex in breastfeeding infants (data Butte, 2000)

As you can see in *Table 3*, one baby's daily caloric needs can be more than double those of another, and yet both are considered normal. If we gave these two babies the same amount, either one would suffer from malnutrition, or the other would become obese. And remember, there are still over 2 per cent of babies that need a little less food, and over 2 per cent that need a little more.

If there is a big disparity between the figures for caloric needs, when it comes to specific nutrients (proteins, vitamins, minerals) the gulf is enormous. By definition, nutrient intake requirements aren't based on the average of the population, but on two standard deviations above the mean. This is usually rounded up to the nearest number to make things neat. So when we are told a person needs 30mg of Vitamin 'X' daily, it is because the experts think (more often than not they don't 'know', they just 'think') that 97.5 per cent of the population needs less than that amount. Officially these aren't called 'needs', but are referred to differently in different countries: in the UK, they refer to RNI (Recommended Nutrient Intake); in Spain CDR (Cantidad Diaria Recomendada) and in America they used to refer to RDA, (Recommended Dietary Allowance), but they now say RDI, (Recommended Daily Intake). In everyday speech we refer to 'needs': 'An adult needs 300mg daily of Vitamin "X"', as if this were a minimum. It would be more accurate to say: 'The vast majority of adults need less than 300mg'.

Just as an example, let us look at the recommendations for one vitamin we assumed had been thoroughly researched: vitamin C. (*Table 4.*)

AGE	UK (1991)	USA (1997)	FAO/OMS (2002)
6–8 months	25	50	30
9–11 months	25	50	30
12–23 months	30	15	30

Table 4: Recommended intake of vitamin C (mg per day) according to various experts.

Not only are the figures different, but the British and the Americans have been unable to agree on whether babies of more than a year old need more or less vitamin C than before.

An even more curious thing happens in the case of another vitamin, niacin. The Americans recommend a daily intake of

2mg for babies of up to six months, and 4mg for those between seven and twelve months. A litre of breastmilk only contains 1.5mg of niacin, and a baby drinks less than a litre a day, which suggests that according to their figures, nursing babies have a niacin deficiency from birth. Their daily intake is barely half the recommended amount. If we followed those recommendations to the letter, nursing babies would need a daily niacin supplement of 1mg. What is going on here? It appears that the experts had no idea how much niacin a baby needs, so they decided the normal intake must be that of nursing babies, as nursing babies don't suffer from any nutrient deficiencies. The recommended daily intake of most vitamins and minerals for the first six months is by definition that of a baby who is exclusively breastfed. However, analyses of breastmilk rarely give the same results, and experts based their calculations on the assumption that one litre contains 1.8mg. Consequently, the baby's daily intake is approximately 1.4mg a day, which if generously rounded up becomes 2mg. The figure of 4mg a day for babies between seven and twelve months comes from a generous rounding up of the average daily niacin intake of a baby that is breastfeeding and on solids.

But let us forget about rounded-up figures and return to the original argument: children need 1mg of niacin a day, because this is the daily intake of a nursing baby. But how can we know whether a baby needs a whole milligram? Is it not reasonable to assume that breastmilk contains a surplus of niacin as a back-up? Is it not possible that the baby would have enough with 0.8, or 0.5 or even 0.1 milligrams? We don't know. And we will never know. In order to find out, we would need to carry out a series of experiments on babies, gradually reducing their niacin intake to see what the minimum necessary amount is to prevent sickness, and for obvious reasons such an experiment is impossible.

What about after six months? At this age, the recommended daily intake doubles from 2 to 4mg. And it is true that breastmilk alone wouldn't supply a quarter of that amount, even if rounded up. Does this prove that after six months, exclusively breastfeeding leads to niacin deficiency, and that the baby needs to eat other foods? Clearly not. These recommendations are based on the baby starting on solids at six months. If solids were introduced at eight months, the recommendations would be: from zero to eight months, 2mg; from eight to twelve months 4mg. This is illogical, a circular argument. We put them on solids because they 'need' vitamins, and they 'need' vitamins because they are on solids.

These are but two examples, and I could provide similar that would apply to almost any vitamin or mineral. To sum up: theoretical calculations of a baby's nutrient requirements are of no use when deciding the best age to start your baby on solids.

→ Dewey, K.G., Brown, K.H. 'Update on technical issues concerning complementary feeding of young children in developing countries and implications for intervention programs', *Food Nut Bull* 2003;24:2-28.

→ Butte, N.F., Wong, W.W., Hopkinson, J.M., Heinz, C.J., Mehta, N.R., Smith, E.O.B. 'Energy requirements derived from total energy expenditure and energy deposition during the first 2 years of life', *Am J Clin Nutr* 2000;72:1558-69

Iron

Iron is a special case. Compared to the other nutrients, for which we only have very debatable theoretical calculations, the data on iron are a little more reliable. And while it is true that nursing babies don't suffer from scurvy (a result of vitamin C deficiency) or pellagra (a result of niacin deficiency), there are quite a high number of cases of babies with anaemia due to iron deficiency.

The iron in breastmilk is low, but it is much easier to absorb than the iron in any other foods. Cow's milk is also low in iron, and moreover it is difficult to absorb. The milk of all mammals that have been tested is low in iron. When a mother is given iron supplements, the level of iron in her milk remains unchanged. This is very interesting, because if we give the same mother aspirin, the level of aspirin in her milk increases. Apparently there is some biological mechanism that actively prevents milk from containing too much iron. Could it be that an excess of iron is bad for nurslings? It has been suggested (although to my knowledge there is no evidence for this) that an excess of iron in the baby's digestive tract can cause diarrhoea, because several of the 'bad' microbes which cause diarrhoea need large amounts of iron in order to thrive, while the 'good' microbes, the lactobacillus that forms the digestive flora in nursing babies, can survive on very little. A couple of studies showed that a group of healthy babies, not suffering from anaemia, who were given a prophylactic iron supplement, weighed slightly less at one year old than the control group who weren't given an iron supplement. It would appear that giving extra iron to a baby who doesn't need it isn't completely harmless, and should perhaps be avoided. (Obviously if your baby does have anaemia and has been prescribed iron then you must give it to him.)

But if milk contains low levels of iron, why don't all babies suffer from anaemia from birth? Where do they get the extra iron? The answer is they don't get it from anywhere; they are born with a supply of iron.

Iron forms part of haemoglobin, the molecule that transports oxygen in the blood. The foetus receives oxygen from the mother's blood through the placenta. Think of the placenta as a net, on either side of which two teams play at passing the ball to each other. The team that keeps the ball wins. But nature can't allow the mother to be the winner; if she kept all the oxygen, her baby would die. And so nature finds a way round it. The foetus's team has more players, all of them professionals. The foetus has a special type of haemoglobin called 'foetal haemoglobin', which binds oxygen more efficiently than normal haemoglobin. And it also has a vast number of red blood cells, more per millilitre than the mother and more even than the father (male adults have more haemoglobin than women, but the foetus has even more).

As a result of this, when a baby is born he has huge numbers of surplus red blood cells. These surplus cells, together with all the others, are quickly destroyed, because the baby no longer needs foetal haemoglobin. At the same time new red blood cells are formed, containing normal haemoglobin. The destroyed haemoglobin turns into bilirubin (which explains why newborns have slightly raised levels of bilirubin, and can be a bit jaundiced). Haemoglobin levels reach their lowest in babies of between one and two months, when hardly any foetal haemoglobin remains, but not enough normal haemoglobin has been produced. The baby then suffers a transitory anaemia, physiologic anaemia of infancy ('physiologic' means it isn't a disease, it is normal).

The iron from the surplus red blood cells is stored, and is gradually used to produce new blood cells. So the important question is, how long does that supply of iron last? Because when it runs out, the small amount of iron in the mother's milk will be insufficient, and the baby will need to eat other foods rich in iron.

A few decades ago, painstaking calculations were carried out and it was concluded that supplies can run out when the baby reaches six to twelve months. This corresponds quite well to reality: at six months you start to see a few cases of babies with anaemia, at eight months a few more, at ten months still more, and so on. Based on these facts, the general consensus is that 'after six months, the iron in breastmilk is insufficient, and babies should therefore be started on complementary foods'. But of course this is only a very exaggerated simplification. It would be more accurate to say: 'After six months, some babies may need complementary foods, while others have sufficient iron to be able to breastfeed exclusively until twelve months' (or possibly even longer). The problem is knowing which baby needs iron and which doesn't.

These calculations were made at a time when it was customary to clamp and sever the umbilical cord immediately after delivery. Today we know it is better to clamp the cord a few minutes after delivery (see page 78), and this reduces the incidence of anaemia in twelve-month-old babies.

The risk of iron deficiency after six months is one of the main arguments in favour of starting babies on complementary foods at that age.

A lot of nursing babies doggedly refuse to eat any solids until eight or ten months, or longer; and when I say 'doggedly', I mean they refuse to eat a single spoonful. Many more will eat three or four spoonfuls, and this brings us to yet another difference in the naming of things. Because when a baby eats three spoonfuls, mothers usually say: 'He doesn't eat'; whereas I say: 'He does eat'.

In my opinion, babies who refuse to eat solids have enough iron, and the moment they lack iron (or any other nutrient) they will begin eating solids. So, all parents need to do is offer their baby iron-rich foods, and they needn't worry whether the baby eats them or not. However, this is only my opinion: as far as I know there is no scientific evidence to back it up.

Others are of the opposite opinion: they believe that iron deficiency makes babies lose their appetite, which is why they refuse to eat. This in turn creates an even bigger iron deficiency, and it becomes a vicious circle. And when this happens, parents should be very concerned. However, this is also just an opinion, and as far as I know there is no scientific evidence to back it up either.

In any event, when a baby refuses to eat there is no way of forcing him. Not only is it ethically wrong (a human being can't be forced to eat against his will), it is also pointless. Thousands of parents spend hours trying to make their children eat, and fail miserably. The (oft heard) advice of 'not nursing him, so that when he's hungry he'll eat solids' is absurd, and it goes against nature: breastmilk is the best food there is; it contains hundreds of ingredients, and depriving your baby of all of them simply to make him eat a little more iron is completely illogical.

There is a much simpler solution. If a baby refuses to eat solids and only wants breastmilk, and his parents or the doctor worry he might have an iron deficiency, they can simply give him a blood test. If the test is fine, then there is nothing to worry about and he can continue not eating solids. And if he does have an iron deficiency, give him a few drops of iron, and he will be fine. If he is breastfeeding and taking an iron supplement, he can go on without eating solids as long as he wants. Another option, to spare the baby a needle prick, is to give iron drops just in case to those babies that reject iron-rich foods.

→ Griffin, I.J., Abrams, S.A. 'Iron and Breastfeeding', *Pediatr Clin N Amer* 2001;48: 401-13

→ Makrides, M., Leeson, R., Gibson, R.A., Simmer, K. 'A randomized controlled clinical trial of increased dietary iron in breastfed infants', *J Pediatr* 1998;133:559-62

→ Idjradinata, P., Watkins, W.E., Pollitt, E. 'Adverse effect of iron supplementation on weight gain of iron-replete young children', *Lancet* 1994;343:1252-4

→ Pisacane, A., De Vizia, B., Valiante, A., Vaccaro, F., Russo, M., Grillo, G., Giustardi, A. 'Iron status in breastfed infants', *J Pediatr* 1995;127:429-31

Empirical data

As we have seen, we can't decide what the ideal age is for starting babies on solids based on their nutritional needs, because we don't know what these needs are. So the decisive arguments are practical in nature: how long can a baby remain healthy when exclusively breastfeeding?

In 1989, Doctor Hijazi published a piece of research entitled: 'The duration for which exclusive breastfeeding is adequate' [sic]. His team studied 331 Jordanian babies of middle-class origin, who had been breastfed for the first month, and whose mothers planned to carry on exclusively breastfeeding them until further notice. The babies were visited at home and weighed fortnightly. A baby's weight was described as 'faltering' when, during two consecutive periods of two weeks, he gained less than the 'minimum' weight he should have gained, according to the growth charts. They stopped studying a baby either when his weight 'faltered' or when the mother stopped exclusively breastfeeding him.

There are many limitations to this type of study. Firstly, by definition, 2.5 per cent of babies gain less than the 'minimum' (which is the second standard deviation under the mean). Secondly, the growth charts are compiled using babies who have begun eating solids. Thirdly, it seems no one advised the mothers in this study how to improve positioning during breastfeeding, or explained about frequent feeds, and no account was taken of whether diarrhoea or other illnesses had contributed to weight faltering. Fourthly, when the mother started her baby on solids of her own accord, while he was still gaining weight nicely, we never knew how the story would have ended: how many months would he have continued gaining weight without eating solids?

How satisfactory the growth charts are is a particularly delicate question. Let us suppose babies who are breastfed and eat solids gain weight more quickly than those who are exclusively breastfed. This is what most people believe, but the fact is it has never been proven (see below). Let us suppose that at ten months, babies who are exclusively breastfed weigh on average 7 kilos, and those who also eat solids weigh 7.2 kilos. Which is better? We still don't know. The decision should be based on other objective facts, such as which babies are generally healthier and which have more advanced psychomotor development, not only at ten months but in the long run. Without these facts, the decision is purely arbitrary: if I decide that it is normal for a baby of ten months to eat solids, then 7.2 kilos is the normal weight and babies who don't eat solids are 200 grams underweight. On the other hand, if I decide that it is normal for a baby of ten months to be exclusively breastfed, then babies who eat solids are 200 grams overweight. Neither theory is based on facts, but rather the facts are interpreted to support the theory.

With all its limitations, Hijazi's study found that fifty-three babies who were exclusively breastfed after six months continued to gain weight normally. Of these, thirteen babies went on exclusively breastfeeding until nine months, one until a year, and another until fourteen months. This is something at least. The study shows that some babies, when they are exclusively breastfed, carry on gaining weight normally for a year or more. What we can't know is whether the same babies would have gained more or less weight, or would have been more or less healthy, if they had also eaten solids.

If we want more reliable results, what we need is an experimental study. The babies are randomly divided into two groups that start eating solids at different ages, in order to see which babies gain more weight and which are healthier. Unfortunately, only two studies of this type have been carried out, both by the same group of American scientists in Honduras in the mid-1990s. Some of the babies started eating solids at four months and others at six. The researchers found no difference in weight or size, or blood zinc levels, or the incidence of diarrhoea, respiratory illnesses, anaemia, or psychomotor development. Mothers who started their babies on solids later lost more weight after the birth. Between four and six months, the babies who ate solids gained the same amount of weight as those who didn't; which shows that they didn't eat more, they simply nursed less to make room for the solids. Because breastmilk is more nutritious than any other food, making this change meant they had fewer nutrients (and had lowered immunity). Based on these two studies alone (none have been carried out in other countries), the world's chief experts (WHO, UNICEF and the American Academy of Paediatrics and other equivalent organisations in nearly all countries) have modified their recommendations; twenty years ago they recommended starting complementary feeding 'between four and six months'; this has now changed to 'around six months'.

Two studies comparing four months to six months show that six months is better. Yet there isn't a single study that compares six months to ten or twelve months. And there never has been, because in the old days recommendations were based on guesswork not on studies. Any parents or professionals who thought that recommendations on infant feeding were based on scientific data or logical processes were mistaken. In fact, it was a bit like musical chairs; everyone ran around in a circle until the music stopped, and then sat down and refused to move. It so happened that when the music stopped (meaning, when the need to carry out proper studies before changing things was accepted) the norm was four months, and it took a long time to increase it from four to six. If the music had stopped a hundred years ago, when the norm was to introduce the first solids at twelve months, those in favour of ten months would have needed to provide solid evidence in order to bring about a change.

→ Hijazi, S.S., Abulaban, A., Waterlow, J.C. 'The duration for which exclusive breast-feeding is adequate. A study in Jordan', *Acta Pædiatr Scand* 1989;78:23-8

→ Cohen, R.J., Brown, K.H., Canahuati, J. y cols. 'Effects of age of introduction of complementary foods on infant breast milk intake, total energy intake, and growth: a randomised intervention study in Honduras', *Lancet* 1994;343:288-293

→ Dewey, K.G., Cohen, R.J., Brown, K.H., Landa Rivera, L. 'Age of introduction of complementary foods and growth of term, low-birth-weight, breastfed infants: a randomized intervention study in Honduras', *Am J Clin Nutr* 1999;69:679-86

Chapter 12
WEANING

For the purposes of this book, weaning means 'weaning from the breast', or 'stopping nursing'. In English the term weaning is also used to mean 'starting solids' so there is sometimes a confusion.

Spontaneous weaning

Sooner or later, all babies are weaned. Believe it or not, your child will stop nursing. If a mother said to me: 'I want to beat the Guinness World Record and breastfeed for fifteen years, how do I do it?' I would have to reply: 'I'm sorry, I don't think you can. Your baby will stop nursing long before, and there's nothing you can do about it'.

There are no reliable studies on spontaneous weaning. Apparently, most children stop nursing between the ages of two and four. Some go on nursing until they are six or seven. Personally, I have never come across a child who was still nursing after the age of seven. I once talked to one of the founders of La Leche League, who has met thousands of nursing mothers over a forty-year career. She told me she had come across two children who had nursed until the age of eight. In his 1542 book *Naufragios* (*Shipwrecks*), Álvar Núñez Cabeza de Vaca refers to a tribe in the area now known as Florida, where children nursed until they were twelve. But the circumstances were very special: the environment the tribe lived in was extremely hostile, and they suffered frequent famines. Núñez was convinced that without this prolonged lactation period, the tribe's children would not have survived.

There are also children who spontaneously wean before they are two, especially if they have been given a lot of solids early on and have consequently missed feeds.

225

Women who breastfeed for more than a year are sometimes faced with incomprehension and disapproval from family, friends and health professionals. It was the same fifty years ago when the first women started wearing trousers. Have patience, they will come round.

There are no limits on breastfeeding. There is no medical, nutritional or psychological reason for a mother to wean her baby at a specific age. Of course, some doctors, nutritionists or psychologists try to establish a time limit: 'Your milk isn't nutritious enough'; 'You are making him dependent' and similar. These assertions have no basis in scientific fact; they are simply prejudices. You don't have to agree with your doctor's opinions on breastfeeding, any more than you have to support the same football team or vote for the same political party.

Some mothers decide to go on breastfeeding until their baby 'tires' of it, or stops of his own accord. Others prefer to take the initiative and wean him before. It is for you to decide.

→ Dettwyler, K.A. 'A time to wean: The hominid blueprint for the natural age of weaning in modern human populations', In Stuart-Macadam, P., Dettwyler, K.A., eds.: *Breastfeeding. Biocultural perspectives,* New York: Aldine de Gruyter, 1995

→ Sugarman, M., Kendall-Tackett, K. 'Weaning ages in a sample of American women who practice extended breastfeeding', *Clinical Pediatrics* 1995; 34:642-7

→ Gonzalez, C., Arauz, F. *Estudio sobre lactancias prolongadas.*

Mother-led weaning

If you want to wean your baby, it is best to do it gradually, reducing the number of feeds over several weeks, or at least over a few days. Sudden weaning is very hard on the baby, the mother and the rest of the family (who have to listen to the baby crying).

Remember that the breast not only provides food, it also provides affection, physical contact, comfort and a human relationship. This is why I had to write a chapter on how to wean. If the breast only provided food, the answer to the question would be ridiculously simple: 'Each time she wants to nurse, give her a glass of milk, or a ham sandwich'. Only it isn't that easy.

In order to wean a baby, you must find other ways of giving

her all of those things: affection, physical contact, comfort. Don't imagine for a moment that weaning means having a rest. A lot of mothers discover that breastfeeding is in fact one of the easiest ways of attending to their child's needs. If you want her to wean you have to play with her more, read her more stories, teach her more songs, admire more of her drawings, listen more patiently when she tries to tell you things, tickle her more, give her more kisses. A child won't give up the breast if she receives nothing in exchange. Of course, unlike with breastfeeding, the father can do all these things, too, but even so, the mother will still have to do more things than before.

And you have to do these things before she wants to nurse. You have to take the initiative, pay attention to her while she is still contented and not demanding anything. Because the moment she gets bored and clamours for attention, she will probably no longer want you to play with her or to tell her a story, she will want to nurse, which is what she is accustomed to. For example, if her dad takes her to the park, and plays with her (not just sitting reading the paper while she gets bored), she is unlikely to say: 'Let's go home, daddy, I want to nurse'. But if she is getting bored at home, while her parents are busy doing other things, and she wants to nurse, then it is best to nurse her immediately. Because by then it is too late to say: 'Take her to the park will you, dear, she wants to nurse again'. The child will quickly understand what is happening and will become more insistent.

Babies weaned before a year old should be given infant formula. After a year old, they can be given full-fat cow's milk. Breastmilk contains more fat than whole cow's milk, so it makes no sense to give an infant semi-skimmed or skimmed milk.

Chapter 13
PRESCRIPTION DRUGS AND OTHER SUBSTANCES

In the perfect, peaceful world we were promised, there would be no need to include a chapter on drugs in a book about breastfeeding for mothers. Any mention of them would be superfluous. The possibility that any drug the mother takes might harm her baby is so remote as to be unworthy of mention. It would be easier to win the lottery (there is always a winner) than to have a problem during lactation due to a drug. And in these extremely rare cases, the doctor who prescribed the drug should know what to do.

However, we live in a crazy world. Drugs cause almost no problems during lactation, and yet the fear of them (on the part of mothers and doctors) causes endless problems, to the point where I feel obliged to write this chapter.

The current situation is bordering on collective hysteria. The same doctor who prescribes a treatment for the baby without thinking twice, believes he must consult thick volumes, and weigh up the pros and cons before prescribing the baby's mother with the same treatment. The same mother who doesn't hesitate to give her baby any drug he is prescribed (and some he isn't!), regards with suspicion anything she herself is prescribed, looks it up on the Internet to make sure it is 'compatible', and consults two or three doctors before deciding whether to take it or not. Why is this? Does the drug somehow become more toxic when dissolved in milk than when it is in pill form? Many patient instruction leaflets that come with drugs warn of supposed dangers, spurious or imaginary. Many medical professionals recommend weaning in cases where the mother has been prescribed a harmless drug, while others consider themselves progressive when they recommend only weaning for as long as the treatment lasts, and then going back to breastfeeding, as if this were as easy as falling off a log. And many mothers have to suffer pain and illness, foregoing treatment simply because they are breastfeeding. Here are a few examples:

- Amaya is forced to wean her baby because she has to take a 'very powerful' antibiotic. The following week, her baby runs a temperature and is prescribed the same antibiotic.

- Silvia has a discal hernia, and is in dreadful pain. Her doctor says to her: 'I can't prescribe you anything because you're breastfeeding'. After months of agony, the doctor tells her she can stop breastfeeding because her milk is 'no longer nutritious', and finally he prescribes an anti-inflammatory. When she reads the instructions, Silvia discovers it is the same drug they gave her son when they vaccinated him, in case he ran a temperature.

- Lola was given a simple chest X-ray, and was told she mustn't breastfeed for twenty-four hours afterwards. Does her doctor think people go luminous green after they have an X-ray, like in the cartoons?

- Lucia is asthmatic. She has had a few mild attacks in recent months, but hasn't been allowed to take any treatment. Can you imagine being exhausted from walking, sleeping only superficially, being unable to breathe properly, being conscious of each breath, knowing that one puff would make you better, and yet not being allowed to use your inhaler? Four days ago the situation became intolerable: 'Wean your baby immediately and use your inhaler every four hours'. Can you imagine having to wean a seven-month old baby from one day to the next, the inconsolable crying, the sleepless nights? After several months of torment, and four days of forced weaning, Lucia discovers that her inhaler is perfectly compatible with breastfeeding, and she could have used it from day one without endangering her baby in the slightest.

- Montse has a urinary tract infection. Although the doctor has told her she can safely take the antibiotic, the instruction leaflet says: "Of unproven safety during lactation". And so, just to be sure, Montse takes two tablets instead of three. Too bad the infection didn't clear up.

The origin of the myth

In my opinion, the hysteria around prescription drugs comes from the failure to differentiate between pregnancy and lactation. And yet they are so obviously different, aren't they? Anyone can see that during pregnancy the baby is inside, and that during lactation the baby is outside. And yet, in the instruction leaflets of every drug you will find a paragraph headed: 'pregnant women and breastfeeding mothers'. Every other circumstance is entitled to a separate explanation: you never see 'children' and 'the elderly' together, or 'operating machinery' and 'kidney failure'. And yet pregnancy and lactation are always lumped together, as if they were one and the same thing.

And they aren't. The difference between pregnancy and lactation is enormous, and not just where the use of prescription drugs is concerned.

During pregnancy, the baby is still developing. Some drugs can cause completely different side-effects in foetuses than in adults. This was never clearer than in the tragic case of thalidomide. Thalidomide was a good analgesic, with very few side-effects, and was therefore widely prescribed to pregnant women. Suddenly babies started being born either with no arms, or with badly deformed arms. Thalidomide affected thousands of babies worldwide. The problem can only occur if the mother takes it exactly when her baby's arms are forming. If it is taken by an adult, an older child, a baby or even an older foetus whose arms are perfectly formed, nothing will happen. Thalidomide doesn't make people's arms drop off.

The effects of any drug taken during pregnancy are completely unpredictable, and have nothing to do with the side-effects they cause in adults. Even if it is considered the most harmless drug in the world, even if the instruction leaflet says: 'Side-effects: rare, may cause mild headaches which are transient and require no treatment', nobody can know whether it will cause deformities. The animal testing laboratories carry out tests on pregnant rats, dogs and rabbits but this is no guarantee, because every species is different. Some drugs are harmful to dog foetuses, but have no effect on rabbit foetuses.

So, when a drug is given to a pregnant woman it is a leap in the dark. No one knows what will happen. It will only be given to her if she is seriously ill and her condition can't be treated using an older, better-known drug. A drug can only be said to be risk-free when it has been given to hundreds or thousands of pregnant women without any adverse effects.

However, when a drug is given to a baby, initially, the side-effects will be more or less the same as in an adult. There may be a few differences: younger babies might be more or less sensitive to particular side-effects, or it may take their liver and kidneys longer to eliminate certain by-products. In any event, if 'sickness, headaches and dizziness' were a drug's worst side-effects, we would happily prescribe it to a baby without any problem, but if it was liable to cause 'fulminant hepatitis, kidney failure, convulsions and coma', we would be as reluctant to give it to a baby as to an adult, and would only use it to treat serious illnesses.

Another significant difference between pregnancy and lactation is the amount of drug the baby receives. Almost all drugs pass easily through the placenta, and the concentration of the drug in the mother's and baby's blood is the same. Meaning, if the drug affects the mother's heart, it will affect the baby's in exactly the same way (as soon as his heart is formed and able to respond). If the foetus has an infection, we can treat it by giving the mother an antibiotic.

But the amount of drug the baby receives through the mother's milk is very small. Some drugs pass with difficulty into breastmilk, and the concentration in the mother's milk is far lower than in her blood. Others pass very easily, and may reach much greater concentrations in the milk than in the blood. This can be measured through the milk/plasma ratio (plasma is what is left after blood is centrifuged and the blood cells removed: red and white blood cells and platelets):

$$\text{Milk/plasma ratio} = \frac{\text{Milk concentration}}{\text{Plasma concentration}}$$

A drug that has a very low milk/plasma ratio is amoxicillin, a widely prescribed antibiotic (in Spain, over-prescribed). The milk/plasma ratio is approximately 0.03. This means that the concentration is thirty-three times higher in the mother's plasma than in her milk. The concentration in her milk is just below 1mg per litre. When the mother takes 1,500mg a day (2.5mg per kilo if she weighs 60 kilos), her baby takes less than 1mg a day (0.3mg per kilo if he weighs 3kg). Amoxicillin is used to treat ear infections in babies, and the dose prescribed is 80mg per kilo. So, if a baby weighing five kilos had an ear infection, he would need to drink 400 litres of milk a day to receive the correct dose of antibiotic.

One example of a drug that passes very easily into milk is ranitidine (trade name Zantac), which is used to treat gastric ulcers. The milk/plasma ratio of ranitidine is ten (this is approximate, as the true ratio fluctuates with time); meaning that the drug is ten times more concentrated in the mother's milk than in her blood. Even so, the concentration in her milk is less than 3mg per litre. So, when the mother takes 300mg a day (about 5mg per kilo), the baby takes a lot less than 1mg per kilo. Ranitidine is a safe drug (meaning it has very few side-effects), and is sometimes administered to babies (to treat reflux) at a dosage of 2-4mg per kilo. Mothers can take ranitidine without any problem.

Ranitidine is one of the drugs that reaches the highest concentrations in milk. In fact there are few cases where the milk/plasma ratio is greater than one.

The reason for all these numbers and figures is to refute a fairly widespread idea. Many people become anxious when they hear things like: 'it reaches a high concentration in breastmilk' or 'ten times higher in milk than in plasma'. 'But this will mean the baby will be taking more of the drug than his mother!' As we have seen, this isn't true. In absolute terms, it is impossible for the baby to receive more of the drug than the mother: if the mother only takes ten she can't have eleven in her milk. The amount that passes into breastmilk is only a fraction of the dose the mother has taken. In relative terms, the dose the baby receives through the milk per kilo in weight is always much smaller than the amount the mother receives. Even when large amounts of the drug pass into the milk, the dose the baby receives is still much smaller (in the case of ranitidine, less than a sixth). When very little of the drug passes into the milk (the vast majority of cases), the dose is incredibly small.

As a consequence, it is impossible to treat a baby who is breastfed by administering the drug to his mother. If mother and baby have the same illness and are treated with the same drug, the baby has to be given a separate dose. The amount that passes into the mother's milk wouldn't be enough even to scratch the surface. Looking at it the other way round, in order to have enough of the drug in her milk to treat her baby, the mother would have to take so much of it that it would probably kill her.

A few general ideas

- Anything that can safely be given to a baby, can also be given to his mother. Hundreds of babies every day are prescribed medicines for common illnesses like coughs, colds and ear infections. Other drugs, like those used to treat tuberculosis, heart failure or epilepsy, are rarely given to babies. Yet when we do prescribe them, nobody gets alarmed and there are usually no side-effects. Generally speaking, these drugs are wholly compatible with breastfeeding. However, when a drug is contraindicated in infants, or used only to treat serious illnesses (such as cancer) because it has dangerous side-effects, it is sensible to look for more information. Even a dangerous drug can be compatible with breastfeeding if it only passes into breastmilk in small quantities; if it passes in large quantities, there could be a problem.

- Any drug that can safely be taken during pregnancy can also be taken during lactation. Some drugs are only prescribed during pregnancy when there is no other alternative, and it is a matter of life or death. But when a drug can be given to a pregnant mother without fear and in complete safety, then it's still safer during lactation. Some experts may disagree on this point: in theory, a drug could be dangerous for a baby but not for a foetus. For example, if it caused respiratory depression; since the foetus doesn't breathe, it can't be affected. But the fact is that, although it could exist in theory, I don't know of any drug that is safe for pregnant women but contraindicated for nursing mothers.

- If the drug isn't absorbed orally, it can't harm the baby. There are no tablets of heparin, insulin and gentamicin, they are only administered by injection. It doesn't matter whether they pass into breastmilk because your baby isn't going to be given an injection of milk. Other drugs are taken orally precisely so they don't get absorbed, because they act directly on the stomach: antacids, many laxatives, some antibiotics used (usually misused) to treat diarrhoea.

- If a drug only has mild side-effects, it doesn't matter whether it passes into breastmilk or not. For example, in the instruction leaflet for omeprazole (used to treat stomach ulcers) it says: 'Is well tolerated. There have been rare reports of nausea, headache, diarrhoea, constipation and flatulence. Rash has been observed in some patients. These symptoms are generally mild and transient'. Even assuming it did pass into breastmilk in large quantities (which it doesn't), what does it matter if the baby gets mild diarrhoea? If he is weaned, he will not only cry inconsolably, he will probably get severe diarrhoea.

- We have more information about older drugs. When a drug is released onto the market, no one knows whether it passes into breastmilk or not, for the simple reason that no mother has taken it. If doctors have a choice between two similar drugs, they will normally prescribe the tried and tested one. But in some cases it will be better to use the new drug, even though it is less well-known, for example if it is safer (has fewer side-effects) than the older drug.

- All drugs for topical use can be safely administered during breastfeeding. 'For topical use' means the drug only acts on the part of the body to which it is applied. For example, penicillin injected intramuscularly so that it is absorbed into the blood and acts on the whole body is not the same as a local anaesthetic, which only numbs a small area around the point of injection. If the anaesthetic doesn't put the mother to sleep completely and only numbs a small area, it is because it hasn't passed into the bloodstream, and therefore doesn't transfer to the breastmilk. There is also a difference between a cream used to treat a skin disease, and nicotine or nitroglycerin patches placed on the skin so that the drug is absorbed and distributed throughout the whole body. (Incidentally, penicillin, nicotine and nitroglycerin are compatible with breastfeeding, not because they are used topically, but for other reasons). Creams, eye drops, eardrops, nasal sprays, bronchial inhalers, vaginal suppositories and the like are safe to use during breastfeeding. It is true that a small amount of these products is always absorbed, but the amount that passes into the bloodstream is already small, and therefore what passes into the milk is miniscule. In short, where possible asthma or allergic rhinitis should always be treated with inhalers, which are much safer than any oral medication.

- As the baby grows bigger, the risks diminish. Newborns still don't have the capacity of grown babies or adults to eliminate certain drugs, because their kidneys and liver aren't yet fully functioning. In addition, newborns will always receive a bigger amount; a six-kilo baby takes more milk than a three-kilo baby, but not twice as much, so the amount of milk (or anything dissolved in the milk, such as medicaments) per kilo, goes down. A nine-kilo baby takes less milk than a six-kilo baby because he is already eating other foods. A twelve-kilo baby takes less milk than a three-kilo baby. Everything written about drugs and lactation has been calculated for the most 'exposed' individual: the newborn. If they say that a certain drug can be administered 'with caution' (so, for example, if the mother takes barbiturates, attention must be paid in case the baby suffers from drowsiness), this refers to newborns. With older children there is usually no need for precautions. It is absurd to tell a mother to wean her two-year-old, who only nurses a couple of times a day, because she is taking a drug, except perhaps in rare cases where the drug is particularly toxic; anyone giving this sort of advice is probably strongly against nursing two-year-olds and is simply using the drug as a pretext.

- By the same token, when the mother takes a drug continuously, the risk diminishes over time. For example, some experts recommend carrying out thyroid hormone tests on nursing babies whose mothers are on anti-thyroid medication. But if we do a test after one month and it is normal, and then we do another after three months and it is also normal, it makes no sense to carry on doing tests.

Any side-effects would occur at the beginning. It makes no sense either to tell a mother who is on permanent medication: 'Nurse her for three months and then wean her'. Again, if there were any danger it would occur within the first few months; if nothing has happened, you can go on breastfeeding for as long as you want.

- Generally speaking, it makes no difference what time a drug is taken during lactation. In a few special cases where drugs can only be administered with caution, your doctor will recommend a specific time. This would be a question of making sure the longest period during which your baby doesn't nurse (which can be at night, but not always) coincides with the peak concentration of the drug in the blood (which differs for each drug). However, with the vast majority of drugs that are wholly compatible with breastfeeding, there is no need to worry about when you take it. What difference does it make if a little more or a little less of the drug passes into the milk when the amounts are incredibly tiny?

- It is extremely irresponsible to withhold treatment from an ailing mother simply because she is breastfeeding. Whatever you do, don't take a smaller dose or stop taking the medication earlier than recommended; your baby will be no worse or better off for taking a slightly more or slightly less of the drug, but both you and your baby will be a lot worse off if you don't get better.

How to find information

Sometimes a mother will ask a paediatrician the following type of question: 'I have ulcerative colitis (or psoriasis, or high blood pressure, or lupus); what can I take for it?' However, the paediatrician doesn't know: only a GP, or in many cases a specialist, can prescribe drugs for these illnesses. It is the specialist who will suggest a treatment (or better still, several alternative treatments). Only then can the paediatrician consult a medical book to see which of the drugs you should take.

In an ideal world, it would be the mother's GP who finds a treatment that is compatible with breastfeeding. In some cases he might consult with her paediatrician about the best treatment.

However, many doctors still forbid breastfeeding for no reason, or they refuse to give the mother the treatment she needs.

In cases like this, ask: 'What drug would you prescribe if I wasn't breastfeeding?' 'Are there any similar drugs that can be used to treat my condition?' Always insist on being given several alternatives, and make a note of their names. This way, a different doctor who is more in favour of breastfeeding will be able to help you choose. In some cases, the mother is forced to find the information herself and take it to her doctor.

Patient information leaflets

The worst place to look for information on lactation is in drug information leaflets for patients. They are truly disastrous, at least in Spain. In nearly all of them they warn of risks, say the drug shouldn't be taken, that it is contraindicated. Many let themselves off the hook with vague qualifications, such as: 'Only use during lactation if the possible advantages outweigh the potential risks, and only under strict medical supervision'; words like these terrify mothers, and yet they are simple platitudes; of course you should only take a drug if the benefits outweigh the risks – the same applies to everyone, whether they are breastfeeding or not.

Doctors will often take great care to ensure that a drug is compatible with breastfeeding. They prescribe it to the mother, who, when she gets home, reads the information leaflet, and is so alarmed she doesn't take it, or she takes a smaller dose, or doesn't finish the course. Don't do this. If you don't take the correct dosage, you probably won't get better. If you are in any doubt, call your doctor and explain what it says in the leaflet. If you can't get hold of him or her, take the medicine, carry on breastfeeding as before, and call again the next day. There will be plenty of time to wean your baby or to stop taking the drug. No prescription drug is so toxic that it will harm your baby if you breastfeed for a few days while taking it. Remember: any drug is more dangerous for the mother who swallows the pill than it is for the baby who only gets it from the milk; if the information leaflet doesn't say: 'Make a will before taking this drug', then there is probably nothing to worry about.

Information online

This excellent page provides a quick reference in English and Spanish:

→ www.e-lactancia.org

You can find a complete monograph on almost every drug on LACTMED, the database of the National Library of Medicine:

→ http://toxnet.nlm.nih.gov/cgi-bin/sis/htmlgen?LACT

PubMed, the mother of all databases

Sometimes, you won't be able to find any information on a specific drug, and your doctor won't find any reference to it in his or her medical books either, or the information given will be insufficient, or you will want to be sure. When this happens, the best solution is to go back to the source: Medline (PubMed).

Medline is an enormous database containing information on thousands of articles in dozens of languages from hundreds of medical journals dating back to the 1950s. The majority are summarised in English, and in some cases it is possible to find the whole text on the Internet. You can find Medline by going to the PubMed website:

→ www.pubmed.gov

Here is a practical example. Supposing you suffer from severe post-natal depression and have been prescribed an anti-depressant called paroxetine. If you type 'paroxetine' and then press 'Enter', over 3,000 articles will come up. Obviously you won't want to trawl through them all just to find the ones about paroxetine and breastfeeding, so after 'paroxetine' type 'breastfeeding' and this time only twenty articles will come up. Scroll through the titles and click on one that interests you. The first (which might not be the first by the time you do your research) is entitled: 'The safety of newer anti-depressants in pregnancy and breastfeeding' and it is a review. It looks promising. But when you read the summary you realise it isn't very specific. In this case, either try to find the whole article in a specialised library, to see whether it is any more instructive, or carry on looking through the other entries.

Article number seven also looks promising: 'Paroxetine during breastfeeding: infant weight gain and maternal adherence to counsel'. This time the summary is detailed: twenty-seven mothers took paroxetine while nursing, and none had any problem.

Article number ten: 'Use of sertraline, paroxetine and fluvoxamine by nursing women'. This looks even better because it says 'Free article', meaning you can read the whole article free online. And it is more conclusive: the babies' blood was tested and no trace of paroxetine was found. So there is no problem with the drug at all, and if necessary you can print out the article and take it to your doctor.

To sum up, you will find several other articles, some of which you can read in their entirety. All of them agree that paroxetine is safe to take during lactation (although not all of them are this explicit, and prefer to say things like: 'No adverse effects have been observed'; 'low concentrations in breastmilk', and so on).

Even then, we may still not have found all the information there is on the subject. Some people write 'breastfeeding', others 'breast feeding' or even 'breast-feeding' (PubMed doesn't mind about the hyphen). There could be articles that don't use the word 'breastfeeding', at least not in the title or in the summary, because they don't refer to babies that breastfeed but rather to the lactation period of the mother. 'Lactation' is also used to refer to animals. And it could be that some articles don't refer to lactation or breastfeeding, but rather to 'paroxetine in human milk or breastmilk'. In order not to miss anything you might want to type the following (word for word, including the brackets):

paroxetine AND (breastfeeding OR breast feeding OR lactation OR milk)

This will bring up all the articles containing the word paroxetine and at least one of the other words. At the time of writing this, there are thirty-one. If you type 'milk' without specifying whether it is breastmilk or not, articles about taking pills with a glass of milk might come up, but in any event it won't take long to scan thirty-one articles.

If you want to do a search using two or more words that make up a sentence, you must put them in inverted commas, and if you also want to look for them separately you must place a comma between them. Medline has an internal dictionary and will recognise some expressions. However, 'paroxetine levels' isn't a dictionary expression, and if you search for it without using inverted commas 388 articles come up, whereas in inverted commas there are only nine.

What if no articles come up? Although we may be unable to find out whether the drug passes into breastmilk or not, we can still discover interesting information. For example if we search for: 'indomethacin infant' more than 1,000 articles come up. A simple glance at the first few will tell you that indomethacin is frequently administered not only to babies but also to premature babies. It is clear from this that the drug is safe to take during lactation.

How many days to take one pill?

The data on drugs and breastmilk can be difficult to understand, even for professionals. For example, a concentration of 0.00096 mg/L digoxin has been found in milk. This is identical to 0.00096µg/ml, or 0.000096mg/100ml, or 0.000096mg/dl, or 0.96µg/L, or 0.096µg/dl, or 96ng/dl, and depending on the book, you will find it explained in other ways. Crazy, isn't it? We can imagine 1kg of rice or 100g of ham, but nobody can imagine 96 nanograms per decilitre. Is this a lot or a little?

Imagine you drop a pill on the floor and your baby finds it and swallows it. Do you think one pill is enough to poison him? Now imagine that instead of swallowing the pill he licks it, hides it, and over the next few days he licks it again. Do you know how many days it would take for him to take the whole pill?

I have worked it out based on the drug's peak concentration in the milk (this is an exaggeration, because the peak is only reached at a precise moment, and the rest of the day the concentration is much lower), and on the assumption that the baby takes 750ml of breastmilk per day (some babies of four of five months will take slightly more, but in fact newborns and older babies who are already on solids take quite a lot less). The following table shows the results for some drugs; the concentrations in milk are taken from Hale's book.

Drug	Concentration in milk (mg/L)	Pill (mg)	Number of days required to take a whole pill
Alprazolam	0.0037	0.5	180
Amoxicillin	1.3	500	513
Atenolol	1.8	50	37
Carbamazepine	2.5	400	213
Cloxacillin	0.4	500	1667
Digoxin	0.00096	0.25	347
Naproxen	2.37	550	309
Nifedipine	0.046	10	290
Paroxetine	0.1	20	267
Pyrazinamide	1.5	250	222
Ranitidine	2.6	150	77

Table 5: Some drugs in breastmilk.

As *Table 5* shows, a baby needs more than a month to take one atenolol (it is better to take propanolol, labetalol or metoproponol); two and a half months to take one ranitidine, almost a whole year to take one digoxin and four and a half years to take one cloxacillin (assuming the mother took cloxacillin every day for all this time). And yet, women are still told to wean their baby if they have mastitis because cloxacillin 'passes into breastmilk'!

When the drug is given to babies, we can also see what dosage would be prescribed, and how many days he would need to breastfeed to obtain the same amount. For example, the usual dosage for digoxin is 0.015mg/kg/d; a five-kilo baby would be prescribed 0.075mg. In order to obtain that amount from his mother's milk he would need to drink 78 litres, which would take him 104 days. He is more likely to drown in milk or be crushed by the weight of it, than to be poisoned by digoxin.

→ Hale, T.W. *Medications and Mothers' Milk*, 11th ed. Amarillo, Texas. Pharmasoft Publishing; 2004

Alcohol

Alcohol passes easily and quickly from the mother's blood into her milk and vice versa, so that the concentration in both liquids is the same. The milk/plasma ratio is 1.

In Spain, the legal alcohol limit for driving is 0.5g per litre of blood, which is the same as 0.05g per 100ml or 0.05 per cent. A few decades ago the legal limit was 0.08 per cent (this is still the legal limit in the UK). If your alcohol level is higher than 0.15 per cent you are unmistakably drunk. If it goes above 0.55 per cent, you simply drop dead. Many die before.

Even habitual drinkers react the same way when they have the same levels of alcohol in their blood. The difference is they eliminate alcohol more quickly, and it takes them longer to reach these levels, but when they have 0.15 per cent alcohol in their blood they are drunk and when they have 0.55 per cent they die like everyone else.

Therefore, it is absolutely impossible for breastmilk to contain more than 0.55 per cent alcohol, and for this to be so, the mother would have to be in hospital suffering from acute alcohol poisoning. Realistically, a mother who is inebriated could have 0.2 per cent or 0.3 per cent alcohol in her milk, but a mother who drinks in moderation won't even have 0.05 per cent.

Wine contains on average 10–14 per cent alcohol. Liqueurs range from 30–40 per cent (sometimes more). Beer contains 4–6 per cent alcohol (sometimes more). Alcohol-free beer can legally contain up to 1 per cent alcohol. Someone with 1 per cent of alcohol in their blood would already be dead. Consequently, even the breastmilk of a completely inebriated mother could be bottled and labelled 'alcohol-free'. And the milk of a mother who has had a small drink, even if her blood contains 0.04 per cent alcohol and in some countries she fails the Breathalyzer test, could still be sold as 'alcohol-free milk', because 0.04 per cent is rounded down to 0.0 per cent(if we are purists, 0.06 per cent is rounded up to 0.1 per cent; I don't know whether beer producers are so rigorous).

To sum up: at worst milk is a very mildly alcoholic drink, and it is almost impossible that drinking alcohol while breastfeeding will harm your baby.

I say 'almost', because newborns are very sensitive to alcohol, they metabolise it very slowly, and moreover they nurse like mad.

Drinking more than half a litre a day when you weigh a little over three kilos is the equivalent of an adult who weighs 60 kilos drinking ten litres a day. A friend of mine who is a midwife told me that in the hospital where she works in Barcelona, a newborn was brought to casualty suffering from excessive drowsiness and hypotonia; the only obvious cause was that the mother usually drank a small beer before each feed. The sad thing was that the mother was teetotal, and was forcing herself to drink beer because someone had told her it would boost her supply of milk.

Alcohol consumption is measured in grams per day, but for practical purposes it is usually measured in 'glasses'. Traditionally, the higher the percentage of alcohol, the smaller the 'glass': beer is consumed from a tankard, wine from a large or small wineglass, liqueurs from a liqueur glass, brandy from a brandy glass and tequila from a shot glass. Each 'glass' of liquid contains more or less the same amount of alcohol. So it can't be said that tequila is any more dangerous than beer, provided the dose consumed is one shot. Naturally, drinking a tankard of tequila would be extremely dangerous.

One study found that children whose mothers drank more than two glasses of alcohol a day showed a slight psychomotor retardation. Based on that information, many books recommend 'a maximum of two glasses of alcohol a day' while breastfeeding. Clearly, this is sensible rule not just during breastfeeding, but in general. Too much alcohol is bad for your health, and it is a good idea for both mothers and fathers not to exceed two glasses.

However, if you are someone who likes to drink three or four glasses a day, and you can't or don't want to stop, I don't think you are harming your child. You are harming yourself, not your baby. Even if the mother drinks three glasses a day, breastfeeding is still better for her baby than bottle feeding. It is very unlikely that this amount of alcohol will affect the baby, and when the same scientists repeated their experiment a year later, they found no link between alcohol consumption and psychomotor development. It is far more likely that many mothers who drink during breastfeeding also drank when they were pregnant, and this is what affected their child's development.

Consuming alcohol during pregnancy is dangerous. Extremely dangerous. No amount of alcohol is considered 'safe' during pregnancy. The aim should be zero consumption, no alcohol at all. Obviously one beer a week isn't as bad as one beer a day, but no one can say with certainty: 'one beer a week is fine'.

If you drink too much at a party one night, it might be wise not to breastfeed while you are visibly drunk, especially if your baby is only a few weeks old. When you sober up, it means the alcohol level in your plasma, and therefore in your milk, has gone down from 0.15 per cent. Remember, alcohol passes from blood to milk and from milk to blood easily; it doesn't accumulate in the breast, so there is no need to express your milk and discard it (unless your breasts are too full and feel uncomfortable). Your milk is 'self-cleaning'.

→ Little, R.E., Northstone, K., Golding, J.; ALSPAC Study Team 'Alcohol, breastfeeding, and development at 18 months', *Pediatrics* 2002;109:E72-2 pediatrics.aappublications.org/cgi/content/full/109/5/e72

Tobacco

Tobacco, like alcohol, is bad for your health. It is better for nursing mothers not to smoke. And for mothers who bottle feed. And for fathers. And for those who don't have children. Smoking is bad for everyone.

However, if you do smoke (or drink), it is still better to carry on breastfeeding, because although smoking is bad, it isn't bad enough to make breastmilk worse than formula.

Children of parents who smoke have more respiratory problems: bronchitis, pneumonia, and ear infections. It has been proven that breastfeeding offers some protection against these illnesses. In other words, being exposed to tobacco smoke and being fed formula is possibly the worst combination for the baby's health. If you can't give up smoking, at least carry on breastfeeding your baby.

Unfortunately, many people (relatives, friends and even some doctors) put pressure on smoking mothers to stop breastfeeding. Perhaps this is why, statistically, mothers who smoke wean their babies earlier.

Nicotine passes into breastmilk. Even some mothers who aren't smokers have nicotine in their milk because they are passive smokers. Bear in mind that nicotine is one of the least harmful substances in tobacco. Nicotine isn't the cause of cancer, bronchitis and emphysema; it is tar and other ingredients in tobacco. This is why nicotine patches are used to stop smoking: because the smoke from tobacco is far more toxic than the nicotine in a patch.

So, if the mother smokes, the danger for the baby isn't 'contaminated milk', it is tobacco smoke. If you never smoke inside the house, your baby will not be exposed to tobacco smoke, and the nicotine in your milk won't do him any harm. However, if you smoke inside the house, your baby will inhale the same amount of smoke whether he is bottle fed or breastfed.

Obviously, the smoke the father or anyone else produces is no less harmful than that of the mother. It is now forbidden to smoke in the workplace in order to protect the health of other workers who aren't smokers. Don't you think your child's health warrants the same level of protection? It isn't enough not to smoke in the same room, because the smoke will easily spread through a small flat or house. Don't let anyone smoke inside the house. If they want to smoke they can smoke outside in the garden or the yard.

And if in order to stop smoking you need patches or nicotine chewing gum, don't hesitate to use them. It is perfectly safe for you to carry on breastfeeding. These patches are designed to release roughly the same amount of nicotine into the blood as when you are smoking, and they therefore pose no threat to your baby.

→ DiFranza, J.R., Aligne, C.A., Weitzman, M. 'Prenatal and postnatal environmental tobacco smoke exposure and children's health', *Pediatrics* 2004;113:1007-15 pediatrics.aappublications.org/cgi/content/full/113/4/S1/1007

Coffee

Caffeine passes into breastmilk, but only in small amounts. In one study, where mothers drank five cups of coffee a day containing 100mg of caffeine per cup, their babies' received less than 1mg per kilo of caffeine per day and their sleep and heart rate were unaffected.

This means you can carry on drinking coffee without any problem. Having said this, it is still conceivable that consuming excessive amounts of coffee, together with cola drinks, chocolate and tea, might affect some particularly sensitive babies. If you think your baby is not sleeping enough or is restless, try drinking decaf and reducing your caffeine intake from other sources.

→ Ryu, J.E. 'Effect of maternal caffeine consumpton on heart rate and sleep time of breastfed infants', *Dev Pharmacol Ther* 1985;8:355-63

Radioactive isotopes

If you are given a scintigraphy (a scan using radioactive isotopes), it may be necessary to stop breastfeeding for a few hours. The United States Nuclear Regulatory Commission has drawn up very strict guidelines on how long breastfeeding must be suspended according to the type and the dose of isotope.

→ www.nrc.gov/reading-rm/doc-collections/nuregs/staff/sr1556/v9/r2/sr1556v9r2-final.pdf

This is a lengthy document, and you will find the information on lactation in Appendix U, pages 395ff. When the third column is blank, it means there is no need to stop breastfeeding. The guidelines have a wide safety margin, so there is no reason to wait any longer. It appears many hospitals are unaware of their existence, and advise mothers to stop breastfeeding for several days, which is completely unnecessary. You can print out these two pages and take them to your doctor.

The use of radioactive iodine to destroy thyroid cells in cases of hyperthyroidism is completely different. The dose is much higher and the baby has to be weaned.

Environmental pollutants

From time to time, a headline in the press (occasionally promoted by an environmental movement) warns of pesticides in human milk, spreading panic among mothers.

Why do scientists look for environmental pollutants in breastmilk? Is it a subject that concerns them? Not exactly. The fact is that some pollutants, such as DDT, dioxins or PCB, accumulate in fat tissue. So a blood test wouldn't be a very effective way of measuring a person's pollutant levels; this would require a biopsy. Breastmilk reflects the level of pollutants in fat tissue, and offers a much simpler method of determining the level of pollutants in a specific sector of the population. This is why dozens of studies worldwide have been carried out on breastmilk: it is a simple epidemiological marker, a way of measuring the problem of pollutants in any given country.

The existence of pollutants in breastmilk is nothing new, and studies of it were already being published decades ago. In fact, the levels of most pollutants (PCBs, DDT and the like) have declined in the last few decades, thanks to legal measures taken to limit or prohibit their use.

The hundreds of studies published in the last few decades showing that breastmilk reduces infections, allergies, diabetes, celiac disease, leukaemia and even global mortality in the United States (see page 308), were carried out on mothers whose milk contained higher levels of pollutants than they would today. Even when it contains pollutants, breastmilk is still much better than formula milk.

Various Dutch studies (Koopman-Esseboom, Boersma, Patandin) prove that exposure to PCBs, especially via the placenta, affects the psychomotor development and intelligence in the medium term. However, breastfeeding partially counteracts these effects, and the development of children who are breastfed, even with milk that contains pollutants, is better than that of children who are bottle fed.

Unless the mother has been exposed to significant accidental contamination, her pollutant levels reflect those of any other person of her age living in the same community. If her baby breathes the same air, eats the same food and drinks the same water as her, when he reaches her age his levels of pollutants will be the same as hers. The fact that he has received a tiny amount of his mother's pollutants will only fractionally increase his own levels. The only way to ensure that our children are less polluted than we are is to fight for a less polluted environment.

Drinking tap water that contains nitrates doesn't increase the concentration of nitrates in breastmilk. However, a baby is more at risk if his bottle is prepared with the same contaminated tap water.

Some mothers are very worried because they work with

chemical products, and have been told they can't breastfeed. This is complete nonsense. Like with any drug, the amount the baby takes through the milk is only a fraction of what the mother is exposed to.

If you are exposed to very large amounts of a substance so deadly that your milk is too toxic to give to your baby, you don't need to wean your baby, you need to look for another job. It is suicide to work for so long in such a hazardous environment. If you aren't in any danger, and you comply with all the safety measures that enable you to carry on working in perfect health until you are sixty-five, then it is safe for you to carry on breastfeeding.

→ Solomon, G.M., Weiss, P.M. 'Chemical contaminants in breast milk: time trends and regional variability', *Environ Health Perspect* 2002;110:A339-47 http://www.ehponline.org/docs/2002/110pA339-A347solomon/abstract.html

→ Landrigan, P.J., Sonawane, B., Mattison, D., McCally, M., Garg, A. 'Chemical contaminants in breast milk and their impacts on children's health: an overview. *Environ Health Perspect* 2002;110:A313-5 http://www.ehponline.org/docs/2002/110pA313-A315landrigan/abstract.html

→ Pronczuk, J., Akre, J., Moy, G., Vallenas, C. 'Global perspectives in breast milk contamination: infectious and toxic hazards', *Environ Health Perspect* 2002;110:A349-51 http://www.ncbi.nlm.nih.gov/pubmed/12055066

→ Koopman-Esseboom, C., Weisglas-Kuperus, N., de Ridder, M.A., Van der Paauw, C.G., Tuinstra, L.G., Sauer, P.J. 'Effects of polychlorinated biphenyl/dioxin exposure and feeding type on infants' mental and psychomotor development', *Pediatrics* 1996;97:700-6

→ Boersma, E.R., Lanting, C.I. 'Environmental exposure to polychlorinated biphenyls (PCBs) and dioxins. Consequences for longterm neurological and cognitive development of the child lactation', *Adv Exp Med Biol* 2000;478:271-87

→ Patandin, S., Lanting, C.I., Mulder, P.G., Boersma, E.R., Sauer, P.J., Weisglas-Kuperus. N. 'Effects of environmental exposure to polychlorinated biphenyls and dioxins on cognitive abilities in Dutch children at 42 months of age', *J Pediatr* 1999;134:33-41

→ Dusdieker, L.B., Stumbo, P.J., Kross, B.C., Dungy, C.I. 'Does increased nitrate ingestion elevate nitrate levels in human milk?', *Arch Pediatr Adolesc Med* 1996;150:311-4

Chapter 14
ILLNESSES OF THE MOTHER

In most cases a mother's illness and the treatment she receives for it won't harm her baby through her milk, nor will breastfeeding harm her. It is quite a different thing if the mother is physically unable, or feels too ill to breastfeed. But each mother must make this decision; her doctor can't decide for her.

Anaemia

Anaemia is very common after delivery because of the loss of blood. Obviously if the mother has anaemia, she must take the appropriate treatment (usually iron supplements, though there are also other types of anaemia). Not only can she carry on breastfeeding, it is good for her to breastfeed for as long she can. The longer she breastfeeds, the longer it will be before her periods come back, and menstruation is the main cause of iron deficiency in women.

The iron that the mother takes doesn't pass into her milk; iron levels in breastmilk remain constant.

Breastfeeding in the delivery room helps prevent anaemia in the mother, because oxytocin makes the womb contract and diminishes blood loss.

It has been observed that acute post-partum anaemia (less than 10mg/dl of haemoglobin) is linked to the early interruption of breastfeeding, which could be due to a reduction in the supply of breastmilk. When a mother tested normal during pregnancy, and has acute post-partum anaemia, it means she has lost a lot of blood during labour. It is thought that this loss of blood can affect the pituitary, leaving her 'confused', and incapable of producing enough prolactin for a few days. However, the problem is frequently transient and can be overcome if breastfeeding is properly handled (correct positioning, breastfeeding on demand, expressing milk where necessary).

Asthma

It is safe to breastfeed, and you can use any type of inhaler to treat your asthma (salbutamol, terbutaline, steroids, ipratropium). The dose you inhale is very low and very little of it passes into the blood, so a puffer is the best solution for both you and your baby (mainly for you; for the baby there is not a big difference). If you need oral steroids, it's still safe to breastfeed. Even when the dosage is high (for example with those used to treat autoimmune diseases) the level of steroids in the breastmilk is far lower than what the baby himself produces every day.

Allergies

It is recommended that babies with a family history of allergies breastfeed for as long as possible. There are several antihistamines (promethazine, loratidine, dexclorfeniramine, cetirizine and others), which are compatible with breastfeeding. Drowsiness in babies has been connected to a few other antihistamines. In any case, nasal steroid sprays are much more effective for treating rhinitis (sneezing and runny nose), and have fewer side-effects (for both mother and baby).

Myopia

I have found no evidence to back up the extraordinary suggestion that myopic women shouldn't breastfeed. Of the eight thousand or more articles on myopia compiled on Medline since 1963, only one (from 1969) mentions lactation. There isn't a single reference to any link between lactation and the development of myopia in any textbook on opthalmology.

Tooth decay

It is commonly believed that pregnancy and breastfeeding cause tooth decay due to decalcification of the teeth. However, tooth enamel contains no blood supply, and therefore can't become decalcified because of metabolic changes affecting the rest of the skeleton. The biggest risk factor for tooth decay, which some studies associated with pregnancy, appears to be due to the changes in the pH (acidity) of the saliva, and this can be prevented by proper dental hygiene.

→ Laine, M.A. 'Effect of pregnancy on periodontal and dental health', *Acta Odontol Scand* 2002; 60:257-64

Epilepsy

Carbamazepine, valproic acid, phenytoine and other drugs are all compatible with breastfeeding. If you have been taking phenobarbital while pregnant, not only can you breastfeed, it is good for you to breastfeed, because it will prevent the newborn from having convulsions (babies who have been receiving the drug in the womb can suffer withdrawal symptoms). There was a case published of a baby girl who suffered convulsions at seven months when her mother (who had been properly monitored in hospital) was wrongly advised by another doctor to force-wean her baby. She was forced to add phenobarbital to her baby's bottle for another year. Weaning should take place gradually over several months, the way it does when a baby naturally starts eating other foods.

Whatever happens, don't stop taking your medication or reduce the dosage without medical advice. Most antiepileptic drugs can't do your baby any harm. However, if you suffer a convulsion when you are holding her or bathing her it can be very dangerous.

→ Knott, C., Reynolds, F., Clayden, G. 'Infantile spasms on weaning from breast milk containing anticonvulsants', *Lancet* 1987;2:272-3

Pain

You can safely take paracetamol, ibuprofen, diclofenac, codeine, and many more.

Colds and flu

There is no treatment. They clear up by themselves after a few days. Unfortunately, in Spain we prescribe too many ineffective drugs, in particular antibiotics. There is only symptomatic treatment, meaning that the illness can't be cured, but you might feel a little better if you were feeling very unwell. If you are running a temperature or have a headache, take paracetamol or ibuprofen. If you have a bad cough and it is keeping you awake, take codeine. Antibiotics, antihistamines, mucolytics and expectorants won't help in these cases, and it isn't worth taking them, whether you are breastfeeding or not (but if you do, they won't harm your baby). Flu vaccines can be administered while breastfeeding.

Stomach ulcers

You can safely take omeprazole, ranitidine, famotidine and antacids. The common treatments for *Helicobacter pylori* (omeprazole, clarithromycin and amoxicillin) are also perfectly compatible with breastfeeding.

Dental fillings

There is a curious myth that fillings are toxic and it is dangerous to have a tooth filled while breastfeeding. This is complete nonsense. If fillings were toxic, the mother would be the one poisoned, as she is the one who will have them in her mouth for the rest of her life, and not her baby who will only be breastfeeding, not sucking her fillings. Local anaesthetic has no effect on babies either. There is no reason why a mother shouldn't breastfeed her baby in the waiting room as soon as she comes out, if her husband is there waiting with the baby.

Diabetes

Diabetic mothers should breastfeed. It has been observed that women with gestational diabetes mellitus (women who have contracted diabetes during pregnancy) are less than half as likely (4 per cent compared to 9 per cent) to become full-blown diabetics if they breastfeed, and in addition their 'good' cholesterol levels go up and their 'bad' cholesterol levels go down. Also, women who were already diabetic before they became pregnant usually require a lower dose of insulin while they are breastfeeding. Control your insulin dose according to your level of glucose, and don't be surprised if you only need three-quarters your usual dose.

Diabetic mothers have normal breastmilk. There may be slight variations, and the supply during the first few days may diminish slightly if the diabetes isn't properly controlled, but if the mother's glucose level is stable, her milk will be completely normal. What is needed is proper glycaemic control, early commencement of breastfeeding, and frequent feeds.

Diabetic mothers, especially when their glucose levels aren't properly controlled, appear more prone to mastitis, and nipple candidiasis. In order to prevent this, it is essential for her to give her baby frequent feeds in the correct position, and not to apply ointment to her nipples.

The newborn baby of a diabetic mother needs to be rigorously observed for the first few days, and given frequent glucose testing. However, these tests can be carried out while he is with his mother. Both skin-to-skin contact and frequent feeds help prevent hypoglycaemia in babies. Hospitalising a newborn, and taking him away from his mother, is not only unnecessary, it is dangerous for the baby of a diabetic mother.

→ Kjos, S.L.; Henry, O.; Lee, R.M.; Buchanan, T.A.; Mishell, D.R. 'The effect of lactation on glucose and lipid metabolism in women with recent gestational diabetes', *Obstet Gynecol* 1993;82:451-5

→ Davies, H.A., Clark, J.D.A., Dalton, K.J., Edwards, O.M. 'Insulin requirements of diabetic women who breast feed', *Br Med J* 1989;298:1357-8

→ Neubauer, S.H., Ferris, A.M., Chase, C.G., Fanelli, J., Thompson, C.A., Lammi-Keefe, C., et al. 'Delayed lactogenesis in women with insulin-dependent diabetes mellitus', *Am J Clin Nutr* 1993;58:54-60

→ Van Beusekom, C.M., Zeegers, T.A., Martini, I.A., Velvis, H.J.R., Visser, G.H.A., Van Doormaal, J.J., Muskiet, F.A.A. 'Milk of patients with tightly controlled insulin-dependent diabetes mellitus has normal macronutrient and fatty acid composition', *Am J Clin Nutr* 1993;57:938-43

→ Ostrom, K.M., Ferris, A.M. 'Prolactin concentrations in serum and milk of mothers with and without insulin-dependent diabetes mellitus', *Am J Clin Nutr* 1993;58: 49-53

→ Ferris, A.M., Dalidowitz, C.K., Ingardia, C.M., Reece, E.A., Fumia, F.D., Jensen, R.G., Allen. L.H. 'Lactation outcome in insulin-dependent diabetic women', *J Am Diet Assoc* 1988;88:317-22

→ Christensson, K., Siles, C., Moreno, L., Belaustequi, A., De La Fuente, P., Lagercrantz, H., Puyol, P., Winberg, J. 'Temperature, metabolic adaptation and crying in healthy full-term newborns cared for skin-to-skin or in a cot', *Acta Pædiatr* 1992;81:488-93

Breast cancer

It is not advisable to breastfeed while undergoing chemotherapy (almost all anti-cancer drugs are contraindicated during lactation). It is also impossible to breastfeed while on tamoxifen, because it is a powerful inhibitor of milk production. However, mothers who have finished their treatment can breastfeed; it has been observed that after having a lumpectomy and radiotherapy mothers are able to breastfeed from the healthy breast, and sometimes even from the sick breast. There is an element of heredity in breast cancer, and women are more likely to get cancer if their mothers had it. Years ago, someone came up with the theory that this could be due to a virus, with which a mother could infect her daughter while breastfeeding. If this were true then mothers with breast cancer shouldn't breastfeed their daughters. But the virus theory was proved false. Heredity is passed on through our genes, not by a virus, and the incidence of breast cancer – malignant or benign – is identical in women who have been breastfed and women who have been bottle fed.

Women who have breastfed for longer are less likely to get breast cancer (see page 311).

→ Helewa, M., Levesque, P., Provencher, D., Lea, R.H., Rosolowich, V., Shapiro, H.M. Breast Disease Committee and Executive Committeee and Council, Society of Obstetricians and Gynaecologists of Canada 'Breast cancer, pregnancy, and breastfeeding', *J Obstet Gynaecol Can* 2002;24:164-80

Cystic fibrosis

More and more female children affected by cystic fibrosis reach adulthood and have babies. Those whose weight is normal and whose clinical situation is stable can breastfeed. The concentration of chlorine and sodium in their blood is normal. Although in some cases the concentration of essential fatty acids in their milk is diminished, most babies who are breastfed by mothers with the disease develop normally. Pregnancy and breastfeeding have no adverse effect on the nutritional or clinical state of patients or on their longevity.

→ Gilljam, M., Antoniou, M., Shin, J., Dupuis, A., Corey, M., Tullis, D.E. 'Pregnancy in cystic fibrosis. Fetal and maternal outcome', *Chest* 2000;118:85-91 chestjournal.chestpubs.org/content/118/1/85full

Infectious diseases

Generally speaking, any infection the mother may have (flu, colds, urinary tract infection, pneumonia, diarrhoea) will not affect the supply or composition of her milk, and won't be transmitted to her baby through her milk, so she can carry on breastfeeding.

In many cases, a few days after she is infected, antibodies to the illness will appear in the milk, which can completely or partially protect the baby. Not only can the baby be breastfed, he should be breastfed.

> → Zavaleta, N., Lanata, C., Butrón, B., Brown, K.H., Lonnerdal, B. 'Effect of acute maternal infection on quantity and composition of breast milk', *Am J Clin Nutr* 1995;62:559-63

Hepatitis B

Hepatitis B is not transmitted through milk. Even before there was a vaccine, this had already been demonstrated. Nor is it transmitted during pregnancy, except in very rare cases, because the virus can't pass through the placenta. Hepatitis can be passed from mother to baby during labour, because the contractions produce tiny tears in the placenta through which the virus can enter. It is therefore possible to prevent infection by treating the baby as soon as he is born, because he will only just have been infected with a few viruses, and these can be destroyed before they cause any harm. If the baby were infected weeks before the birth, this wouldn't work.

All pregnant women are tested for hepatitis B. When a mother is a carrier, the newborn is immediately given immunoglobulin and vaccinated against the virus. It is essential that this is done within twenty-four hours, and if possible within twelve hours. If it is left any later, it might not work.

You can safely breastfeed both before and after your baby is vaccinated.

> → Giles, M.L., Sasadeusz, J.J., Garland, S.M., Grover, S.R., Hellard, M.E. 'An audit of obstetricians' management of women potentially infected with blood-borne viruses', *Med J Aust* 2004; 180:328-32 www.mja.com.au/public/issues/180_07_050404/ gil10614_fm.html

Hepatitis C

Several studies have shown that hepatitis C can't be transmitted through breastmilk. In general, the virus is rarely transmitted from mother to baby.

For example, S. L. Thomas and his colleagues examined eleven studies carried out in different countries. In six of them, there wasn't a single case of infection among 227 babies, 168 of whom had been breastfed. This means the babies weren't infected either in the womb or during delivery or during breastfeeding. In the other five studies (involving 197 babies, 114 of whom were breastfed) there were a few cases of infection, which must have occurred during pregnancy or delivery, because they were evenly distributed between those who were breastfed and those who were bottle fed.

It is possible to measure the amount of virus present in a carrier's blood: if the level is high it means they are highly contagious. Mothers with a high level of the virus are sometimes advised not to breastfeed. But there is no reason for this. In a small study carried out in Hong Kong, out of eleven highly contagious mothers who breastfed, not a single baby was infected.

There are also those who say that a mother who has cracked nipples shouldn't breastfeed, because if they bleed the baby could be infected. This sounds logical, but there is no evidence to back it up. In contrast, when we say that hepatitis C can't be transmitted through breastmilk, we aren't basing our argument on theories, we aren't saying: 'the virus isn't present in breastmilk' or 'it is destroyed by gastric juices' or anything of the sort. We say it because actual studies have been carried out on hundreds of nursing mothers whose babies have not been infected. It is reasonable to assume some of these mothers had cracked nipples, and yet their babies weren't infected. Whether you carry the hepatitis C virus or not, it is sensible to try to avoid cracks (no one likes having cracks), and I have explained how to do this in the chapter on correct positioning. But even if you do have cracks, you can still breastfeed.

The one exception is mothers who are carriers of both hepatitis C and HIV. In this case, hepatitis C can be transmitted during pregnancy and during breastfeeding. It is as though the two viruses were friends, each helping to transmit the other.

→ Thomas, S.L., Newell, M-L., Peckham, C.S., Ades, A.E., Hall, A.J. 'A review of hepatitis C virus (HCV) vertical transmission: risks of transmission to infants born to mothers with and without HCV viraemia or human immunodeficiency virus infection', *Internat J Epidemiol* 1998;27:108-17

→ Lin, H.H., Kao, J.H., Hsu, H.Y., Ni, Y.H., Chang, M.H., Huang, S.C. et al. 'Absence of infection in breastfed infants born to hepatitis C virus-infected mothers', *J Pediatr* 1995;126:589-591

HIV/AIDS

HIV/AIDS is transmitted through breastmilk. About 15 per cent of the children of carrier mothers are infected during pregnancy, labour and delivery, and 15 per cent more during breastfeeding. As a result, breastfeeding is inadvisable in countries where there are adequate alternatives (access to formula milk, and drinking water) as there are in Europe.

In some countries, the mortality rate from malnutrition and infectious diseases among babies who don't breastfeed is so high that breastfeeding is seen as the lesser of two evils.

Administering antiretroviral drugs (anti-HIV/AIDS medicine) during lactation lowers the infection rate, but doesn't prevent it completely.

One study suggests that mixed feeding is the cause of HIV transmission. Apparently microbes and alien proteins in other foods cause tiny lesions in the baby's digestive tract, which allow the virus to pass. But further studies are necessary for this to be established as fact. In any case, it would require exclusive breastfeeding; the baby shouldn't be given a single bottle, not even water, during the entire breastfeeding period, and he should be weaned from one day to the next, because gradual weaning or introducing solids constitutes mixed feeding.

Studies have also been undertaken to examine the possibility of expressing milk, and treating it with heat or chemicals to disinfect it before feeding it to the baby.

In short: there is no safe way of preventing infection. In developed countries, breastfeeding with HIV is inadvisable.

Tuberculosis

Tuberculosis isn't transmitted through breastmilk, except perhaps in cases of breast tuberculosis, a disease now very infrequent in developed countries. The more common form of the disease, pulmonary tuberculosis, has respiratory transmission. The baby can become infected whether he is breastfed or bottle fed. So the question is not whether the baby can nurse, but whether he should remain with his mother.

Occasionally, a diagnosis of tuberculosis can be delayed due to an unwillingness to take X-rays during pregnancy. This is a serious mistake. Untreated active tuberculosis represents a far greater danger to both mother and foetus than the tiny amount of radiation from a chest X-ray. If a pregnant woman is suspected of having tuberculosis, she must have a chest X-ray and start treatment.

If, at the moment of delivery, the mother has been receiving treatment for several weeks, she is no longer contagious and there is no risk for the baby. If on the other hand tuberculosis is diagnosed a few days after the baby is born (for example, when she is admitted to hospital someone notices the mother has a persistent cough, gives her the tuberculin test, waits three days for the result, gives her a chest X-ray, waits another couple of days...), the baby will already have been exposed, and there is no point in taking him away from his mother. This baby will need to take isoniazid for at least ten weeks, whether he is with his mother or not.

If, when the baby is born, the mother has been receiving treatment for less than two months, separating the baby from her in order to prevent infection could be a consideration. However, the psychological cost to the family as a whole is very high, and it would also be necessary to make sure those looking after the baby haven't been infected (have other members of the infected mother's family also been tested?) For this reason, WHO recommends keeping the baby with the mother and giving him isoniazid. Obviously, if the baby remains with his mother, he can nurse.

If the tuberculosis is renal or skeletal, there is no need to stop breastfeeding, as neither form is contagious.

→ Division of Child Health and Development. 'Breastfeeding and maternal tuberculosis', UPDATE 1998;23

Diarrhoea

Normally speaking, the mother won't need any medication (except in special cases where an antibiotic is prescribed, usually after a culture is made). However, she will need to drink more to compensate the loss of liquid. Some women with acute diarrhoea who don't consume enough liquid notice a slight decrease in milk supply. If the diarrhoea is serious, take an oral rehydration solution, and continue breastfeeding.

It would be unwise for a mother to wean her baby when she has diarrhoea, because it is the most dangerous time: how did she get the diarrhoea? Is there an epidemic? Perhaps the water is contaminated? What would she use to prepare the baby's bottle?

Chicken pox/shingles

The same virus causes chicken pox and shingles. When we are infected with chicken pox, the virus remains hidden in our body, and can take advantage of a lowered immune system to re-emerge as shingles many years later.

In the early stages of pregnancy (before the twentieth week), chicken pox can cause malformations. Chicken pox is a serious, and often fatal, illness for a newborn. However, for a baby of one month old or more, it is a mild illness, the same as in an older child. This is why very strict precautions are taken when a pregnant woman has chicken pox.

The following is a list of rules taken from the Australian Society for Infectious Diseases, which you can look up in its entirety on the Internet, and if necessary print out and take to your doctor.

- Zoster immunoglobulin (ZIG) should be offered to pregnant women who have not had chicken pox within seventy-two hours after significant exposure to chicken pox. Remember that chicken pox is already contagious before the lesions appear, so if you discover that your little nephew whom you played with the day before yesterday has chicken pox, contact your midwife or obstetrician immediately. If you don't know for sure whether you have had chicken pox or not they will give you a test.
- In some cases you may need to be given an anti-viral treatment.

- If the mother contracts chicken pox seven or more days before giving birth, she will have had enough time to produce anti-bodies which will pass through the placenta and protect her baby. There won't be any problem.

- If a mother develops chicken pox up to seven days before delivery or up to twenty-eight days after delivery, zoster immunoglobulin (ZIG) should be given to the baby within seventy-two hours (better still within twenty-four hours) of being born or exposed. This is an emergency. It means that if you contract chicken pox less than twenty-eight days after you give birth, you must call your doctor immediately or have someone take your baby to casualty so that he can be given an injection. But don't whatever you do go to maternity, because you may infect other pregnant women.

  (A reassuring fact: if you get chicken pox twenty-nine or thirty-two days after you give birth, don't panic and don't insist your baby is given an injection 'to be on the safe side'. We doctors are extremely cautious in these situations, and the 'safe side' has already been taken into account in the twenty-eight days. In fact, the real risk is in the first two weeks. So if a doctor who appears to know what she is doing, says: 'There's no need, we only give injections up to 24 days,' you can trust her.)

- If you get shingles during or after pregnancy, there is no need to worry; it means you had chicken pox years ago, and your baby has already received antibodies through your placenta. Neither the foetus nor the newborn are in any danger.

- A mother with chicken pox or shingles doesn't need to be isolated from her own baby, and breastfeeding of babies infected with or exposed to chicken pox is encouraged, although mother and baby might need to be isolated in the hospital from other mothers and babies.

→ Heuchan, A.M., Isaacs, D. 'The management of varicella-zoster virus exposure and infection in pregnancy and the newborn period', Australasian Subgroup in Paediatric Infectious Diseases of the Australasian Society for Infectious Diseases. *Med J Aust* 2001;174:288-92 www.mja.com.au/public/issues/174_06_190301/heuchan/heuchan.html

Herpes simplex

In the newborn (younger than fifteen days) herpes simplex can cause a potentially fatal generalized infection. Infection normally takes place during delivery, but a few cases of infection through breastmilk have been reported. During the first month, where herpes simplex lesions appear on the nipple, breastfeeding is inadvisable until they are healed. The baby can carry on nursing from the other breast. Likewise, people who have cold sores shouldn't kiss a newborn. For a month-old baby, herpes simplex is no longer serious, and babies frequently infect their mothers with herpes simplex. There is no reason to stop breastfeeding.

→ Lawrence, R.A. *La lactancia materna*, Barcelona: Mosby-Doyma, 1996

Hyperthyroidism

This disease is usually treated with anti-thyroid drugs such as carbimazole and methimazole. Many doctors prefer to prescribe pregnant mothers with propylthiouracil. There are a lot of published studies about nursing mothers who take methimazole, some for more than a year, and their baby's hormone levels are normal.

It isn't always easy to give the correct dose to each patient, and regular tests should be carried out to determine whether to increase or decrease the dosage. However, even during periods when the dosage was too high, and the mother was suffering from hypothyroidism, nothing happened to the baby.

Many recommend regular testing of the baby's hormone levels. This is probably an unnecessary precaution. In any event, it would only have to be done for the first few months, because as the baby grows bigger he takes less and less milk per kilo of bodyweight (and therefore less of the drug). If he was fine during the first few months there is no reason for him not to be later on.

If a doctor tells you not to breastfeed, get a second opinion. If necessary, print out the relevant article below and take it to your doctor.

→ Azizi, F., Khoshniat, M., Bahrainian, M., Hedayati, M. 'Thyroid Function and Intellectual Development of Infants Nursed by Mothers Taking Methimazole', *Clin Endocrinol Metab* 2000;85:3233-8 jcem.endojournals.org/cgi/content/full/85/9/3233

Hypothyroidism

Hypothyroidism is treated with thyroid hormones. The aim of the treatment is to restore the thyroid hormone levels to those of a healthy person. It follows that a mother who is being treated for hypothyroidism will have the same levels of hormone in her milk as any other mother. She can breastfeed without any doubt. Thyroid hormone is a normal component of breastmilk.

Can it harm her baby if the mother takes too much of the hormone for a while? No. The amount of hormone in the milk is so small that even if it were doubled or trebled it would still be insignificant. Too much thyroid hormone produces very visible symptoms: nervousness, hyperactivity, tachycardia and so on. The mother would realise she was altered, would lower the dose, and the baby would be oblivious.

Hypothyroidism (and to a lesser extent hyperthyroidism) may cause the milk supply to decrease (see page 151), but with the proper treatment it can be re-established.

Hypertension and heart disease

Occasionally a mother who has heart disease is forbidden to breastfeed because it might put a 'strain' on her heart.

This is untrue. Many years ago, it was shown that there is no difference in heart rate, heart output (the amount of blood the heart pumps in one minute) or blood pressure between mothers who breastfeed and mothers who bottle feed. Breastfeeding therefore doesn't put any strain on the heart. And the drugs used in these cases are usually compatible with breastfeeding.

Diuretics like thiazide and furosemide pose no threat to babies, although some think that in certain cases they reduce the milk supply. This is unlikely, but we should be vigilant; probably the baby's response would be to feed more, which would increase the milk supply again.

Depression

During the first few weeks after childbirth, the majority of mothers experience moments of depression, irritability or tearfulness: what is commonly known as 'the baby blues'. Full-blown post-natal depression is a serious condition that requires treatment. A mother suffering from post-natal depression doesn't respond properly to her baby: she talks to him less, smiles at him less, is incapable of paying attention to him or comforting him, and this in turn affects the baby's development.

Social support plays an important role in preventing post-natal depression. It isn't good for a mother to be alone with her baby most of the day. Visits from the baby's grandmothers or other family members and friends can be a great help, as well as going to breastfeeding support groups, or post-natal gym classes. It has been shown that a simple weekly home visit from a nurse helps prevent and treat depression.

Depression is no reason to wean a baby. There have been cases where mothers have taken their own lives after being told to wean their baby. Of course, this could be coincidental, but it is easy to see why weaning won't improve a mother's state of mind. Depression is characterised by feelings of inadequacy and failure, so if a depressed mother is also told she has to stop breastfeeding because she is doing it wrong, because her milk isn't good for her baby…

There are a number of antidepressants that are perfectly compatible with breastfeeding. The most suitable ones are probably paroxetine, sertraline and nortriptyline. Others considered as safe are amitriptyline, desipramine, clomipramine and dotiepine. A few (mildly) adverse side-effects have been observed in some newborns whose mothers were taking doxepine or fluoxetine. In the case of fluoxetine (Prozac), this is a little vague; it has been shown that the amount of drug that passes into the milk is very low, and many believe it is compatible with breastfeeding, and that the supposed adverse affects are due to it being by far the most widely prescribed antidepressant on the market.

→ Gjerdingen, D. 'The effectiveness of various postpartum depression treatments and the impact of antidepressant drugs on nursing infants', *J Am Board Fam Pract* 2003;16:372-82 www.jabfp.org/cgi/reprint/16/5/372

Prolactinoma

Prolactinoma is a benign, sometimes microscopic, tumour on the pituitary gland, which secretes prolactin. It can cause amenorrhea (absent menstruation) and galactorrhea (spontaneous flow of milk from the breast in someone who isn't breastfeeding). In cases of amenorrhea, it is necessary to treat the woman with lactation suppressants so that she is able to ovulate and have children.

Breastfeeding doesn't aggravate the illness or cause the tumour to grow. If your doctor tries to dissuade you from breastfeeding, you can recommend these articles:

→ Hölmgren, U., Bergstrand, G., Hagenfeldt, K., Werner, S. 'Women with prolactinoma – effect of pregnancy and lactation on serum prolactin and on tumour growth', *Acta Endocrinol (Copenh)* 1986;111:452-9

→ Pasinetti, E., Schivardi, M.R., Falsetti, L., Gastaldi, A. 'Effetti della terapia e della gravi- danza nella iperprolattinemia da adenoma ipofisario. Caso clinico', *Minerva Ginecol* 1989;41:157-60

→ Zárate, A., Canales, E.S., Alger, M., Forsbach, G. 'The effect of pregnancy and lactation on pituitary prolactin-secreting tumours', *Acta Endocrinol (Copenh)* 1979;92:407-12

Admission to hospital

If a mother is admitted to hospital (for example, due to an accident, or to have a gallbladder removed), her baby should go with her, whether he is being breastfed or not. It is very traumatic for children under three to be separated from their mother, especially if the separation lasts for several days. This isn't simply about sustaining breastfeeding; it isn't enough for the mother to express her milk and for someone else to feed it to her baby. The baby needs milk, but he needs his mother much more.

Sometimes babies aren't allowed on hospital visits for fear they may catch germs. But if hospitals are such dangerous places, why do they allow babies to be born or admitted there when they are ill? Separation would only be justified in special cases; for example, if the mother has to be quarantined because she has a serious infectious disease. Otherwise, a baby should be allowed to visit his mother for as long as her physical state allows (not based on the hospital staff's preconceptions or how convenient it is for them).

A caesarean section is a full-blown abdominal operation. If a mother who has given birth by caesarean is able to have her newborn baby in the room and to nurse him, a woman who has undergone surgery for appendicitis, gallstones or an ovarian cyst can also have her baby of four or fifteen months in her room and nurse him.

Also, if the mother can see her baby frequently, she will probably relax more than if she is away from him for several days.

If you have undergone surgery, you will be able to breastfeed as soon as you come round from the anaesthetic (which means you have already metabolised nearly all of the drug).

If you are scheduled to go into hospital, besides trying to be admitted as late as possible, you can express your milk a few days in advance, and leave it in the freezer for those moments when it is impossible for you to breastfeed (with an older baby who is on solids you probably won't need to express milk). Ask around the various hospitals where you live, and try to find one where they provide the facilities for you to be with your child. If they have needless restrictions, this is the time to speak with the hospital manager, the head of department, or whoever it is you need to see in order to demand your rights.

If it will be physically impossible for you to breastfeed for a few hours (because you are in the operating theatre, or the recovery room, or undergoing tests), it is important for your milk to be expressed so your condition isn't further complicated by engorgement or mastitis. Your relatives should remind the nurses of this.

Ulcerative colitis (how to find information online)

It isn't within the scope of this book to list every illness a mother might have while she is nursing, so you need know how to look for information yourself. I will use ulcerative colitis as an example.

The Internet is an inexhaustible source of information. Unfortunately, it allows anyone to publish all sorts of nonsense, and it is important to know how to find and identify accurate information.

In order to learn more about this disease, a good place to start is Medline Plus, an American government search engine for non-professionals. It only lists accurate information:

→ www.nlm.nih.gov/medlineplus

Other pages provide detailed information for medical professionals. Remember that the language used is a little opaque, and not exactly designed to reassure patients; it is very easy to fall prey to 'medical student syndrome', and to imagine you have all the symptoms you read about.

For example, www.emedicine.com provides excellent, detailed articles:

→ www.emedicine.com/med/topic2336.htm

It is possible that so far you have been unable to find the exact answer to the question 'is it safe to breastfeed?' This is a highly specialised query, which many textbooks on gastroenterology won't even touch on. In this case, we will need to go to the source, and search on Medline (see page 238). Type in:

ulcerative colitis AND (breastfeeding OR breast feeding OR lactation)

You will find thirty articles (or more). If you read through the summaries, you will see that it is safe for you to breastfeed if you suffer from ulcerative colitis, that there are many studies of women who have breastfed, and that the majority of drugs used to treat it are compatible with breastfeeding. You will also discover that breastfeeding reduces the risk of ulcerative colitis and Crohn's disease in babies, and you should keep this in mind when anyone happily tells you that you shouldn't breastfeed. You can print out the most relevant articles and show them to your doctor.

Chapter 15
SPECIAL CIRCUMSTANCES

Twins

It is perfectly possible to breastfeed twins. In fact, there are many known cases of mothers exclusively breastfeeding triplets, and even quadruplets.

Any mother can produce enough milk to breastfeed two babies. The secret, as with one baby, is to start as soon as possible, to nurse frequently and in the correct position. The biggest obstacle to nursing your baby isn't a lack of milk, it is the number of people (including health professionals) who will tell you that it is impossible.

To start with, especially with first-time mothers, it is probably easier to nurse them separately. Once you have mastered the technique, you may find it more comfortable to nurse them at the same time. They may alternate between breasts, but sometimes each baby has his or her favourite breast, which needn't be a problem (some old books warn mothers that if a baby always nurses from the same breast, he will always look at her through the same eye, which will develop more quickly than the other. This sort of advice seems absurd and speculative; the baby has the whole of the rest of the day to look at his mother through both eyes).

Obviously, having twins is exhausting, whether you breastfeed or bottle feed them. It is easy enough to find somebody who will bottle feed them while you do the shopping, but ideally you need somebody to do the shopping (and cooking and cleaning) while you breastfeed. This is most important in the early days, because you will have very little free time. If you discover you are having twins, try to contact some mothers' groups, and speak to other women who have had twins. Also, think about who could help you with chores. If none of your family can help, think about hiring someone. It will be money well spent.

There are specific support groups for mothers with twins, triplets, and quadruplets and you can find groups local to you using an Internet search (in the UK, try TAMBA www.tamba. org.uk). Some breastfeeding supporters also specialise in helping mothers of multiples to breastfeed.

Premature babies

When a mother gives birth before term, her milk is different. For several weeks it contains more proteins, calcium, sodium and other nutrients than ordinary breastmilk. It is specially adapted to the needs of the premature baby.

It is a good idea to express milk a few hours after delivery, as soon as you feel physically able. It works better if you express several times a day (six to eight), but for shorter periods. Within a few days, you will probably have too much milk, because premature babies nurse very little. The left over milk can be frozen and kept for later.

In the old days, premature babies weren't allowed to nurse at the breast until they could drink from a bottle without any problem. Now we know this was a mistake. Breastfeeding is much easier than bottle feeding, and a premature baby's heart rate, respiratory rate and blood oxygen level is closer to normal when he nurses, so he should start much sooner. Many hospitals practise the kangaroo method (hopefully this will one day apply to all hospitals): the baby is taken from the incubator, and placed skin-to-skin with his mother. This has been done successfully with premature babies of less than twenty-six weeks who weigh less than 600 grams. Premature babies that remain in skin-to-skin contact their mothers are warmer, they breathe more easily, gain weight more quickly, have fewer infections and their psychomotor development is better. The mother feels much more assured, and she produces more milk.

If your hospital doesn't practice this method, insist and give them information. Set yourself workable, short-term objectives: 'I'm not suggesting you change the care you give premature babies, but could I hold my baby for a few hours this afternoon?'

In Germany, Sontheimer and his colleagues transported

premature newborns in skin-to-skin contact with their mothers as far as 400km without using any incubators, and with excellent results. One important advantage of this form of transportation is that the mother is able to travel with her baby: too often she has to remain in a small local hospital, alone and anxious, while her sick child is transported to a large hospital.

→ Ludington-Hoe, S.M., Ferreira, C., Swinth, J., Ceccardi, J.J. 'Safe criteria and procedure for kangaroo care with intubated preterm infants', *J Obstet Gynecol Neonatal Nurs* 2003;32:579-88

→ Ludington-Hoe, S.M., Anderson, G.C., Swinth, J.Y., Thompson, C., Hadeed, A.J. 'Randomized controlled trial of kangaroo care: cardiorespiratory and thermal effects on healthy preterm infants', *Neonatal Netw* 2004;23:39-48

→ Feldman, R., Eidelman, A.I., Sirota, L., Weller, A. 'Comparison of skin-to-skin (kangaroo) and traditional care: parenting outcomes and preterm infant development', *Pediatrics* 2002;110:16-26 pediatrics.aappublications.org/cgi/content/full/110/1/16

→ Hurst, N.M., Valentine, C.J., Renfro, L., Burns, P., Ferlic, L. 'Skin-to-skin holding in the neonatal intensive care unit influences maternal milk volume', *J Perinatol* 1997;17:213-17

→ Sontheimer, D., Fischer, C.B., Buch, K.E. 'Kangaroo transport instead of incubator transport', *Pediatrics* 2004;113:920-3 pediatrics.aappublications.org/cgi/content/full/113/4/920

→ Closa Monasterolo, R., Moralejo Benéitez, J., Ravés Olivé, M.M., Martínez Martínez, M.J., Gómez Papí, A. 'Método canguro en recién nacidos prematuros ingresados en una Unidad de Cuidados Intensivos Neonatal', *An Esp Pediatr* 1998;49: 495-8.

→ Cattaneo, A., Davanzo, R., Uxa, F., Tamburlini, G. 'Recommendations for the implementation of Kangaroo Mother Care for low birthweight infants', *Acta Pædiatr* 1998; 87: 440-5

→ Humane neonatal Care Initiative. www.hnci.eu

→ Fundación Canguro http://fundacioncanguro.co/en.html

Chapter 16

INFANTS' DISEASES

Jaundice

In jaundice, the skin and mucosa (in particular the whites of the eyes) turn yellow due to a build-up of bilirubin.

Bilirubin is a derivative of haemoglobin. The red blood cells (or erythrocytes) that contain haemoglobin have a life-span of only four months. They die and are replaced by new ones. When haemoglobin isn't contained inside the red blood cell it is toxic, and the body breaks it up. The protein part is removed, and so is the iron (which is recycled to make new red blood cells), and what remains is turned into bilirubin. A lot of work for nothing, because bilirubin is still toxic and has to be excreted from the body.

Bilirubin is fat soluble, and therefore can't be excreted through the urine or the bile, both of which are made up of water and water-soluble substances. Fortunately, the liver is able to combine (conjugate) the bilirubin with other substances; the conjugated bilirubin can then be dissolved in water and excreted in the bile. It is bilirubin that gives faeces its distinctive colour (and explains why some liver diseases cause white stools).

Conjugated bilirubin can't be absorbed in the intestine. But inside the intestine, part of the bilirubin becomes fat-soluble again, and is reabsorbed. This is the enterohepatic cycle of bilirubin.

All of this occurs in both children and adults, but not in foetuses. The foetus can't expel bilirubin through the bile (foetuses don't poo inside the womb, though this can occur during delivery, and is a sign of foetal distress), and so foetal bilirubin passes through the placenta and is excreted into the mother's liver. In order for the bilirubin to pass through the placenta it has to be fat-soluble.

The liver of a foetus can't conjugate bilirubin, because if it did, the conjugated bilirubin would remain in the foetal blood, unable to pass through the placenta, and would gradually build up until it killed the foetus.

When the baby is born, everything changes: his lungs, which were full of water, now have to fill with air. He was receiving all his food through the placenta, now he has to eat, digest and metabolise. His kidneys, which haven't had to expel any toxic substances (the amniotic fluid is basically the foetus's urine, only it is non-toxic because the foetus has to drink it), now have to start eliminating them. And at the same time, his liver has to begin conjugating bilirubin. The majority of newborns make all of these changes quickly and simultaneously without any problem.

It takes a while for the baby's liver to start working at full capacity, and for a few days there is a build up of bilirubin and the baby becomes slightly jaundiced. This slow activation of the liver probably isn't a design fault, but rather it happens on purpose. Bilirubin isn't good for adults, but for the newborn it acts as an antioxidant. It is good for newborns to be slightly jaundiced. But not too much; very high levels of bilirubin can cause serious brain damage (kernicterus).

Nature couldn't predict that we would separate the newborn from his mother, stick dummies and bottles in his mouth, and only allow him to nurse every four hours. Babies who don't breastfeed very much poo less, and so the conjugated bilirubin that has been excreted into the bile remains in the gut for many hours and is reabsorbed. The liver is unable to conjugate all the bilirubin that has come back from the intestine, and the baby becomes more jaundiced. This is what is known as 'breastfeeding jaundice', although some suggest 'jaundice due to lack of breastfeeding' would be more apt. The best way to prevent the baby from becoming more jaundiced is to start breastfeeding properly: the baby's first feed is in the delivery room, the baby stays with his mother round the clock, is breastfed on demand, and nurses and midwives are there to help the mother position her baby correctly.

Because a small amount of bilirubin is good for the baby, breastmilk contains a substance that helps bilirubin to de-conjugate in the intestine. In babies who are bottle fed, jaundice disappears completely in a about a week, while babies who are breastfed can remain visibly yellow for several weeks, and even as long as two or three months. This is what is known as 'breastmilk jaundice'. It is terribly misleading, and I would like to think that one day some American scientist will change the name, but for the moment this is what we have to work with.

Some paediatricians, who have little experience of normal nursing babies (up until a few years ago there were so few of them), are alarmed when presented with prolonged jaundice, and insist on doing tests, tests, and more tests. This is unnecessary. If the baby looks very yellow, you do a blood test, if the result is high (18mg/dl) it is sensible to wait a couple of days and do another test to make sure it hasn't gone up. But if the second test shows it has gone down, then there is no need to do more tests to make sure it has gone down from 16 to 13 to 11 to 8.5 to 7, and so on. We already know it will continue to go down gradually, and that this can take several weeks.

Almost a third of healthy babies who remain jaundiced for more than a month have Gilbert's syndrome – a hereditary condition caused by a faulty gene that affects the conjugation of bilirubin in the liver (this is not an illness, and people with Gilbert's syndrome can live until they are a hundred). Adults with Gilbert's syndrome can experience intermittent episodes of mild jaundice, which often coincide with other illnesses such as flu. The problem is that when this happens, the doctor panics and orders blood tests, thinking you might have hepatitis. It is a relief to know what you have, and that there is no need to worry. If there are any known cases of Gilbert's syndrome in your family (or suspected cases; people who occasionally suffer from jaundice and the doctor can't find anything wrong with them), tell your paediatrician.

As bilirubin is eliminated through the liver and not the urine, drinking more water has no effect. Dextrose solution is useless in preventing or treating jaundice.

When bilirubin levels are very high, phototherapy is used. The light from special lamps acts on the skin, destroying the bilirubin. There is no need for a baby to be placed in the neonatal intensive care unit if all he needs is phototherapy; phototherapy lamps are mobile, and can be wheeled into the mother's room. Insist on them letting the baby stay with you. He has to be breastfed as often as possible, firstly so that his bilirubin goes down, and secondly because the heat of the lamps means he needs more liquid (more frequent feeds should do the trick, but in some cases he may need to be given water). Decades ago, it was thought that if a baby had jaundice, he should not be breastfed for a day or two. Some doctors still recommend this, even though it has been shown to be unnecessary. In cases where jaundice is caused by another illness, or is due to Rh incompatibility, breastfeeding should not be discontinued either.

In rare cases where the levels of bilirubin are so high that the baby is at serious risk, he has to be given an exchange transfusion; all his blood must be taken out and replaced with fresh blood. This is extremely rare in cases of 'normal' jaundice, which are due to the baby simply not nursing enough – what we call physiological or paraphysiological ('almost normal') jaundice. However, jaundice has many other causes: problems with blood group compatibility (Rh and ABO), liver problems, infections and so on. Depending on the baby's age and other symptoms, the hospital will carry out the appropriate tests to make sure it is nothing serious.

Nowadays, healthy babies of three to four days old aren't usually given phototherapy unless their bilirubin reaches 20, and will only be given an exchange transfusion if it reaches 25. In the old days, phototherapy was given a lot sooner, but this has been shown to be unnecessary. However, jaundice is much more dangerous in babies that are ill or premature, and it has to be treated much sooner.

These days, babies leave hospital so soon they haven't yet turned yellow. Check your baby's colour when you leave the hospital; his face, his feet, his eyes. If after a few days at home he definitely looks more yellow, go to your nearest health centre, or return to the hospital. You must always check the colour in natural daylight, as artificial light is often yellowish and can be very deceptive.

Many doctors and nurses still advise mothers to put their babies in the sun to reduce jaundice. This is a mistake. When a baby is given phototherapy in hospital, he is under the lamp around the clock (he is only taken out to be fed). However, a baby shouldn't be exposed to the sun for more than ten minutes without a sun protection factor of at least thirty; if he is left in the sun for an hour without any sunscreen he could get severe sunburn, but the jaundice won't have reduced because an hour isn't enough. Take no notice. Either your baby needs phototherapy (which has to be done in hospital, or sometimes at home with a hospital-grade phototherapy lamp) or he doesn't (in which case he doesn't need to be in the sun). What he needs is frequent breastfeeding.

→ American Academy of Pediatrics Subcommittee on Hyperbilirubinemia, 'Management of hyperbilirubinemia in the newborn infant 35 or more weeks of gestation', *Pediatrics* 2004;114:297-316 aappolicy.aappublications.org/cgi/content/full/pediatrics;114/1/297

→ Johnston, R.V., Anderson, J.N., Prentice, C. 'Is sunlight an effective treatment for infants with jaundice?', *Med J Aust* 2003;178:403 www.mja.com.au/public/issues/178_08_210403/joh10652_fm.html

Down's syndrome

Babies with Down's syndrome may have difficulty nursing. They suffer from hypotonia, which means they can't latch on to the nipple properly, and will slip off easily if they aren't firmly held. They have big tongues (macroglossia), which can mean the breast won't fit properly into their mouth. Many also suffer from heart disease, and get tired while nursing.

And yet, breastfeeding is particularly beneficial for these babies: it protects them against infection (to which they are prone), and it strengthens the emotional bond with the mother (it is hard to give birth to a malformed child, and many mothers experience feelings of rejection. There is no shame in this. It is normal. You will get over it by holding your baby and giving him lots of affection). Moreover, babies with heart disease get tired while breastfeeding, but they get even more tired while bottle feeding (and this affects their heart rate, oxygen saturation and so on).

It is very important to find the best position possible when breastfeeding babies with Down's syndrome. Nursing can take a long time, and compressing your breast while your baby is feeding might prove useful (see page 87). On a bad day, you may have to express your milk and feed it to her from a cup or with a dropper. The weight gain of babies with Down's syndrome is never normal, and doesn't conform to growth charts. As adults they are smaller than average, so don't be alarmed if people say she isn't gaining enough weight as a baby. It isn't a reason to wean her. You can find special growth charts for Down's syndrome babies at:

→ http://www.fcsd.org/tablas-de-crecimiento-espec%C3%ADficas-para-ni%C3%B1os-con-el-sd_21453.pdf

→ www.fcsd.org/cas/revista/downloads.htm

→ Breastfeeding & Down's Syndrome Resources. www.kellymom.com/babyconcerns/down-syndrome.html

Cleft lip

Cleft lip is a split in the upper lip, below the nose. Sometimes the hole can be quite large. It presents few problems during breastfeeding. In the majority of cases, the breast itself fills the hole when the baby is nursing. When the hole is large, and the breast can't fill it properly, air can pass through the hole making it difficult for the baby to create a vacuum (the baby swallows air and can't exert enough pressure to keep the nipple in place); you can usually solve this problem yourself by placing your thumb over the hole during the feed.

Patients with cleft lip can undergo surgery during the first weeks, and your baby will be able to nurse as soon as she comes round from the anaesthetic. It isn't necessary or desirable for her to abstain from nursing for several hours (see 'cleft palate' below). The sooner she begins breastfeeding after the operation, the sooner she will gain weight and go home.

→ Weatherley-White, R.C., Kuehn, D.P., Mirrett, P., Gilman, J.I., Weatherley-White, C.C. 'Early repair and breastfeeding for infants with cleft lip', *Plast Reconstr Surg* 1987;79: 879-87

→ Childrens Hospitals and Clinics. 'Breastfeeding an infant with cleft lip', xpedio02.childrenshc.org/stellent/groups/public/@manuals/@pfs/@nutr/documents/policyreferenceprocedure/018722.pdf

Cleft palate

Sometimes, while the foetus is still developing, the two plates that form the palate don't fuse properly, leaving a gap between the mouth and the nasal cavity. In many cases of cleft palate there is also cleft lip. The problem is that food can be inhaled through the hole into the lung, causing aspiration pneumonia.

It has been shown that babies with cleft palate who breastfeed suffer fewer ear infections (to which they are also prone). Moreover, if food is inhaled, formula is a foreign substance that can easily trigger an infection, whereas breastmilk is full of antibodies and white blood cells, which make it less likely to cause pneumonia.

It is essential for a newborn with a cleft palate to be fed on breastmilk, by whatever method.

Some babies manage to breastfeed if they are placed in an upright position (sitting astride their mother's knee). They are more likely to be able to nurse if the hole is covered by a soft orthopaedic plate (a Hotz plate – a sort of made-to-measure silicone patch that covers the fissure). If no one suggests this, ask your doctor about it. You can print out the article referenced below (it is on the internet) and take it along with you.

Other babies find it impossible to nurse; they have to be fed through a tube, or using a specially adapted bottle, or sometimes a normal bottle. All these methods have their problems and drawbacks. If your baby chokes less with a bottle, then feed her with a bottle, but make sure it contains breastmilk. You can breastfeed her later, once she has had surgery to correct the cleft palate.

Babies with a cleft palate tend to gain less weight because they find feeding difficult. If your baby is breastfeeding but not gaining much weight, express more milk and try to feed it to her using other methods. You will soon see that you are expressing more milk than your baby can drink, and you will have a surplus of milk. So formula isn't the solution. Moreover, an underweight baby will have further problems if he catches viruses, diarrhoea and ear infections, which occur more frequently in babies fed with artificial milk.

After surgery, it was the custom to feed these babies with a spoon, or through a tube, for fear the stitches would come out with all the movement involved in breastfeeding or bottle feeding. However, the stitches are far more likely to come out if the baby cries. So, in order to stop her from crying it is best to place your breast in her mouth as soon as she wakes up from the anaesthetic. It has been shown that babies can nurse immediately after the operation, and this way they gain weight more quickly and the stitches don't come out.

→ Roberts, J., Hawk, K. 'Cleft Lip and Palate' *New Beginnings* 2002;19:88 www.llli.org/NB/NBMayJun02p88.html

→ Kogo, M., Okada, G., Ishii, S., Shikata, M., Iida, S., Matsuya, T. 'Breast feeding for cleft lip and palate patients, using the Hotz-type plate', *Cleft Palate Craniofac J* 1997;34:351-3

→ Darzi, M.A., Chowdri, N.A., Bhat, A.N. 'Breast feeding or spoon feeding after cleft lip repair: a prospective, randomised study', *Br J Plast Surg* 1996;49:24-6

Phenylketonuria

This is an extremely rare metabolic disorder. Babies suffering from it have to be given special milk that doesn't contain the amino acid phenylalanine, but they must also receive a certain amount of normal milk, because a certain amount of phenylalanine is essential to human life. Breastmilk contains less phenylalanine than cow's milk, and so these babies need less special milk when they are breastfed than when they are bottle fed.

→ Cornejo, V., Manríquez, V., Colombo, M., Mabe, P., Jiménez, M., De la Parra, A., Valiente, A., Raimann, E. 'Fenilquetonuria de diagnóstico neonatal y lactancia materna', *Rev Med Chil* 2003;131:1280-7 www.scielo.cl/pdf/rmc/v131n11/art08.pdf

Jaw deformities

Some babies are born with a small lower jaw (retrognathia and micrognathia), as in Pierre Robin syndrome. It is difficult for these babies to breastfeed because they are unable to take a good mouthful of the breast to be able to position their tongue correctly. Sometimes it is necessary to express milk and feed it to them from a cup. The mother may also be able to help her baby by placing him in an upright position and holding his jaw between her thumb and forefinger, while supporting her breast with the palm of her hand, and compressing her breast while he is nursing.

→ Landis, J. Pierre Robin Sequence. *Leaven* 2001;37:111-112 www.llli. org/llleaderweb/LV/LVOctNov01p111.html

Neurological problems

Hypotonia, hypertonia, or lack of coordination can make breastfeeding difficult. Babies suffering from hypotonia usually nurse better if they are placed in a horizontal position on a cushion, their head and bottom almost level. It can help if the mother holds his jaw between her thumb and forefinger, while supporting his chest with the palm of her hand, and compressing her breast while he is nursing.

→ Childrens Hospitals and Clinics, 'Breastfeeding an infant with neurological problems' xpedio02.childrenshc.org/ stellent/groups/public/@Manuals/@PFS/@Nutr/documents/ PolicyReferenceProcedure/018724.pdf

Congenital heart disease

Babies with congenital heart disease have a more stable oxygen saturation when they are breastfed than when they are bottle fed. In other words they tire more easily at the bottle than the breast. It can be helpful to compress the breast while the baby is nursing.

→ Marino, B.L., O'Brien, P., LoRe, H. 'Oxygen saturations during breast and bottle feedings in infants with congenital heart disease', *J Pediatr Nurs* 1995;10:360-4

Diarrhoea

When I was a child, every type of diarrhoea was treated with antibiotics. There wasn't even any need to see a doctor, as they were available over the counter in Spain. I even remember the name of the one my father used to give me. It was called Sulfathalidine®, and tasted horrible. My parents would never have dared give me an antibiotic for tonsillitis without seeing a doctor, but everyone knew what to do in cases of diarrhoea. You took the pill and that was that.

When, years later, Spanish doctors wanted to convince people (as well as some of their most reticent colleagues) that antibiotics are useless for treating diarrhoea, and in some cases can even be harmful, they apparently felt obliged to offer them something in exchange: *the astringent diet*. This diet was nothing new, but there is no doubt that Spanish doctors in the 1970s and 1980s greatly contributed to its dissemination. 'What, you don't give him antibiotics for diarrhoea?' 'No, Madam, the best thing is a strict diet, you'll see how quickly his diarrhoea clears up', sounds a lot better than: 'No, Madam, he doesn't need anything, diarrhoea clears up on its own'. If it weren't for the diet, half of the mothers would have gone to the chemist, disgruntled, and bought the antibiotic themselves (as they could in Spain at that time). Eventually, many doctors ended up believing in the diet.

Basically (there are a few variations) the diet consisted of fasting for twenty-four hours (only drinking the broth from boiled rice and boiled vegetables), and then eating rice and boiled carrots, poached or grilled chicken, poached fish, baked apple, ripe banana and toast. Decades ago, American and British doctors used to prescribe the BRAT diet: banana, rice, apple sauce and toast.* No milk, and certainly no breastmilk (which, as we all know, is toxic). I never understood why the chicken couldn't be roasted or fried, or why the apple couldn't be raw, or why the bread had to be toasted, but this was the way it was. For protracted bouts of diarrhoea, the diet was even stricter, cutting out the chicken and fish, and possibly the toast.

The result was that the wretched child was famished, because he wasn't given enough food, and the small amount he was given was low in fats and proteins, and so bad-tasting it would have been a struggle to eat when he was healthy, let alone when he felt unwell and had an upset stomach. The upshot of all this was that the child lost weight (inevitable when you don't eat) and, ironically, his diarrhoea got worse. The diet was based on the well-known principle: 'Out of nothing, comes nothing', or 'if you don't eat, you won't poo': only things aren't that simple. When you have diarrhoea, the cells in the intestinal mucosa are destroyed, and in order for them to be renewed they need raw material in the form of proteins and nutrients.

Nowadays, the correct treatment for diarrhoea is:
- If the baby is nursing, continue breastfeeding him without any delays or stoppages, the more the better. Try making him nurse more frequently by offering him your breast even when he isn't asking for it.

---

* See en.wikipedia.org/wiki/BRAT_diet and www.diet-weight-lose.com/detox-diet/astringent-diet.php

- If you are bottle feeding him, continue giving him the bottle and prepare them the way you usually do (don't put more water or less powder in them, or prepare them with rice water or any liquids other than water). In some cases your doctor might prescribe lactose-free formula, but to begin with ordinary infant formula is usually fine.
- If the baby's diarrhoea is moderate to severe (some people see three small poos and call it 'diarrhoea'), besides breast or formula milk, feed him oral rehydration solution (ORS). It comes in sachets and is available at chemists. Mix it by following the instructions on the packet. If he refuses to take it (and looks healthy), he probably doesn't need it.
- If he is on solids, continue to give him the same foods. He doesn't need to eat rice; he will get better just as quickly if he eats pasta or lentils. If he has a stomach-ache, he won't have a big appetite, so try offering him small amounts more frequently. Don't try giving him rice, rice water, or carrots unless he usually eats them, as it isn't a good idea to introduce new foods when the child has diarrhoea.
- If he vomits, it doesn't matter. Keep breastfeeding him and giving him ORS. If he takes 100ml and vomits 80ml at least he is keeping down 20ml. If he takes nothing, he is keeping down nothing. If his stools are copious and he is vomiting a lot, go to the doctor (but keep breastfeeding him and giving him ORS on the way).

→ Román Riechmann, E., Barrio Torres, J. 'Diarrea aguda (Protocolo de la Asociación Española de Pediatría)' www.aeped. es/protocolos/gastroentero/2.pdf

Lactose intolerance

Lactose intolerance has nothing to do with milk allergy. There is no such thing as an allergy to lactose. A milk allergy is an allergy to the proteins in milk, and can be a very serious illness. Some children who show symptoms of milk allergy test negative for milk allergy, and some doctors call this 'milk protein intolerance', which is a way of saying: 'I think he has an allergy, but I can't prove it'.

Lactose intolerance isn't an allergy. After weaning, lactose intolerance is perfectly normal; the abnormal ones are those of us who as adults are able to drink milk due to a genetic mutation (see page 165). However, in babies and small children secondary lactose intolerance can sometimes occur when they have diarrhoea. This is a mild condition and goes away after a few days. When the baby is bottle fed, he may be given lactose-free formula, but if he is nursing there is usually no problem. Carry on breastfeeding him as usual.

The lactose in breastmilk doesn't depend on whether the mother drinks milk or not. Lactose isn't absorbed (which is the reason for the intolerance; lactose is either digested and broken down, or it isn't able to be absorbed); the mother can drink litres and litres of milk and she won't have a single lactose molecule in her blood. The lactose in breastmilk is produced in the breast, regardless of whether the mother drinks milk or not.

There are some cases of primary lactose intolerance, a very rare congenital illness that can be treated by feeding the baby lactase enzyme mixed with breastmilk.

Galactosemia

Galactosemia is an extremely serious congenital disease (cataracts, jaundice, mental retardation, cirrhosis, low weight gain, vomiting, hypoglycaemia). It affects one in every 50,000 newborns.

Babies with galactosemia can't breastfeed, nor can they be fed on ordinary infant formula. They have to drink 100 per cent lactose free milk. It is an absolute contraindication.

Galactosemia has nothing to do with secondary lactose intolerance, which is a mild and transient condition compatible with breastfeeding. The only reason for mentioning galactosemia in this book is to prevent readers from confusing the two (or being misled by someone who has confused them), because with (secondary) lactose intolerance you can breastfeed without any problem.

Milk and other food allergies

A baby can have an allergic reaction to something his mother has eaten. Cow's milk is the most common cause, but it can also be fish, soybeans, nuts, or any other food. The symptoms range from a rash through to inconsolable crying, diarrhoea, blood in the stools and breast refusal. Sometimes the baby seems insatiably hungry; he feeds for two minutes, then lets go of the breast crying, and after a few moments he wants to feed again because he hasn't had enough, he feeds for two minutes then lets go again, and so on. He appears to be fighting with the breast.

It is wrong to lay the blame for every problem on allergies. I am not referring to the occasional upset, but to intense crying or continual breast refusal at almost every feed, for days or weeks.

If a mother suspects her baby has an allergy, she should stop drinking cow's milk for at least seven to ten days. Cow's milk protein has been found in breastmilk up to four days after being eliminated from the mother's diet. If the baby shows no improvement, then it isn't the milk (if there are clear symptoms of allergy, try eliminating other foods). If the baby improves (this can be immediate, or it can take a few days), milk could be the cause, or it might be a simple coincidence. It is necessary to corroborate this by drinking some milk. Too many mothers stop drinking milk or eating other foods for months or years without any justification because they haven't carried out this test. If the mother drinks milk again and the baby is all right, then it was a coincidence and she can go back to drinking milk. If the symptoms come back, she should try to avoid the food in question for several years. Talk to your doctor about it (he or she may decide to run a few allergy tests on your baby).

Where allergies are concerned, there are no half measures. Drinking less milk won't make any difference; the baby probably won't improve, and you will never be sure. When you stop milk, you have to stop completely. Read the label on everything you drink or eat: lots of biscuits, margarine, processed meats and cakes contain milk (it can be described variously as 'milk solids', 'whey protein', 'milk proteins', 'lactoprotein', 'casein', 'milk whey' etc). When you do the test by going back on milk again, it is no good drinking a thimbleful, because it may not be enough to cause any symptoms. Drink one or two glasses a day.

Some babies are sensitive to several foods at once, so it is often worth eliminating milk, eggs, fish, soybeans and nuts at the same time (when you stop drinking cow's milk don't replace it with soymilk or almond milk, as they can also cause allergies) as well as any other foods you might suspect (if the baby's father is allergic to strawberries, or if the day you ate peaches the baby seemed to get worse). If your baby improves, go back to eating or drinking the eliminated foods one by one, leaving a week in between, until you discover which one is causing the symptoms.

If a baby shows no improvement after his mother eliminates milk from her diet, some doctors recommend weaning him and feeding him hydrolyzed milk formula. This is complete nonsense; before taking this extreme measure, other possible causes of the allergy have to be ruled out. Some babies are allergic to several different foods at once. A few are allergic to a lot of different foods. I came across a baby once who was allergic to milk, eggs, fish, chicken, beef, rice, wheat and other foods. He only got better when his mother took the hydrolyzed milk prescribed for her baby, and nothing else for several days (if you take enough of it, it is a complete food). For several months afterwards, the mother ate a diet of hydrolyzed milk, carrots, potatoes, lentils and horsemeat (these foods aren't particularly hypoallergenic, they were simply the ones the baby tolerated, and they could cause an allergic reaction in others).

The term 'cow's milk protein intolerance' is used when the symptoms suggest milk allergy, but the allergy tests are negative. This situation occurs more frequently in digestive problems such as colitis (bloody diarrhoea). Milk should be avoided, exactly as it is when the allergy test is positive. It shouldn't be confused with lactose intolerance.

In some instances, chronic constipation, even in babies who are exclusively breastfed, can be due to a genuine IgE-mediated cow's milk allergy.

It goes without saying that if something the baby's mother eats disagrees with him, it will disagree with him even more if he eats it himself. Allergy to cow's milk usually goes away between the ages of two and four; don't feed your baby any dairy products until your doctor says so. Make sure the nursery school and your family know about it. If a baby is allergic to a specific food, special care must be taken when giving him complementary foods. They should always be introduced into his diet in small quantities, one at a time, so that any problem can easily be detected.

Many doctors aren't aware that an allergy to cow's milk can cause constipation; they think it only causes diarrhoea. Some doctors may even tell you that it is impossible for your baby to be allergic to something his mother has eaten. Several scientific studies are referenced below, in case you need to convince anyone.

→ Tormo, R. 'Alergia e intolerancia a la proteína de la leche de vaca (Protocolo de la Asociación Española de Pediatría)' www.aeped. es/protocolos/gastroentero/1.pdf

→ Pomberger, W., Pomberger, G., Geissler, W. 'Proctocolitis in breast fed infants: a contribution to differential diagnosis of haematochezia in early childhood', *Post-grad Med J* 2001;77:252-4 pmj.bmjjournals.com/cgi/content/full/77/906/252

→ Clyne, P.S., Kulczycki, A.' Human breast milk contains bovine IgG. Relationship to infant colic?', *Pediatrics* 1991;87:439-444

→ Iacono, G., Cavataio, F., Montalto, G., Florena, A., Tumminello, M., Soresi, M. et al. 'Intolerance of cow's milk and chronic constipation in children', *N Engl J Med* 1998;339:1100-4

Surgery

Before an operation, a patient has to go without food for several hours. The idea is for the stomach to be empty so the patient can't choke on his or her own vomit while under anaesthesia. However, breastmilk is digested far more quickly than a helping of beef stew, and it is wrong to make a baby go that long without milk before an operation.

According to the American Society of Anesthesiologists, children of any age can drink clear liquids (water, juice, camomile tea) up to two hours before being anaesthetised; breastmilk up to four hours before, and artificial milk and light meals (without meat or fat) up to six hours before. Many experts believe that breastmilk can be given as little as two hours before anaesthetic. If your baby has to have an operation, ask how long she needs to go without food. If they tell you too many hours, print out the referenced document from the Internet and take it to the anaesthetist, the surgeon or both.

→ American Society of Anesthesiologists Task Force on Preoperative Fasting and the Use of Pharmacologic Agents to

Reduce the Risk of Pulmonary Aspiration. Practice guidelines for preoperative fasting and the use of pharmacologic agents to reduce the risk of pulmonary aspiration: application to healthy patients undergoing elective procedures, 1999. www.asahq.org/ publicationsAndServices/npoguide.html

Gastroesophageal reflux

All babies vomit. Consequently they all have gastroesophageal reflux (which is what vomiting is: the contents of the stomach flowing back towards the oesophagus). They improve at around the age of one. If they are healthy and happy and not in any pain and are gaining weight, gastroesophageal reflux isn't a problem and doesn't require any treatment.

In a few cases, gastroesophageal reflux is a genuine illness, and causes oesophagitis (inflammation of the oesophagus due to the acid from the intestine) or respiratory problems (due to aspiration). Breastfeeding is specially recommended in these cases, because it reduces the duration of these reflux episodes.

In contrast, thickened feeds (such as anti-regurgitation milks) are almost useless for treating reflux. It is a serious mistake to wean your baby in order to feed her one of these products.

→ Heacock, H.J., Jeffery, H.E., Baker, J.L., Page, M. 'Influence of breast versus formula milk on physiological gastroesophageal reflux in healthy, newborn infants', *J Pediatr Gastroenterol Nutr* 1992;14:41-6

→ Aggett, P.J., Agostoni, C., Goulet, O., Hernell, O., Koletzko, B., Lafeber, H.L., Michaelsen, K.F., Milla, P., Rigo, J., Weaver, L.T. 'Antireflux or Antiregurgitation Milk Products for Infants and Young Children: A Commentary by the ESPGHAN Committee on Nutrition', *J Pediatr Gastroenterol Nutr* 2002;34:496-8 www. meb.uni-bonn.de/kinder/espghan/position_papers/con_15.htm

→ Spitting Up, Reflux and Breastfeeding, www.kellymom.com/ babyconcerns/reflux.html

Infant dental caries

The habit of putting a baby to sleep with a bottle in his mouth, especially if it contains juice or sweetened liquids, can cause multiple dental caries in the incisors, so-called 'nursing bottle caries'. In 1983, Brams and Maloney were astonished to find a few cases of 'nursing bottle caries' in babies who were exclusively breastfed. Since then, this type of tooth decay has been given several names: 'nursing caries', 'rampant caries' and so on. The definition is imprecise; normally there should be multiple caries, and yet a single dental cavity in one milk tooth before the age of six is sufficient for a diagnosis of 'early childhood caries'.

The link between breastfeeding and dental caries is unclear, because the disease is multi-causal. While reviewing earlier studies, Valaitis and colleagues found that they weren't rigorous enough, and therefore didn't allow any conclusions to be drawn. In its 2003 recommendations, the American Academy of Pediatric Dentistry was somewhat non-committal: they reiterate that breastfeeding is best, that frequent night-feeds can produce dental caries, and that more research is needed.

In their study of 3,000 babies aged eighteen months, Hallonsten and colleagues found that only sixty-one were still breastfeeding. Of those still breastfeeding, 19.7 per cent had dental caries compared to 1.7 per cent of those who had been weaned; but the babies who had dental caries (whether they breastfed or not) ate more cariogenic (that promote tooth decay) foods than those who didn't have dental caries. The authors believe that there is a link and that babies who are breastfed for longer are 'more likely to establish inadequate eating habits'.

Weerheijm and colleagues found dental caries affected 14.5 per cent of a group of Dutch babies (with an average age of twenty months), whose mothers attended La Leche League meetings. They concluded that 'breastfeeding on demand doesn't increase the percentage of dental caries', but that frequent feeds and a low consumption of fluoride contributed to the appearance of dental caries.

Erickson left teeth soaking in breastmilk and found that it does not produce decay in the laboratory.

It is interesting to compare the extent of dental caries in different countries. In Tanzania, in a study of 2,000 children aged four, Matee and colleagues found that 6.8 per cent had nursing caries, ranging from 1.5 per cent to 12.8 per cent according to region. Bottles were rarely used, and there weren't many sweets. Sleeping with the breast in the mouth and hypoplasia (an enamel defect that is probably due to an intercurrent disease during pregnancy while the teeth are being formed) were linked to dental caries. Note here that this is not about whether the baby nurses during the night (which is probably true of all Tanzanian babies), but that he sleeps with the breast in his mouth all night. In any event, the incidence of nursing caries is extremely low.

In India, which is a more westernised country, but where breastfeeding is still widespread, Jose and King found 44 per cent dental caries among children between the ages of eight and forty-eight months; 99 per cent of them were still breastfeeding, usually on demand. The risk factors they identified were poor dental hygiene, the consumption of sweets and poverty.

Among the Canadian Inuits, where breastfeeding has reached alarmingly low levels, Houde and colleagues found 72.2 per cent of baby bottle tooth decay in 244 children aged between two and five.

An important factor in preventing dental caries could be the saliva transfer between mother and baby (for example, from kissing on the mouth) prior to teething, possibly because it produces immunity to the *Streptococcus mutans* in the maternal saliva. In a cohort study, Aaltonen and Tenovuo divided fifty-five seven-month-old Finnish babies into two groups, according to whether their saliva transfer was frequent or infrequent. The children aged between five and seven years with greater saliva transfer had fewer dental caries in their canines and first premolars (19 per cent compared with 56 per cent), despite eating more sweets.

In conclusion, infant dental caries can be prevented by kissing, breastfeeding, avoiding bottle feeding (in particular bottles containing juice, sugar or honey, and bottle feeding at night), avoiding sweets and sugary foods, by practicing dental hygiene as soon as the baby's first teeth appear, and administering fluoride after six months depending on the levels of fluoride in the drinking water (your doctor will tell you about this). If in spite of everything, your baby develops dental caries (which could be due to a particular sensitivity or a family predisposition), it might be helpful not to let her spend all night with the breast in her mouth, but rather to have her nurse and then release the breast before going to sleep (Elizabeth Pantley's book gives some useful pointers on how to achieve this, see below).

→ Brams, M., Maloney, J. '"Nursing bottle" caries in breastfed children', *J Pediatr* 1983;103:415-6

→ Valaitis, R., Hesch, R., Passarelli, C., Sheehan, D., Sinton, J. 'A systematic review of the relationship between breastfeeding and early childhood caries', *Can J Public Health* 2000;91:411-7

→ American Academy of Pediatric Dentistry. Policy on Breastfeeding. 2003. www.aapd.org

→ Hallonsten, A.L., Wendt, L.K., Mejare, I., Birkhed, D., Hakansson, C., Lindvall, A.M., Edwardsson, S., Koch, G. 'Dental caries and prolonged breastfeeding in 18-month-old Swedish children', *Int J Paediatr Den* 1995;5:149-55

→ Weerheijm, K.L., Uyttendaele-Speybrouck, B.F., Euwe, H.C., Groen, H.J. 'Prolonged demand breastfeeding and nursing caries', *Caries Res* 1998;32:46-50

→ Erickson, P.R., Mazhari, E. 'Investigation of the role of human breast milk in caries development', *Pediatr Dent* 1999;2186-90

→ Matee, M., van't Hof, M., Maselle, S., Mikx, F., van Palenstein Helderman, W. 'Nursing caries, linear hypoplasia, and nursing and weaning habits in Tanzanian infants', *Community Dent Oral Epidemiol* 1994;22:289-93

→ Jose, B., King, N.M. 'Early childhood caries lesions in preschool children in Kerala, India', *Pediatr Dent* 2003;25:594-600

→ Houde, G. Gagnon, P.F., St Germain, M. 'A descriptive study of early caries and oral health habits of Inuit pre-schoolers: preliminary results', *Arctic Med Res* 1991;Suppl:683-4

→ Aaltonen, A.S., Tenovuo, J. 'Association between mother-infant salivary contacts and caries resistance in children: a cohort study', *Pediatr Dent* 1994;16:110-6

→ Pantley, E. *The No-Cry Sleep Solution*, McGraw-Hill Contemporary, 2002

Chapter 17
MISCELLANEOUS QUESTIONS

'I mix feed my baby. Can I stop bottle feeding her?'

Yes. Milk supply adapts to demand. If you bottle feed your baby, she will take less milk from the breast, and you will produce less. If you stop bottle feeding her, she will nurse more and you will produce more milk.

Of course, we must take into account why bottle feeding was introduced in the first place. If there was no good reason; for example if you were told that gaining 150 grams a week wasn't enough (when in fact it is perfectly adequate), or if the baby's weight wasn't the issue, and they told you to bottle feed her 'to make her sleep more', or because you are on prescription drugs, or for some other strange reason, obviously your breasts are in perfect working order and will resume working. But if they advised you to bottle feed because there was a genuine problem, for example if your baby really was losing weight, or gaining very little weight, then you might ask: 'Is it because my milk supply is really that low? Will I always have to mix feed my baby? Or was it a question of incorrect positioning or scheduled feeding, and now that I'm doing things differently everything will be fine?' On the other hand, stopping supplementary bottles is not something you can do without thinking. You must weigh your baby every few days. Her weight may stagnate for three or four days and then go up again. However, if she starts losing weight, or if after several days she doesn't start catching up, you will have to reduce the amount of formula more slowly, and you may not be able to stop using it completely.

If your baby only takes a small amount from the bottle, less than 200ml per day, you can probably wean her off it in one go. Just stop. For a day or two she will want to nurse all the time, and then things will go back to normal.

You can also do it gradually, by reducing the amount in the bottle from 180ml to 150ml, then 120ml and so on. With some babies you can phase them out completely in less than a week; with others you have to do it more gradually. In the meantime, of course, you have to check your baby's weight, and make sure you prepare her bottles with the correct ratio of milk powder to water. Don't dilute them, because she won't get enough nourishment, but won't be able to breastfeed to compensate because her tummy will be full of liquid.

Another way of doing it is to try reducing the number of bottle feeds on demand. Offer her your breast, compressing it if she isn't nursing properly (see page 87). Then offer her the other breast (if she wants it). If she seems reasonably calm and contented don't give her the bottle. If after twenty minutes she cries and wants to feed again, offer her your breast again. Keep doing this as often as necessary. Only give her a bottle if she has just finished the second breast and she is still hungry. But give her less than usual, only a tiny amount, 30 or 60ml. If she finishes this, and is still hungry, give her another 30ml, and then another, until she stops, but if she seems fairly calm don't give her any more. And if after twenty minutes she wants to feed again, offer her the breast. This means, if your baby is crying because she is genuinely hungry, you will be giving her (in instalments) the same amount of formula that she always has. But if she manages on less, you will be giving her less. The idea is, that instead of breastfeeding and bottle feeding every three hours, she breastfeeds every hour, or hour and a half, and only bottle feeds every four to five hours. Within a few days you will have weaned her off bottles completely.

I keep referring to bottle feeding. What I am really talking about is infant formula, administered by any means. If you really have no choice but to feed your baby a supplement, it is best not to use a bottle, because in many cases, the baby will become confused and will start nursing incorrectly. Try to feed her using a cup or a dropper. However, if you have been bottle feeding her for several days, and you want to stop, there is little point in starting now to feed her from a glass. You can try; but if it's difficult, it isn't it worth it for you or your baby when in a few days time she will stop that too.

Besides breastfeeding her at all hours, is it worth expressing milk in order to stimulate milk production? If your baby is nursing at all hours, you will scarcely have the time. And if your baby is nursing properly (or if compressing your breast works well for her) there won't be much left to express. However, if your baby is not nursing properly, or compressing your breast isn't working, it is a good idea to express your milk and feed it to her as a supplement, after breastfeeding her, and before giving her formula milk.

'I stopped breastfeeding weeks ago, can I start again?'

Yes. It's possible to stop giving supplementary bottles and go back to exclusive breastfeeding, even if you haven't breastfed for weeks or months, or have never breastfed.

It could be that your baby was born premature, or was too ill to breastfeed. Or that you decided you didn't want to breastfeed, and now you have changed your mind. Perhaps you were told she wasn't gaining weight, and you have realised that even with the bottle she is still gaining the same or even less.

The process is usually referred to as relactation, and it requires two things: you have to produce milk, and the baby has to suckle. The two are related, and yet relatively separate. The baby will probably nurse better if some milk comes out, but not necessarily; dummies don't secrete anything, yet babies still suck them, so why wouldn't they suck a breast that has no milk? Similarly, you will secrete more milk if your baby nurses, but this isn't obligatory: you can also stimulate milk secretion by expressing your milk, either by hand or using a pump.

Obviously very little (or no) milk will come out to begin with. Be patient and don't give up. But don't pulverise your breasts; it is better to spend five or ten minutes trying to express milk eight or ten times a day (or more, if you have the time and the energy) than to insist for half an hour and then nothing comes out. Various different drugs have been used to try to stimulate milk supply, but generally speaking they aren't very effective; it is possible to achieve relactation without drugs.

Producing milk is relatively easy. If you persist it will eventually come out. Another thing is getting your baby to nurse, because of course this doesn't depend on you. If your baby doesn't want to nurse, she won't. The younger the baby, the more likely she is to end up nursing. With babies under four months the success rate is very high. With babies over four months it is less straightforward. Some mothers produce milk but can't get their baby to nurse; they have to express their milk and feed it to the baby from a cup, or mixed with cereal. But there are also cases of one-year-olds who have gone back to breastfeeding, so it is definitely worth a try.

Sometimes it is enough just to place your baby on your breast, and she will happily begin nursing, even though she hasn't done it for weeks. But often a baby will become used to the bottle, and will refuse the breast, or not know what to do with it. Don't try to force your baby to nurse by withholding food. Firstly because it is disrespectful, and secondly because it won't work: the hungrier she is the more upset and fractious she will become, and the more unlikely it is she will nurse properly. The best thing is to feed her (preferably with milk from a cup, but if she has been bottle feeding for weeks or months, a few days more won't make any difference), and then, when she has calmed down again, make sure you have plenty of skin-to-skin contact with her. Lie down on the bed, naked from the waist up, your baby wearing only her nappy. Hold her on top of you with her head between your breasts, like you did after she was born. Say loving things to her, caress her, relax. Many children, after half an hour, or longer, will go to the breast themselves and begin nursing. And if not, at least you have had some time to relax and enjoy your baby, and you can try again another day. If, on the other hand, you spend that time trying to make her take your breast (turning her this way and that, forcing her mouth open when she won't latch on, then trying again), mother and baby will probably both end up in tears, and in addition, the unpleasant experience will probably ensure that next time she has even less desire to nurse.

Many mothers succeed in going back to exclusive breastfeeding. Others don't. Some mothers have to mix feed for a few months, because if they try to stop giving their baby formula milk, her weight stagnates or drops. If this is the case, when you start your baby on solids, you can begin substituting formula milk with solids, so that at nine or ten months, your baby will only be taking breastmilk and solids, as if she had never been bottle fed.

'I took pills to dry up my milk...'

You can still go back to breastfeeding even if you have taken drugs to dry up your milk. Years ago they used bromocriptine (Parlodel®), and before that estrogens. The effect of these drugs was very limited, and it was enough to stop taking them, and to breastfeed normally for the milk to come back. Bromocriptine is hardly used nowadays, and in the United States it is no longer legal to use it as a milk suppressant, due to the side-effects. Nowadays, the drug used to dry up breastmilk is cabergoline (Dostinex®). Unfortunately, the effects are longer lasting; I know some mothers who have changed their minds and managed to breastfeed again, but it took them two weeks or more to produce a few drops. Precisely because almost no milk comes out, you can start breastfeeding your baby immediately. Don't listen to anyone who says the drug will have passed into your milk. What milk?

'Can I breastfeed an adopted baby?'

In some cultures, when a mother dies during childbirth, it is normal for her mother or sister to breastfeed the newborn. In our culture, many mothers breastfeed their adopted children.

The process is the same as going back to breastfeeding your own baby. The younger the baby, the easier it will be for her to take to it. You will need to breastfeed or express your milk ten times a day or more. If you know exactly when your adopted baby is going to arrive, you can start stimulating your milk a few months before. If you are starting from scratch, it could take from a few days to a week for the first few drops to appear, and if you are successful you could be breastfeeding exclusively in three or four weeks. It is easier when a woman has already breastfed children of her own. If you have a hormone problem that prevents you from having children, you may also have difficulty breastfeeding.

In any case, even under the most favourable circumstances, not all mothers succeed in breastfeeding exclusively. Many mothers have to mix feed, and some only manage to produce a few symbolic drops of milk. It is not good to dwell on the amount of milk you produce; the most important thing about this adventure is the special relationship you have with her, the amazing feeling of her pressed against your body.

On the following webpage from WHO there is an interesting document about relactation:

→ www.who.int/maternal_child_adolescent/documents/who_chs_cah_98_14/en/

Caesarean section

Women who give birth by caesarean section usually breastfeed for a shorter time than women who have given birth vaginally. But it shouldn't be like this. During a caesarean, they operate on the belly, not the breasts, which continue to work perfectly. The problem is that in many hospitals lactation begins very differently after a caesarean. In some hospitals, babies born by caesarean begin nursing within an hour. In some hospitals, the baby is already in skin-to-skin contact (and nurses if he wants) while the surgeon is still stitching the mother up. But in others, babies born by caesarean are separated from their mothers for six or twelve hours (or more!), and mothers aren't helped to find a position in which to breastfeed that doesn't irritate the incision. What begins as a minor difficulty can snowball into a big problem: if breastfeeding is delayed, in the meantime the baby will have been given a bottle, she won't latch on properly, the mother will get cracked nipples, and so on.

Hair loss

Hair doesn't just keep growing. Each hair has a cycle where it sprouts, grows and falls out. Dozens of our hairs fall out every day, and others grow in their place. In many animals, the hairs grow all at the same time: they have a beautiful coat in winter and they moult in the summer. In humans, each hair does its own thing, and our hair looks the same all year round.

However, during pregnancy, a lot of hairs decide simultaneously to go into inactive mode, meaning that women experience very little hair loss during pregnancy. And it is true that with their thick locks, their soft, smooth skin, and their proud smiles, women are dazzlingly beautiful when they are pregnant. The downside is that their hairs have all become synchronised, and between one and five months after they give birth, they enter the falling-out phase. This is a completely normal phenomenon known as telogen effluvium. However many hairs appear in your brush every morning, you aren't going bald! Six to twelve months after you give birth, things will return to normal.

Post-partum hair loss isn't due to breastfeeding, and there is just as much hair loss among women who bottle feed. Nor is it due to an iron deficiency (if you have had a blood test and your iron levels are low then of course you must take an iron supplement, but taking iron won't prevent hair loss), or any other nutrient deficiency. A few kind souls will insist on telling you that you are 'sacrificing your health', or 'wearing yourself out' because of your ridiculous obsession with breastfeeding. Ignore them. Alarmed by the prospect of going bald (why are women so afraid of going bald? It is understandable in men, but not in women. How many bald women do you see walking around?), many mothers resort to buying lotions, supplements and treatments from the chemist or the health food shop, which claim to slow the rate of hair loss. And at least in this case there is some truth to it: six to twelve months after giving birth, everything will return to normal, just as it would have done had you done nothing. The only difference is that you will have spent a small fortune that could have been employed more usefully.

→ American Academy of Dermatology, 'Expecting a baby? expect some changes in your skin, hair and nails'. www.aad.org

→ American Academy of Dermatology, 'Hair today, gone tomorrow: early diagnosis is the key to treating hair loss in women'. www.aad.org

X-rays

X-rays are electromagnetic radiations, like light, and they travel at the speed of light. A few seconds after the X-ray is taken, they have already travelled further than the moon. They don't stay inside us. They don't make us radioactive or make us go luminous green like in the cartoons. They don't affect the breasts or breastmilk in any way. You can have all the X-rays you need during lactation, including chest X-rays and mammograms, and you needn't wait five hours or even five minutes after you leave the hospital before you breastfeed, nor do you need to express your milk and discard it. Your milk is perfectly normal after a mammogram.

The same goes for contrast X-rays. Intravenous iodinated X-ray contrast dye is non-toxic (it is injected into your vein, and nothing happens), it doesn't affect the thyroid gland for better or worse (the iodine in it is inseparable from the molecule of which it forms a part), almost none of it passes into breastmilk, and almost none of it is absorbed orally. A barium meal, which is used to take X-rays of the stomach or intestine, is also non-toxic, and can't be absorbed orally, making it impossible for it to pass into breastmilk. Newborns are given contrast X-rays without any risk. You can breastfeed your baby two minutes after they inject you with the contrast dye; there is no need to wait, and no need to express your milk and discard it.

Similarly, it is safe to have ultrasound, CT scans and MRI scans, and breastfeed immediately. Only a tiny amount of the two contrast dyes sometimes used with MRI scans (gadopentatate and gadoteridol) are absorbed orally or pass into breastmilk, and they are used on newborns because they are non-toxic. In order to give a newborn the amount of gadopentatate necessary for an MRI scan, we would have to inject her with several thousand litres of breastmilk. And yet, many people still recommend expressing milk and discarding it for twenty-four hours. This is completely crazy. Breastfeeding after an MRI scan with gadopentatate poses no risk. And I don't mean 'not very much', I mean none whatsoever. In contrast, stopping breastfeeding for twenty-four hours does, as does not giving an MRI scan to a mother who needs one, and leaving her illness undiagnosed and untreated for months because she is breastfeeding.

→ Kubik-Huch, R.A., Gottstein-Aalame, N.M., Frenzel, T., Seifert, B., Puchert, E., Wittek, S., Debatin, J.F. 'Gadopentetate dimeglumine excretion into human breast milk during lactation', *Radiology* 2000;216:555-8

Hair dyeing

I have frequently hear people quote the urban myth that you shouldn't dye your hair when breastfeeding because the dye can transfer to your breastmilk, but I have no idea where it comes from.

You aren't swallowing the dye, you are putting it on your hair. How much of it is absorbed through your skin and transferred to your bloodstream? To be honest, I don't know and I don't care. Maybe a hundredth or a thousandth of the dye is absorbed, I don't know, but it is possible. And maybe a hundredth of what is absorbed into the blood passes into milk; I don't know that either. In any case, one thing is certain: if the dye were toxic, the first person to be poisoned would be the hairdresser, who spends all day handling hair dyes, and breathing in their fumes. Even though they use gloves, we would still see thousands of cases of hairdressers poisoned by hair dye. The second person would be the mother, who is the one with all the dye on her hair. Rest assured that if toxic hair dyes ever existed, they would have been banned years ago. And if the dye is harmless for you, it is even more harmless for your baby.

Physical exercise

You can practise any kind of sport during breastfeeding. Your milk will be equally nourishing and equally abundant.

Some babies don't like the taste of sweat around the nipple. You can clean the area with a damp towel before breastfeeding.

Occasionally, after an intense physical effort, some babies refuse the breast for a few hours. It is thought this may be due to an increase in lactic acid (responsible for muscle stiffness) in the breastmilk. I am talking about hardcore exercise, the sort practised by professional sportspeople, not an hour spent in the local gym, and in any case it isn't a big problem. Lactic acid isn't toxic (it is found in yoghurt), and if the baby refuses the breast, he can feed later. You can safely carry on working out and breastfeeding.

Exercising during breastfeeding can contribute to the mother's mental and physical well-being, without in any way affecting the composition of her milk or harming her baby. It is perfectly safe for a mother who is breastfeeding to practice any type of sport.

→ Lovelady, C.A., Hunter, C.P., Geigerman, C. 'Effect of exercise on immunologic factors in breast milk', *Pediatrics* 2003;111:e148-52 pediatrics.aappublications.org/cgi/content/full/111/2/e148

→ Wright, K.S., Quinn, T.J., Carey, G.B. 'Infant acceptance of breast milk after maternal exercise', *Pediatrics* 2002;109:585-9 pediatrics.aappublications.org/cgi/content/full/109/4/585

Hair removal creams

Depilatory creams are very caustic. Ingesting them causes far more serious burns than drinking bleach. Make sure you wash scrupulously before holding your baby, and that you keep them in a very safe place, because small children could mistake them for toothpaste. In fact, to be on the safe side it is better not to have depilatory creams in a house where there are small children. However, they aren't absorbed by the skin, they don't pass into the blood, and still less into breastmilk. It is safe to use depilatory creams while breastfeeding. It is also safe to use wax, laser treatment or any other method.

UVA rays

The ultraviolet rays used in tanning parlours are bad for your skin. Overuse can cause skin cancer (the same as staying too long in the sun). For years, the American Academy of Dermatology has recommended banning UV sunlamps.

In any case, only the mother is exposed to harm. She can even use a UV sunlamp on her breasts and breastfeed immediately afterwards. There is no danger for the baby.

→ American Academy of Dermatology 'Tanning Salon Exposure Can Lead to Skin Cancer' www.aad.org/public/News/NewsReleases/Press+Release+Archives/Skin+Cancer+and+Sun+Safety/Exposure.htm

Chapter 18
BREASTFEEDING AND FERTILITY

The contraceptive effect of breastfeeding

Some might have heard people say that breastfeeding acts as a contraceptive and think they mean: 'You can't get pregnant while breastfeeding'. Of course you can. If you breastfeed for three or four years, and engage in sexual relations without using a contraceptive, you are almost certain to get pregnant.

The truth is that it is more difficult to get pregnant while breastfeeding. Not impossible, just more difficult. Especially at the beginning.

This is logical. For millions of years, our ancestors had no form of contraceptive, and almost no restriction on sexual activity. Women simply got pregnant as many times as they could. If a Palaeolithic woman had given birth every ten months from the age of puberty, she would probably have died along with all her children. There had to be a natural contraceptive. Natural selection favoured women who gave birth every three or even four years; this way they were able to take better care of their offspring, and in the long run they had more descendants from fewer births.

Nowadays, many women have a second child a year after their first, sometimes sooner. What became of the natural contraceptive? We stopped using it. That contraceptive was breastfeeding.

It is one of these elegant, deceptively simple yet remarkably adaptable solutions nature comes up with when it has millions of years in which to work. If contraception had a fixed duration: 'Women can't get pregnant for "x" number of years after giving birth', it wouldn't be able to adapt to circumstances, to the pace at which the baby develops, and above all to the child's survival.

We have become accustomed to taking it for granted that babies survive, and yet during the whole history of humanity, up until the twentieth century, infant mortality was extremely high. And it still is in a large part of the world, much to our shame. It isn't in nature's interest for a mother to lose her child and take three more years to have another. If the child dies, the mother has to get pregnant again as soon as possible.

This is why nature's contraceptive isn't inflexible, but rather depends on lactation: a woman can get pregnant when the sudden cessation of lactation indicates that her baby has died, or when its gradual decrease suggests that her baby is eating solids, and therefore no longer exclusively dependent on his mother's milk. During the first few months, when the baby is nursing a lot, all the time, getting pregnant is almost impossible. As the frequency of feeds and the production of milk diminish, so the possibility of getting pregnant increases. Babies of the !Kung bushmen breastfeed very frequently for the first few years, several times an hour, and eat very little complementary food (what can you eat in a desert?). The women get pregnant roughly every four years. Other people, who live in less harsh environments, and are more able to give their small children other food, usually get pregnant every two or three years. In our culture, a lot of children are already eating plenty of solids at six months, and many nursing mothers get pregnant within a year (and therefore give birth again eighteen months after their last child). Mothers who don't breastfeed can get pregnant within two months.

This decrease in fertility is caused by three mechanisms:

1. For several months the mother has no periods. This is known as 'amenorrhea', cessation of menstruation. It is possible for menstruation to occur without ovulation. But it is impossible for ovulation to occur without menstruation. Each time a woman ovulates, one of two things can happen: either she gets pregnant, or she has a period after two weeks. In fact, the woman who knows when she is ovulating (because she checks her temperature), and who doesn't have a period in the twenty days that follow, can be sure she is pregnant. For women with irregular periods, it is the first part of the cycle,

between menstruation and ovulation, which varies. The second phase, between ovulation and menstruation, is always very regular.

Therefore, if a woman has her first period eight months after she gives birth, it can mean only one of two things: either she ovulated fifteen days before, or she didn't ovulate at all. The later a woman begins menstruating again, the more likely it is that she has ovulated. A woman who has a period four months after she gives birth almost certainly hasn't ovulated. A woman who has her first period after fifteen months almost certainly has ovulated. It is possible to get pregnant before your first menstruation occurs.

2. Secondly, when the woman's menstruation returns, it is common for her to have several menstrual cycles without ovulation. The earlier her menstruation returns, the more likely this is.

3. Thirdly, when the woman starts ovulating again, she may have several infertile cycles, where the fertilized egg isn't able to implant itself.

In some cases, the woman may have one or more months of luteal insufficiency. The *corpus luteum* (Latin for 'yellow body') is the part of the ovary from which the egg emerges. It produces large amounts of hormones, which allow the fertilized egg to embed itself in the womb and start to gestate. When the *corpus luteum* disappears, menstruation starts. If the *corpus luteum* disappears too quickly and menstruation starts in less than ten days after ovulation, pregnancy is no longer possible.

Breastfeeding is the most widely used contraceptive on the planet, and the one that prevents the most pregnancies. In the majority of cases it is used unwittingly, yet it helps space out pregnancies and reduces the number of children each woman has during her lifetime. Hundreds of millions of women use no other form of contraception; if women in certain countries stopped breastfeeding, there would be a huge increase in the birth-rate.

LAM

Another question is whether breastfeeding can be used on an individual basis as a safe form of contraception. In 1988, making use of the information available at the time, a group of experts met in Bellagio (Italy) and came up with the 'Lactational Amenorrhea Method' (LAM).

A woman is less than 2 per cent likely to get pregnant if she fulfils all three of the following criteria simultaneously:

1. Her baby is less than six months old.
2. She breastfeeds exclusively, or almost exclusively.
3. Her periods still haven't returned.

The subject of menstruation sometimes creates confusion following childbirth. For the first fifty-six days after giving birth, it is by definition impossible for a woman to have a period. Any loss of blood during that time is referred to as 'lochia' (normal blood loss that occurs after childbirth). After fifty-six days, a distinction is made between normal blood loss (bleeding) and minimal blood loss (spotting). Just as the first swallow doesn't signify the arrival of summer, in order to call it menstruation we need at least two consecutive days of bleeding, or one of bleeding and two of spotting, or three days of spotting.

'Almost' exclusive breastfeeding refers to a tiny amount of supplement given occasionally (once a week), even if it is the mother's own milk (for example if she goes to the cinema and leaves some of her milk in the fridge for the grandmother to feed the baby with).

The more spaced out the feeds, the greater the chances of getting pregnant. One interval of ten hours or two intervals of six hours a week are permissible (when your baby sleeps through the night, for example), but if she sleeps eight hours every night without feeding (which fortunately is very rare) the method can fail.

Several subsequent studies have found that LAM works even better than expected. Out of a hundred women who fulfill all three criteria, one or none is likely to get pregnant. This is slightly less efficient than the pill, but on a par with the IUD, and a lot more efficient than condoms. In addition, the method is relatively robust: even if it is not followed to the letter (for example, when a mother gives the baby one too many bottles, or when she still has no period and isn't using any other form of contraception a year after she gives birth), the percentage of women who get pregnant increases, but it doesn't shoot up (unlike, say, with condoms, where forgetting once is enough).

When she no longer fulfils these criteria, meaning if her periods come back (this is unlikely before six months if she is exclusively breastfeeding, but of course it can happen), or she starts mix feeding her baby, or giving him solids, or she is working and therefore unable to breastfeed for long periods, or when her baby is six months old, and she doesn't want to get pregnant, she should think about using a different method.

LAM is not only a method for developing countries. Several different studies found that the failure rate in developing countries is higher than in Europe and the United States. As with all types of contraception, LAM works better for women who are more educated, and have access to professional advice. You can find more information at

→ www.fhi360.org

Other methods of contraception

I use the word contraception in a broad sense. Strictly speaking, a contraceptive is something that prevents conception, the union of ovule and sperm (either by coming between them, or by preventing ovulation). However, some contraceptives can work by preventing nidation, meaning that they prevent the embryo from implanting itself in the mucosa of the womb a few days after conception. Some consider this differentiation hair-splitting; for others it is fundamental. It all depends at what point you think human life begins. This is for you to decide. Emergency contraception, or 'the morning after pill', usually prevents nidation, although sometimes it can prevent ovulation. Contraceptives that only contain gestagens, whether oral or, like the IUD, implanted, usually prevent ovulation, but quite often they prevent nidation as well. Oral contraceptives (gestagens and estrogens) are almost always anovulatory, but in some cases they prevent nidation.

Condoms and diaphragms (with or without spermicidal creams) as well as the intrauterine device or IUD (with or without hormones) can be used safely during breastfeeding, as can oral contraceptives containing only gestagens (derived from progesterone), or implants containing gestagens. Needless to say, sterilisation (male or female) is also wholly compatible with breastfeeding.

Oral contraceptives containing estrogens (the majority) were said to reduce milk production. This hasn't been clearly demonstrated, and many are unconvinced. However, to be on the safe side, women are usually advised not to use them until the baby is six months old and has started eating solids. If for some reason it is considered necessary for you to use them before this, go ahead and see what happens. I suspect nothing radical will happen; if your milk supply decreases, your baby will be hungrier and if she feeds more frequently, your milk production will increase again. A problem would only arise if the mother were breastfeeding to a strict schedule, every three or four hours, in which case the baby would be unable to 'order' more milk from the dairy. Maybe this explains why in the past, when a lot more women breastfed to a schedule, there appeared to be a problem, whereas now that women breastfeed on demand there doesn't.

In any case, the only possible harmful side effect of contraceptives is a reduction in milk supply. There isn't the remotest possibility that the hormones might harm your baby or your child. The first contraceptive pills, produced decades ago, contained higher levels of oestrogen than those on the market today, and studies show that the children who were breastfed in those days, while their mothers were on the pill, have grown up to be completely normal. The boys don't become feminised or anything strange like that.

The so-called 'morning after pill' can also be taken while breastfeeding. Although the dose of hormones it contains is very high, it is only taken for a short period, and doesn't harm the breastfeeding baby. It isn't necessary (or desirable) to stop breastfeeding for a few hours.

→ Larimore, W.L., Stanford, J.B. 'Postfertilization effects of oral contraceptives and their relationship to informed consent', *Arch Fam Med* 2000;9:126-133 archfami.ama-assn.org/cgi/content/full/9/2/126

Breastfeeding and pregnancy, tandem feeding

Many babies wean themselves more or less voluntarily when their mothers are pregnant. This is due to a combination of three different factors:

- The time is right. They have to be weaned one day, and when the mother gets pregnant again it means the baby isn't such a baby anymore.
- Halfway through the pregnancy, the mother's milk supply decreases and the taste changes, or at least so they say. Some children say 'Ugh!' and don't want any more.
- A lot of mothers find their nipples hurt during pregnancy, so they pull a face when the baby nurses, and the baby takes the hint.

However, many other babies overcome all these obstacles. They ignore the hints, spoken or unspoken (or perhaps their mothers' nipples don't hurt), they want to carry on nursing, and if they notice any change in the taste, it seems not to bother them. A lot of women go on breastfeeding throughout the pregnancy, and then breastfeed both babies. This is known as tandem nursing.

There is still a great deal of prejudice attached to this, and no doubt more than one person will say you must wean your older baby immediately. Here are a few answers to some of the arguments they might use:

- Can breastfeeding cause miscarriages? No. It is true, as I already mentioned, that when the menstrual cycle begins again, there might be a period of luteal insufficiency for a few months, during which the embryo will be unable to implant itself, because by the time it reaches the womb menstruation will have already started. In these cases, the mother won't suspect she is pregnant; her period isn't late, it is early. Once the embryo is implanted, and the mother knows she is pregnant, breastfeeding can't cause miscarriage. It was believed it could because oxytocin produces contractions in the womb. However, the womb only responds to oxytocin towards the end of pregnancy; oxytocin isn't used to induce abortion because it doesn't have any effect in early pregnancy. Remember that sexual activity also produces oxytocin, and it isn't forbidden during pregnancy.

- Can breastfeeding cause premature labour? To my knowledge, this has never happened, although in theory it could. If a pregnant woman is prescribed complete bed rest because she is in danger of going into premature labour, she won't be able to work or even go out because walking might cause premature labour. Women who aren't in danger of going into premature labour can walk, work, and climb stairs right up until their due date. If you have a normal pregnancy, you can breastfeed and walk without any problem. If you have been prescribed complete bed rest then you must find out whether breastfeeding is harmful or not. Oxytocin only survives in the blood for a few minutes, before being quickly eliminated. This is why when oxytocin is used during delivery it is administered via infusion; there is no point in injecting it every hour and a half to two hours. So, if breastfeeding produces contractions, this has to occur at the moment when your baby is nursing, exactly when, months before, you experienced cramping, and your other breast leaked milk. If you have been put on complete bed rest because you are in danger of going into premature labour, and you notice strong contractions when you breastfeed, it is best if you stop breastfeeding. However, if the contractions don't coincide with the feed, but occur twenty minutes or two hours afterwards, you can safely breastfeed.

- Won't breastfeeding during pregnancy 'wear you out'? No. Being pregnant with twins, not to mention quadruplets, wears you out far more. Compared to the amount of physical energy it takes to be pregnant, breastfeeding only uses up a fraction more. Besides, European women nowadays rarely have more than three children. Think of our great-grandmothers, who often had between five and seven children, and who frequently breastfed when pregnant, at a time when not everyone could eat every day. Simply eat what you need to gain weight normally.

- When breastfeeding in tandem, doesn't the older baby

take milk from the younger one? No. You will have enough milk for both babies. In fact, it is possible that thanks to the older baby, who sucks harder, the breast will be better stimulated, resulting in more milk for the younger one. To begin with, it is sensible to feed the newborn first, but after a few weeks it probably doesn't make any difference.

- Won't the older baby pass on his viruses to the newborn by leaving his saliva on the nipple? The older baby will pass on his viruses to the newborn, whatever you do. It is usually enough for them to be in the same house, but on top of this, older brothers and sisters are prone to smothering newborns with kisses. Fortunately, breastmilk contains a permanent stockpile of antibodies to the viruses that are 'in vogue' in the family. In fact, it isn't uncommon for the rest of the family to have a cold while the baby is unaffected. There is no need to disinfect your breast between one baby and the next.

Of the children who are weaned while their mother is pregnant, some will want to nurse again when they see their baby brother or sister nursing. The best thing is just to let them: they usually give it a try, don't remember how, and are surprised by the almost forgotten taste. 'This milk is for babies!', they declare, and don't ask to nurse again. They were probably only asking as a way of testing your love, to make sure their mummy isn't rejecting them. Other children will go back to nursing for a few months: this is perfectly normal, too.

Some mothers are happy breastfeeding in tandem, but some mothers don't enjoy it. This is also normal. Remember, you have the right to do it, and you have the right not to do it.

Chapter 19
BREASTFEEDING AND HEALTH

As I mentioned in the introduction, I lost interest in the 'benefits' of breastfeeding long ago. Many people extol the virtues of human milk because they believe it will encourage more mothers to breastfeed. But the truth is, mothers have been breastfeeding for millions of years without being aware of any benefit; and yet it is precisely in the period and in the countries where these benefits were discovered that breastfeeding has been on the point of dying out.

Moreover, many experts criticise those who espouse 'the benefits of breastfeeding', as if they considered artificial feeding normal, and breastfeeding a bonus. In fact, breastfeeding is normal, and should be the yardstick for any other sort of feeding. It would therefore be more accurate to talk of the 'risks of artificial feeding', in the same way we talk of the 'dangers of smoking'. However, even though the beneficial effect breastfeeding has on health isn't what makes women breastfeed (and still less what makes babies eager to suckle), it is important for you, dear reader, to be aware of some of the benefits of breastfeeding. Because mothers are all too frequently advised to wean their babies for the strangest reasons, because of the most remote or imaginary dangers. As if artificial feeding were perfectly safe, while breastfeeding is always threatening to harm their baby. Well it isn't: artificial feeding is far from safe, and people should think twice before advising mothers to wean their babies.

Breastfeeding and infant health

According to Ball and Wright's calculations, comparing a group of 1,000 babies who weren't breastfed with a group of 1,000 babies who were exclusively breastfed for the first three months, there would be a difference of sixty cases of respiratory illness, 580 middle ear infections and 1,053 cases of gastroenteritis during the first year, which would generate 2,033 visits to the doctor, 212 days of hospitalisation, 609 prescriptions and 51 X-rays totalling (in 1990) $330,000. The study only took into account three months of breastfeeding, three illnesses and the cost of doctors' bills, (not the number of working days missed by parents, and the suffering, which can't be measured monetarily).

UNICEF calculates that one and a half million babies die each year because they aren't breastfed. We have been used to thinking that all these deaths occur in the Third World, and that in developed countries, thanks to hygiene and medical attention, although artificial feeding might cause a few mild cases of diarrhoea, surely it wouldn't affect the mortality rate. Of course, there were exceptions, for example in the case of premature babies. In Britain, in 1990, Lucas and Cole attributed 100 premature baby deaths a year from necrotising enterocolitis to artificial feeding.

However, in a recent revision, Chen and Rogan found that breastfeeding is also associated with a significantly lower infant mortality rate in the United States. They compared 1,204 baby deaths in 1988 with a control group of 7,740 children. In order to avoid any confusion due to inverse causality (meaning that the child didn't nurse because he was ill), they discounted deaths in the first month, or deaths caused by congenital malformations or malignant tumours. They found a dose-response relationship: the longer the period of breastfeeding, the lower the mortality rate. If the relationship is causal, they reckon that promoting breastfeeding could prevent 720 deaths a year in the United States of babies between one month and twelve months of age.

Breastfeeding doesn't only prevent minor illnesses. Artificial feeding is also associated with a heightened risk of meningitis due to *Haemophilus influenzae*, leukaemia and SIDS (Sudden Infant Death Syndrome, often known as 'cot death').

Long-term effects on infant health have also been observed: for years after they are weaned, children who were breastfed continued to have fewer respiratory illnesses, less obesity and a higher IQ. Prolonged breastfeeding protects against diabetes mellitus type 1 (insulin-dependent), probably because it delays the introduction of cow's milk and other dairy products (such as formula milk).

A revision by PAHO (Leon-Cava), which is available in its entirety on the internet, gives more detailed information about the effects of breastfeeding on the health of both mother and baby.

→ Ball, T.H., Wright, A.L. 'Health care costs of formula-feeding in the first year of life', *Pediatrics* 1999;103:870-6 pediatrics. aappublications.org/cgi/content/full/103/4/S1/870

→ Lucas, A., Cole, T.J. 'Breast milk and neonatal necrotising enterocolitis', *Lancet* 1990;336:1519-23

→ McGuire, W., Anthony, M.Y. 'Donor human milk versus formula for preventing necrotising enterocolitis in preterm infants: systematic review', *Arch Dis Child Fetal Neo-natal Ed* 2003;88:F11-4 fn.bmjjournals.com/cgi/content/full/88/1/F11

→ Chen, A., Rogan, W.J. 'Breastfeeding and the risk of postneonatal death in the United States', *Pediatrics* 2004;113:e435-9 pediatrics.aappublications.org/cgi/content/ full/113/5/e435

→ Silfverdal, S.A., Bodin, L., Olcen, P. 'Protective effect of breastfeeding: an ecologic study of Haemophilus influenzae meningitis and breastfeeding in a Swedish population', *Int J Epidemiol* 1999;28:152-6 ije.oxfordjournals.org/cgi/content/ abstract/28/1/152

→ Bener, A., Denic, S., Galadari, S. 'Longer breastfeeding and protection against childhood leukaemia and lymphomas', *Eur J Cancer* 2001;37:234-8

→ Shu, X.O., Linet, M.S., Steinbuch, M., Wen, W.Q., Buckley, J.D., Neglia, J.P. et al. 'Breast-feeding and risk of childhood acute leukemia', *J Natl Cancer Inst* 1999;91:1765-72 jncicancerspectrum.oupjournals.org/cgi/content/full/ jnci;91/20/1765

→ Alm, B., Wennergren, G., Norvenius, S.G., Skjaerven, R., Lagercrantz, H., Helweg-Larsen, K., Irgens, L.M. 'Breast feeding and the sudden infant death syndrome in Scandinavia, 1992-95', *Arch Dis Child* 2002;86:400-2 adc.bmjjournals.com/cgi/ content/full/86/6/400

→ Wilson, A.C., Forsyth, J.S., Greene, S.A., Irvine, L., Hau, C., Howie, P.W. 'Relation of infant diet to childhood health: seven year follow up of cohort of children in Dundee infant feeding study', *Br Med J* 1998;316:21-5

→ Von Kries, R., Koletzko, B., Sauerwald, T., von Mutius, E., Barnert, D., Grunert, V., von Voss, H. 'Breast feeding and obesity: cross sectional study', *Br Med J* 1999;319:147- 50 bmj.bmjjournals. com/cgi/content/full/319/7203/147

→ Angelsen, N.K., Vik, T., Jacobsen, G., Bakketeig, L.S. 'Breast feeding and cognitive development at age 1 and 5 years', *Arch Dis Child* 2001;85:183-8 adc.bmjjournals.com/cgi/content/full/85/3/183

→ Ziegler, A.G., Schmid, S., Huber, D., Hummel, M., Bonifacio, E. 'Early infant feeding and risk of developing type 1 diabetes-associated autoantibodies', *JAMA* 2003;290:1721-8

→ León-Cava, N., Lutter, C., Ross, J., Martin, L. 'Cuantificación de los beneficios de la lactancia materna: reseña de la evidencia', Washington, Organización Panamericana de la Salud, 2002

→ www.paho.org/Spanish/HPP/HPN/Benefits_of_BF.htm

→ www.ibfan-alc.org/nuestro_trabajo/apoyo_lm.htm

Breastfeeding and maternal health

Frequently, mothers who breastfeed hear remarks like: 'You're wearing yourself out,' or 'You're ruining your health'. Not so long ago, similar arguments were used to insist that women shouldn't work, practise sport, or study (it would wear out their brains!).

And yet, breastfeeding is also beneficial to the mother's health. Earlier on in this book I mentioned that breastfeeding reduces the risk of fractures due to osteoporosis (see page 173) and iron deficiency (see page 249), and that it doesn't cause hair loss (see page 294). But the biggest advantage of breastfeeding is probably the prevention of breast and ovarian cancer.

After re-analysis of data from forty-seven studies carried out in thirty different countries, on more than 50,000 cases of breast cancer and more than 90,000 controls, it has been concluded that in developed countries alone, with every twelve-month increase in the average length of time spent breastfeeding, 50,000 cases of cancer a year could be prevented. Note that what we usually think of as breast cancer prevention – regular mammograms – is in fact nothing more than early diagnosis. You already have cancer, and it remains to be seen if it can be cured. On the other hand, breastfeeding allows genuine prevention, meaning that some women who would otherwise have got cancer will not develop the disease as a direct result of having breastfed their children.

→ Collaborative Group on Hormonal Factors in Breast Cancer, 'Breast cancer and breastfeeding: collaborative reanalysis of individual data from 47 epidemiological studies in 30 countries, including 50302 women with breast cancer and 96973 women without the disease', *Lancet* 2002;360:187-95

→ Tung, K.H., Goodman, M.T., Wu, A.H., McDuffie, K., Wilkens, L.R., Kolonel, L.N., Nomura, A.M., Terada, K.Y., Carney, M.E., Sobin, L.H. 'Reproductive factors and epithelial ovarian cancer risk by histologic type: a multiethnic case-control study', *Am J Epidemiol* 2003;158:629-38

→ Rosenblatt, K.A., Thomas, D.B. 'Lactation and the risk of epithelial ovarian cancer. The WHO Collaborative Study of Neoplasia and Steroid Contraceptives', *Int J Epidemiol* 1993;22:192-7

→ Labbok, M.H. 'Effects of breastfeeding on the mother', *Pediatr Clin North Am* 2001;48:143-58

→ León-Cava, N., Lutter, C., Ross, J., Martin, L. 'Cuantificación de los beneficios de la lactancia materna: reseña de la evidencia', Washington, Organización Panamericana de la Salud, 2002

→ www.ibfan-alc.org/nuestro_trabajo/apoyo_lm.htm

Chapter 20
LEGAL PROTECTION

Throughout the twentieth century, a multitude of causes have led to breastfeeding being abandoned: interference during and after childbirth, social changes, work, and so on. However, the advertising campaigns of producers of artificial milk deserve a special mention.

In 1981, WHO adopted an International Code of Marketing of Breast-milk Substitutes, the main provisions of which are:

- It should apply to all breast-milk substitutes, including those that are inadequate (juices, herbal teas etc.) as well as to bottles, teats, and dummies.
- Manufacturers should not distribute educational material (leaflets, books, videos etc.) without health authorities having requested it in writing; and even then, the content of such material is limited, and must include a warning about the dangers of bottle feeding and not name any particular brands.
- There should be no advertising or other forms of promotion to the general public, including offers and discounts.
- Information provided by manufacturers to professionals should be restricted to scientific and factual matters.
- There should be no contact between marketing personnel and mothers or pregnant women.
- There should be no free samples given to mothers, pregnant women, infants and young children, or health facilities.
- Health facilities should not be used to display products, placards or posters.

- The words 'humanised' or 'maternalised' or similar terms should not be used, or any images that idealize these products.

Subsequent resolutions from WHO clarify or modify some of these points. The texts are all available on the Internet. The degree to which different countries have implemented the Code varies widely.

These rules are designed to protect mothers and babies against misleading marketing. To allow you to decide freely, without being subjected to pressure or brainwashing, how you want to feed your baby.

Advertising uses clever strategies. The posters, calendars and leaflets the industry produces usually depict a beautiful, smiling baby (what has she been eating that makes her look so healthy?) alone and in close up. Images of babies on their own didn't appear in our culture until the twentieth century. Up until then, babies were always depicted sitting on their mother's lap. When the industry produces an advert or leaflet featuring a baby nursing, the baby is always very small, almost a newborn (this contrasts with classical depictions of the Virgin Mary breastfeeding, where the baby Jesus is usually about two years old). In these images and promotional leaflets, the mother who is breastfeeding is usually shown in her bedroom, wearing a nightdress, or with almost nothing on, and her clothes and hair look frumpish. In contrast, the mother who is bottle feeding is dressed more stylishly, in street clothes, and gives the impression of being an active, energetic woman. The language used always suggests that breastfeeding is difficult ('Try, as soon as you are able', 'If for some reason your breast-milk is inadequate or insufficient...').

IBFAN is an international network of groups that defend the right to breastfeed. Take a look at their website, you will find a lot of interesting things on it.

→ http://www.unicef.org/nutrition/files/nutrition_code_english.pdf

→ IBFAN, 'International Baby Food Action Network' www.ibfan.org

→ IBFAN 'América Latina y Caribe' www.ibfan-alc.org/

Chapter 21
SEPARATION AND DIVORCE

Some Spanish judges, it appears, are only able to conceive of one form of shared custody in divorce cases: alternate weekends and two weeks in the summer holidays, regardless of the circumstances or the children's age. I have seen a one-year-old baby subjected to this type of regime, forced to separate from his mother and spend a weekend (and shortly after that two whole weeks) with a father who abandoned the family home while the mother was still pregnant. It is easy to imagine (but some appear to have no imagination) how much the child must have suffered. After each separation, he spent the first few hours crying, and the next few days in a daze, he lost weight, and when he returned home he as soon clung to his mother as rejected her. He regressed in his speech and his autonomy, and woke screaming.

Some mothers try to argue that they are breastfeeding, and therefore can't be separated from their baby for this long. To no avail. Occasionally, judges have been advised that the question of breastfeeding isn't a problem, because the mother can express her milk and give the father a cool bag full of frozen milk, which he can use during the two-week period, after which the baby can resume breastfeeding as though nothing had happened. More often than not, the mother discovers that the father has also brought up the subject of breastfeeding with the judge, but with the opposite idea in mind: to show that this mother who is still breastfeeding is clearly unhinged, is abusing her child, causing him psychological trauma, as well as creating a dependency, and that it is imperative the child be taken away from her. There are still those in our society who are ready to believe this sort of reasoning.

These separations are distressing for the child and painful for the mother, but they are also distressing for the father. If what he wants is to build a normal, loving relationship with his child, is this the right way to go about it? If every visit with his father is a nightmare, the child will learn to loathe him.

Out of respect for the love you once had for each other, and for the love you both profess to feel for your child, I implore you not to do this. Whatever the judge may decide, try to reach an alternative, more sensible agreement, better adapted to the needs of your child. You will both need to compromise, and to make an effort.

A baby can't build a relationship based on alternate weekends. It is impossible. He needs much more frequent contact. An hour or two a day, or every other day. To begin with, this contact should take place with the mother present, because at the slightest separation, the baby will start to cry and reject the father. I realise you are divorced and don't want to live together, but what harm is there in meeting for a while in the park, or going to watch a puppet show together? During these few hours, the father will need to make an effort to establish a bond with his child by playing with her, sitting next to her, pushing her on the swing, reading her stories. Don't fall into the absurd trap of trying to 'win the child over' with toys and presents; what the child wants and needs are cuddles and words. In time, she will be able to spend time alone with her father. Her responses and behaviour will tell you if she is ready, or if it is still too soon. Perhaps the father can pick the child up from nursery, take her to the park for an hour and then leave her at her mother's house. If by the time the child is three, the relationship has been constant and satisfactory for a few months, the child is probably ready to spend the night with the father. Be prepared the first time to take the child back to her mother before midnight if you see she is unhappy, and if this is the case, don't repeat the experiment again for another three or four months.

Holidays spent with the father can be introduced gradually. When the child is six or seven, she may be ready to spend two weeks with her father, but she will probably prefer to do one week, and then later another. A very interesting book on this subject is Brazelton, T.B., Greenspan, S.I. *The Irreducible Needs of Children*, Perseus Publishing, Cambridge MA, 2000.

Chapter 22
GUILT

When, as an inexperienced young doctor (I am currently an inexperienced middle-aged doctor), I became interested in the subject of breastfeeding, I was surprised by the response of many of my teachers, bosses and colleagues: 'Be careful not to make mothers feel guilty'. We were advised to say things like: 'Nothing compares to breastfeeding, but artificial feeding is just as good', or 'Don't worry if you can't breastfeed, nowadays babies who bottle feed do just as well'. I even went so far as to write in a draft pamphlet, which never saw the light of day, words to the effect: 'better to bottle feed with love than to breastfeed with bitterness'.

We doctors aren't usually this considerate in other cases. Tobacco causes cancer, and we spell it out in big letters, unreservedly, and if the smoker feels guilty, then too bad. And this isn't only because a lot of doctors have bottle fed their children; doctors who smoke have no qualms about telling people that smoking causes cancer.

It appears obligatory, when recommending breastfeeding, to prepare an escape route. A recent pamphlet published in Spain about how to prevent cot death (SIDS) included the following advice: 'Place your baby on his back', 'Don't smoke anywhere near him' and 'If possible breastfeed him'. Why is only breastfeeding optional? Why not: 'If possible place your baby on his back' or 'Try not to smoke anywhere near him'?

The fact is, generally speaking, women feel guilty about a lot of things, or at least they do in our culture. I am not sure whether this is genetic or purely cultural (are they really like that, or do they learn to be like that from when they are small?), but there is something in this. Diane Wiessinger, a breastfeeding specialist, explains that she has put the following scenario to many people:

'You are a passenger on a light aircraft, and the pilot has a heart attack. You have taken one flying lesson; you try landing the plane and you crash it. Would you feel guilty?' A common response from men is: 'Guilty? Of course not! Flying a plane is really hard, I did what I could…' In contrast, women often say they would, that they should have paid more attention during their first lesson, that it was their fault that the plane crashed. One of them even felt guilty about feeling guilty: 'Well, I know I shouldn't feel guilty, but I think I would.'

When a woman becomes a mother, her guilt feelings seem to intensify, and not just about breastfeeding. I have a doctor/patient column in a magazine, and many of the letters I receive speak openly about guilt.

Many mothers feel guilty not about things that have happened, but about things that could have happened. And not only serious things, like 'My child nearly died and I'm to blame', but for things anyone else would consider trivial. Marta, for example, feels guilty because her daughter won't eat meat: 'I feel slightly guilty when I think I might be exposing my daughter to the risk of anaemia by not giving her meat.'

Someone once said: 'If we have done what we can, explained what we know and given all that we can, no more can be expected of us'. But guilt feelings aren't rational. Beatriz blames herself for having been wrongly informed (instead of blaming those who gave her wrong information): 'I am the mother of a one-month-old baby girl. I have been breastfeeding and bottle feeding her because I didn't have the right information when I needed it (*mea culpa*).'

Is it possible to suffer an unexpected stroke of bad luck and to feel guilty instead of feeling you are the victim? If you are a mother, yes. Ibone feels guilty because she suffered from depression: 'I don't think I've given my little girl the security and happiness every child needs, especially when they are small. I feel guilty and I'm afraid it might affect her personality, or her brain or her development.'

It is also true that unjustified feelings of guilt are one of the symptoms of depression. Full-blown post-natal depression is relatively rare, but many mothers suffer from a mild from of depression referred to as the baby blues.

Mothers manage to feel guilty about what they 'do badly', but also about what they fail to do, or about what others do, or even about what they 'do well'. Julia has been strongly criticised for picking her baby up and 'spoiling' him… '…They even make me feel guilty for loving him so much.'

If mothers feel guilty about almost everything else, is it a surprise that they also feel guilty about not breastfeeding? Laura sometimes feels guilty because she breastfeeds her baby: 'Wouldn't it be better to stop breastfeeding, even though I'd regret it, because I'm passing on my anxiety and depression to my baby, and my milk isn't doing her any good?'

Isabel feels guilty because she is breastfeeding her baby on demand, despite her doctor telling her to breastfeed him only twice a day: 'The fact is I feel slightly guilty for going against what the paediatrician says.'

Montse feels guilty because she takes her son into the bed with her when he cries at night. She says she is glad she read my book *Kiss Me:* 'After reading your book I feel less guilty.' (That accursed word!).

But I am not taking any credit for this; I know other mothers who left their first born to cry, and who felt guilty after reading my book…

Why is it that everyone tries to shield us from feeling guilty about some things but not others? The same doctor who would never say: 'If you don't breastfeed your baby, he won't have as much immunoglobulin' (which is perfectly true), won't hesitate to tell a mother: 'If you don't feed your baby meat, she will have an iron deficiency' (which is only sometimes true), or even: 'If you don't give him fruit, he will have a vitamin C deficiency' (which is completely untrue). If at a family gathering you say: 'I feel guilty leaving him at a nursery when he's still so young', they will all try to reassure you: 'Don't worry, they love being at the nursery'. On the other hand, if you dare to say: 'I feel guilty about letting him sleep in our bed', how many people will tell you: 'Don't worry, they love sleeping in your bed?' Some mothers who bottle feed their babies feel bad when they read a magazine article about the advantages of breastfeeding; but at least those articles aren't directed at them personally, and if they don't want to read them they don't have to. In contrast, the mother who breastfeeds for two years is more than likely to be openly subjected to criticism from family, friends or health professionals, some of which can be hostile or insulting.

Of course, I am not suggesting that those of us who are in favour of breastfeeding are kinder and more respectful of others. The fact is, the way things stand, bottle feeding and leaving babies to cry are overwhelming trends in our society. Breastfeeding for more than a year and co-sleeping are considered eccentricities, which only 'weirdos' indulge in. Some people are by nature kind and respectful of others, they respect the majority and the minority alike, those who think as they do, and those who think differently. But many people only pretend to respect others. In fact, they look up to those in power and they despise ordinary people. They are cowards when they are in a minority and grow bolder when they have the backing of a group. It is possible that within a few decades, if breastfeeding continues to become more widespread, some people will begin to openly criticise mothers who don't breastfeed. I hope, dear reader, that you won't be one of those criticising.

I suspect that sometimes, through our efforts not to make mothers feel guilty, we achieve the exact opposite. Imagine for example that you are in a car accident and your three-year-old daughter suffers a broken arm. Which of the following remarks would make you feel most guilty?

(a) A broken arm? The poor thing! I hope it mends soon.

(b) Don't blame yourself. I often drive my son without using the child safety seat too. I'm sure it won't leave a scar, whatever people say, breaking an arm isn't a big thing nowadays. And kids love wearing a cast.

The fact is that the mother who wanted to breastfeed her baby, and for whatever reason was unable to do so, can't help but feel bad. It isn't logical to feel guilty when you are the victim due to a lack of information, or assistance, or due to simple fate. However, nor is it logical to feel good when you want something and can't achieve it. We feel bad when we fail an exam, or are given a parking ticket, or if it rains when we go to the beach. And breastfeeding is something far more important; it is a special gift the mother wanted to give her baby, because she thought it was the best thing for him, and because it is part of her sexual cycle, part of life.

For many women, the end of breastfeeding is a sort of mourning process, similar (though less intense of course) to when a loved one dies. I have known mothers who feel bad when they wean their child of one and a half or four years old; mothers who feel they have lost something important they will never get back. Although it is something they expected, accepted, and even chose to make happen, they still feel bad. How must a mother feel when she is forced to wean against her will, in the first few weeks, after much pain and suffering?

Unfortunately, our society doesn't seem to understand this sort of suffering. Well-meaning people insist on denying it, eliminating it, blanking it out. I think this is a mistake. Imagine if you went deaf, and that your doctors and friends all tried to deny your pain: 'Don't worry, hearing aids are very advanced these days'. 'At least you can relax now you know what the problem is'. 'An aunt of mine went deaf, and she said it was better than before because she had more inner peace.' 'Well, when you think of the sort of stuff one has to hear...' 'I don't know why you bother; if you're deaf you're deaf, you just have to accept it'. Wouldn't you be incensed?

In addition to the pain they feel at not being able to breastfeed, many mothers have to put up with being misunderstood. Rather than a lot of false reassurances, what they need to hear is a sensible, compassionate voice: 'You really wanted to breastfeed, didn't you? I'm really sorry it didn't work out for you...'

→ Wiessinger, D. 'Watch your language!' *J Hum Lact* 1996;12:1-4children

Chapter 23
HOW TO CHANGE THE WORLD

If breastfeeding has been something of an obstacle course for you, if you have been forced to argue with doctors and nurses, mothers and mothers-in-law, friends and family, or all these people at once, you may want to do something to help change things, to pave the way for others after you. If so, here are a few suggestions.

The power of the pen

You may not believe this, but you can achieve a lot by writing a letter, if you bear in mind a few important things:

- The recipient. Are they in the habit of receiving a lot of letters, possibly hundreds or thousands? The fewer they receive the more likely they are to read your letter, and to act on it. How will they feel when they read it? Be careful not to offend the person you hope to win over to your cause, don't be aggressive if you haven't first tried being polite. Who is the key person you need to address in this particular case?
- Presentation. The letter has to be formal, especially if it is a complaint. A proper letter in an envelope with a stamp on it makes a far deeper impression than an email (some people fire off emails willy-nilly, and join any fashionable cause. A letter shows that a person is truly concerned about something, and has taken some trouble and even spent some money). Use writing paper, not paper torn out of a notebook. Be careful about spelling and syntax, language and margins. When you are making a complaint or a demand, it is important to show that you are a reasonable, educated person.

- The tone. Always be polite and moderate, never insulting or offensive. One letter of thanks will always achieve more than ten complaints. But even when you are complaining, remain civil. It is no good making enemies if you want to change things.

- Sign the letter. An anonymous letter would only be justified if you were in the gravest danger ('forgive me for not telling you my name, but the mafia is after me…'). Give your name and address, especially if the letter is a complaint. No one takes any notice of an anonymous letter. Don't forget to give your name in your emails as well.

- Praise should be circulated as widely as possible. If someone goes out of their way to help you, you might write them a personal thank you letter, which they will treasure for the rest of their lives. But, out of modesty, they probably won't show it to many people. However, an open letter to a head of department, a hospital manager or a health authority would persuade a lot of people. A letter to your local newspaper will inform other mothers about what to expect and what demands they can make (newspapers don't publish all letters; if yours doesn't appear for a couple of weeks, send it directly to the person concerned).

- On the other hand, it is best to limit the circulation of a complaint (if the complaint is absolutely necessary); speak directly to the doctor or nurse in question, and only if they are rude or unhelpful talk to their superior. Never go directly to the press with a complaint before writing to the hospital. If you go public with your complaint, those involved might feel betrayed, as if you had trampled on them: 'If she had a problem, why didn't she come to us, instead of telling tales?'

- Think about what you aim to achieve; what effect your complaint might have on the recipient, his or her colleagues, on the public at large. Remember this person also has feelings. Complaining is rarely a good idea; praise achieves far better results.

Imagine a hospital where for years many people have been working hard to try improve care for breastfeeding mothers. A representative from a laboratory has brought a box of free formula milk samples. The head nurse has hidden them in a cupboard in order to return them the following week, because the hospital doesn't accept or distribute free samples. A well-meaning student nurse finds them, and has the idea of giving a few away. Two weeks later, the director of the hospital receives a letter from the health authority demanding a written report because they have received an irate letter complaining that the hospital is handing out free formula milk samples, which is prohibited by law. Can you imagine the recriminations this would unleash, the frayed tempers? Do you think it will make the staff any more favourable to breastfeeding? Surely it would have been far more effective to write a friendly letter to the person responsible.

A complaint can be very counterproductive. For example: 'I had to insist on being allowed to have my baby with me at night, and they gave me funny looks. Luckily one of the nurses helped me position my baby correctly, so I could breastfeed despite having cracked nipples, but the advice I got from the other staff was meaningless and contradictory'.

A lot of people will think you are exaggerating and complaining for no reason ('She's complaining because they gave her funny looks?' 'They let her keep her baby with her, helped her with the cracked nipples and still she complains?') The complaint will probably be looked into, and this could prove very unpleasant for all the staff. The director will ask to see the head of department, the ward supervisor or both, and will demand an explanation. Possibly in writing. And they in turn will demand an explanation from those concerned. They will look at the patient's file, find out which doctors and nurses were on duty that day. If it turns out somebody made a mistake, they will receive a severe reprimand and will feel very annoyed. The nurse who acted correctly would rather die than be singled out for praise amid a stream of complaints, and it might cause a rift between her and her fellow nurses. Those who have been trying hard to improve the situation, and have actually been doing things a lot better than the year before, will feel disillusioned, almost betrayed ('You look after them, and this is the thanks you get'). Those who have made no effort at all, and who think breastfeeding and the mother and baby relationship is a lot of nonsense, will look at their colleagues with a superior smile ('I told you it was a waste of time').

Alternatively, this mother could have written a thank you letter:

Dear Sir/Madam,

I gave birth in your hospital on 12 March. I would like to congratulate you on the excellent care I received. It was a joy to be able to hold my baby in my arms in the delivery room, and to be able to breastfeed her as soon as she was born. And being allowed to have her with me in the room day and night made things much easier for me. It was a huge improvement on four years ago, when I had my eldest. They used to take him away at night to the nursery, and I would spend the whole night worrying about him. I understand the enormous effort these changes must have required, but they have certainly paid off.

Everyone was very kind to me, and gave me a lot of assistance with breastfeeding. One of the nurses on night duty spent half an hour showing me how to position my baby correctly, and I am sure that thanks to this I haven't cracked nipples. Also, I found it very reassuring when the paediatrician gave my baby a check-up in the room with me, and explained everything so clearly.

Please would you be so kind as to thank all the staff on the maternity ward for me, and encourage them to keep up the wonderful work.

Kind regards,
Martha Pritchard

You may wonder how talking about what they are already doing will change anything. You can't begin to imagine the waves it will make. To start with, it is very likely that these changes didn't have unanimous approval. Some of the nurses, doctors and possibly even the hospital manager will have considered it all a lot of nonsense. And, because people often prefer to grumble rather than to show gratitude, some mothers might even have complained about not being able to sleep because they left her baby in the room with her. And so a letter like this (or several!) will encourage those who were pushing for change, it will convince those who were in two minds, and it will silence the naysayers. As managers generally receive more complaints than letters of thanks, his secretary will no doubt place your letter on top of the pile so as to brighten his morning and put him in a good mood. She might even say: 'Look at this letter that arrived today'. The manager will read it, mention it to the head of the maternity service and the nursing supervisor when he next sees them, whether at a formal meeting or if he bumps into them in the staff café. Someone will stick a photocopy of it up on the notice board in the nurses' station, and one sarcastic nurse will say: 'What a surprise, finally someone remembered to thank us!' while another will add: 'Martha Pritchard, wasn't she that nice blonde woman in room 312?' The nurse who helped her for half an hour will know she is the one referred to in the letter, and it will put her in a good mood for the rest of the day, while the others will try to guess who it was: 'I wonder who helped her with her breasts for half an hour?' 'It must be Magda, they always call her when one of them is having difficulty nursing, and, honestly, she has the patience of a saint...'. The supervisor, who probably doesn't know the night staff so well, will overhear the conversation and make a mental note that Magda is a good member of the team. The paediatrician who gives the babies their check-ups in front of the mothers will be overjoyed, and his colleague, who takes them away to examine them in the nursery, might decide to try it...

Our actions change the world; never doubt it. Through your words, your example, your patience and your good humour, you pave the way for other mothers after you.

INDEX

MINI INDEX

'Everything's going well!'
Dip into main index or contents page to find
something you're interested in, or read cover-to-
cover. Enjoy!